Herbal Medicine in Yemen

Islamic History and Civilization

Studies and Texts

VOLUME 96

The titles published in this series are listed at brill.nl/ihc

Herbal Medicine in Yemen

Traditional Knowledge and Practice, and Their Value for Today's World

Edited by

Ingrid Hehmeyer
Hanne Schönig

with the collaboration of

Anne Regourd

BRILL

LEIDEN • BOSTON
2012

Cover illustration: Medicinal herbs for sale in the Khamīs Banī Saʿd market (druggist Muḥammad Saʿīd b. Saʿīd Ḥawbānī) (photograph by Hanne Schönig, 2000). With kind permission of the Orient-Institut Beirut of the DGIA.

Library of Congress Cataloging-in-Publication Data

Herbal medicine in Yemen : traditional knowledge and practice, and their value for today's world / edited by Ingrid Hehmeyer, Hanne Schönig ; with the collaboration of Anne Regourd.
p. cm. — (Islamic history and civilization, ISSN 0929-2403 ; v. 96)
Includes index.
ISBN 978-90-04-22150-5 (hardback : alk. paper) — ISBN 978-90-04-23207-5 (e-book)
1. Herbs—Therapeutic use—Yemen (Republic) 2. Traditional medicine—Yemen (Republic) 3. Medicinal plants—Yemen (Republic) 4. Materia medica, Vegetable—Yemen (Republic) 5. Medicine, Arab. I. Hehmeyer, Ingrid. II. Schönig, Hannelore. III. Regourd, Anne. IV. Series: Islamic history and civilization ; v. 96.

RM666.H33H4673 2012
615.3'2109533—dc23

2012022110

This publication has been typeset in the multilingual "Brill" typeface. With over 5,100 characters covering Latin, IPA, Greek, and Cyrillic, this typeface is especially suitable for use in the humanities. For more information, please see www.brill.nl/brill-typeface.

ISSN 0929-2403
ISBN 978 90 04 22150 5 (hardback)
ISBN 978 90 04 23207 5 (e-book)

This book is printed on acid-free paper.

CONTENTS

FOREWORD

I am delighted to present this foreword to a book on traditional medicine in Yemen. The individual contributions are based on lectures given at an interdisciplinary workshop hosted by Martin Luther University Halle-Wittenberg in September 2009 that I had the pleasure to attend in my capacity as Cultural Counsellor of The Embassy of the Republic of Yemen in Germany. As a graduate of this university in chemistry, the topic is of great academic interest to me and besides, being a Yemeni, I am proud to have this international attention focused on the cultural heritage of my country.

The value of traditional medicine is well-recognized by international organizations such as the World Health Organization. Yemen has an ample repertory of medical knowledge and practice utilized in the prevention, diagnosis, and treatment of illness that has been shaped by local experience and beliefs from ancient times. Most of the medicinal substances are plant-based, a reflection of the country's rich vegetation.

Traditional medical knowledge along with its practitioners survive in Yemen in our time and have an important function, especially when modern Western medicine is not affordable or where it may not be available at all. It also plays a significant role in alternative healing methods that a patient may resort to, either because these usually involve a more holistic approach to healing and encompass the entire body including the mind, not just the afflicted part, or where modern Western medicine fails.

However, while it is true that since the 1960s Yemen has made enormous progress in terms of becoming a player in the modern world, it is a sad reality that some of the very effective medicinal measures that were used by people in the past are increasingly being abandoned because it is felt that by modern standards they are no longer appropriate. Modern Western medicinal substances and practices are supplanting traditional medical lore, a process that began in the urban centres but is now having an impact on rural areas as well. At the same time, some plant resources have become critically endangered in Yemen, with consequences for their availability—or rather the lack thereof—as medicines.

The authors of this book on traditional herbal medicine in Yemen have documented and evaluated knowledge and practices that are increasingly under threat. By doing this, they contribute to helping preserve a significant aspect of Yemen's cultural heritage, while opening avenues for future research on a topic that has so far received little attention.

Prof. Dr. Sheikh A. Bawazir
Cultural Counsellor
Embassy of The Republic of Yemen, Berlin

ACKNOWLEDGEMENTS

The editors would like to offer their warmest thanks to His Excellency, Prof. Dr. Sheikh A. Bawazir, Cultural Counsellor at the Embassy of The Republic of Yemen in Berlin, for enthusiastically supporting and patiently overseeing the workshop whose results we are delighted to publish in this volume. He not only consented to open the event, but also contributed greatly by attending and showing deep interest in its success. Finally, and very graciously, he accepted our invitation to write the foreword to the book that we are happy to present here.

The workshop, "The Use of Herbs in Yemeni Healing Practices: An Interdisciplinary Workshop on Traditional Knowledge and Cultural Concepts in Scientific Perspective," took place in Halle (Germany), in September 2009. The Centre for Interdisciplinary Area Studies—Middle East, Africa, Asia (ZIRS, of the Martin Luther University Halle-Wittenberg), kindly hosted the two-day event. We would like to thank all the members of the audience for the insights we gained from their questions and comments.

The workshop could not have taken place without generous financial assistance from an international array of funders: Ryerson University and the Royal Ontario Museum Yemen Program Fund (both of Toronto, Canada), Martin Luther University Halle-Wittenberg, the National Center for Scientific Research (CNRS, UMR 7192, Collège de France, "Proche Orient, Caucase, Iran: continuités et diversités"), and the École Pratique des Hautes Études, section des Sciences historiques et philologiques (EPHE, both of Paris, France); we warmly thank them all. In particular we are grateful to the Office of the Dean of Arts and the Office of the Vice President, Research and Innovation, at Ryerson University, for their confidence in our project, and François Déroche, EPHE, who, from the very beginning, affirmed our faith in the interest and value of our area of study.

We would like to thank all the contributors to this volume for their enthusiastic cooperation, the timely submission of their chapters, and their prompt responses to our queries.

During our preparations for publication we have incurred a large debt of gratitude to the copy editors, Eileen Reilly, Charles Whitmer, Peter Nix, and in particular Miranda Morris. They checked the English of the articles and introductory material written by non-native English speakers. Antje Seeger, ZIRS, took the photographs during the workshop and prepared the illustrations for the book. Heike Heklau (Institute of Biology, Department of Geobotany and Botanical Garden, Martin Luther University Halle-Wittenberg) gave generously of her time to guide us through the botanical garden of Halle, answering our many questions with patience and erudition. She also helped us confirm the scientific names of many of the plants described in this volume. Special thanks are due to Marie-Claude Simeone-Senelle, CNRS, UMR 8135, "Langage, langues et cultures d'Afrique noire" (LLACAN) for checking the transliteration of Modern South Arabian. Brandon Jacoby, Department of Geography, and Michelle Sawka, Environmental Applied Science and Management Program, Ryerson University, prepared the maps. Edward J. Keall, Department of World Cultures, Royal Ontario Museum, Toronto, never failed to provide extensively researched and authoritative answers to the series of Yemen-related questions the editors posed to him.

The Centre for Interdisciplinary Area Studies—Middle East, Africa, Asia, Martin Luther University Halle-Wittenberg, and especially the Royal Ontario Museum Yemen Program Fund, the Office of the Dean of Arts and the Department of History, Ryerson University, gave generous financial support for the publication of this book. We are sincerely grateful to them.

Finally, we wish to thank Professors Wadad Kadi (Chicago) and Sebastian Günther (Göttingen) for accepting this book in Brill's *Islamic History and Civilization* series.

ABOUT THE AUTHORS

MOHAMMED AL-DUAIS, Assistant Professor of Phytochemistry at the University of Ibb (Yemen). He received his PhD in Biochemistry in 2009 from the Friedrich Schiller University, Jena (Germany).

JACQUES FLEURENTIN, Pharmacist, Adjunct Professor of Biology of Plants and Pharmacognosy at Paul-Verlaine University, Metz (France) (1995–2001); president of the Société Française d'Ethnopharmacologie, Metz. He received his PhD in Pharmacy in 1983 from the University of Metz.

AMIN AL-HAKIMI, Professor of Plant Breeding at the University of Ṣan'ā' (Yemen), and head of the Yemeni Association for Sustainable Agriculture Development (YASAD). He received his PhD in Plant Breeding in 1995 from the École Pratique des Hautes Études, Montpellier (France).

INGRID HEHMEYER, Associate Professor of History of Science and Technology at Ryerson University, Toronto (Canada). She received her doctorate in Agriculture in 1988 and a Master of Science (equiv.) in Pharmacy in 1990, both from the Rheinische Friedrich Wilhelms University, Bonn (Germany).

GOTTFRIED JETSCHKE, Adjunct Professor and Lecturer for Theoretical and Plant Ecology at Friedrich Schiller University, Jena (Germany). He received his PhD in Physics in 1979 and his habilitation in Mathematics in 1989, both from the University of Jena.

EFRAIM LEV, Professor of History of Medicine and Ethnopharmacology at the University of Haifa (Israel). He received his PhD in History of Medicine and Pharmacology in the Medieval Levant in 1999 from the Bar Ilan University, Ramat Gan (Israel).

ULRIKE LINDEQUIST, Professor of Pharmaceutical Biology at Ernst Moritz Arndt University, Greifswald (Germany). She received her PhD in 1977 and her habilitation in Pharmaceutical Biology in 1987, both from the University of Greifswald.

MIRANDA MORRIS, Honorary Research Fellow at the University of St. Andrews (United Kingdom). She received her PhD in Modern South

Arabian Languages in 1979 from the School of Oriental and African Languages, London (United Kingdom).

ESTER MUCHAWSKY-SCHNAPPER, Curator in the Forchheimer Department of Jewish Ethnography in the Israel Museum, Jerusalem (Israel). She received her Master's degree in Art History and Folklore in 1987 from the Hebrew University, Jerusalem, and is currently completing her dissertation in Ethnology at the University of Haifa (Israel).

FRÉDÉRIC PELAT, Country Officer and Project Director in Yemen for the French NGO Iddeales that he created in 2003. He received his Master's degree in Tropical Agronomy in 1998 from the Institut des Régions Chaudes (IRC), Centre International d'Études Supérieures en Sciences Agronomiques (SupAgro), Montpellier (France).

MIKHAIL RODIONOV, Professor of Arabian Studies at St. Petersburg State University (Russia) and head of the Department of South and Southwest Asia at the Peter the Great Museum of Anthropology and Ethnography. He received his PhD in Social Anthropology in 1976 from the Peter the Great Museum and his habilitation in 1991 from the Institute of Oriental Studies, Russian Academy of Sciences, St. Petersburg.

PETRA G. SCHMIDL, Researcher at the Department of Islamic Studies, Rheinische Friedrich Wilhelms University, Bonn (Germany). She received her PhD in History of Science in 2005 from the Johann Wolfgang Goethe University, Frankfurt (Germany).

HANNE SCHÖNIG, researcher at the Centre for Interdisciplinary Area Studies, Martin Luther University Halle-Wittenberg (Germany). She received her PhD in Oriental Languages and Islamic Studies in 1984 from the Johannes Gutenberg University, Mainz (Germany).

DANIEL MARTIN VARISCO, Professor of Anthropology at Hofstra University, Hempstead, New York (United States of America). He received his PhD in Anthropology in 1982 from the University of Pennsylvania (United States of America).

ANHAR YA'NI, Secretary General of the Yemeni Association for Sustainable Agriculture Development (YASAD). She received her Master of Science in Genetics in 2007 from the University of Ṣan'ā' (Yemen).

A NOTE ON TRANSLITERATION CONVENTION

Arabic
Transliteration of Arabic generally follows that of the *Encyclopaedia of the Qurʾān* (Jane Dammen McAuliffe, general ed., Brill: Leiden, 2001–6).

ا	ā	ذ	dh	ظ	ẓ	ن	n
ب	b	ر	r	ع	ʿ	ه	h
ت	t	ز	z	غ	gh	و	w, ū
ث	th	س	s	ف	f	ي	y, ī
ج	j	ش	sh	ق	q	ء	ʾ
ح	ḥ	ص	ṣ	ك	k	ى	ā
خ	kh	ض	ḍ	ل	l	ة	-a(t)
د	d	ط	ṭ	م	m		

Short vowels are rendered as *a, i, u*, the *nisba* as *-ī/-iyya*. Diphthongs are rendered by *aw* and *ay*. Vocalization of the Arabic plant names can be at variance due to local dialect.

The Arabic article (al-) takes no alphabetic precedence in the bibliography and index listings, e.g. al-Malik al-Muẓaffar is listed under the letter 'm.' Some exceptions to this rule may occur in the usage of modern personal names, where the article is also capitalized.

Other languages
Transliteration of Modern South Arabian languages follows the system of the Seminar for Arabian Studies, London:
<http://www.arabianseminar.org.uk/ArabianSeminarLatestGuidelines2010.pdf>

Transliteration of Hebrew follows Brill guidelines:
<http://www.brill.nl/default.aspx?partid=162>

LIST OF ILLUSTRATIONS AND MAPS

MAPS

FIGURES

[1] H = manuscript Huntington 233, Bodleian Library, see Petra Schmidl's chapter in this volume, 45.

Mikhail Rodionov

Mohammed Al-Duais and Gottfried Jetschke

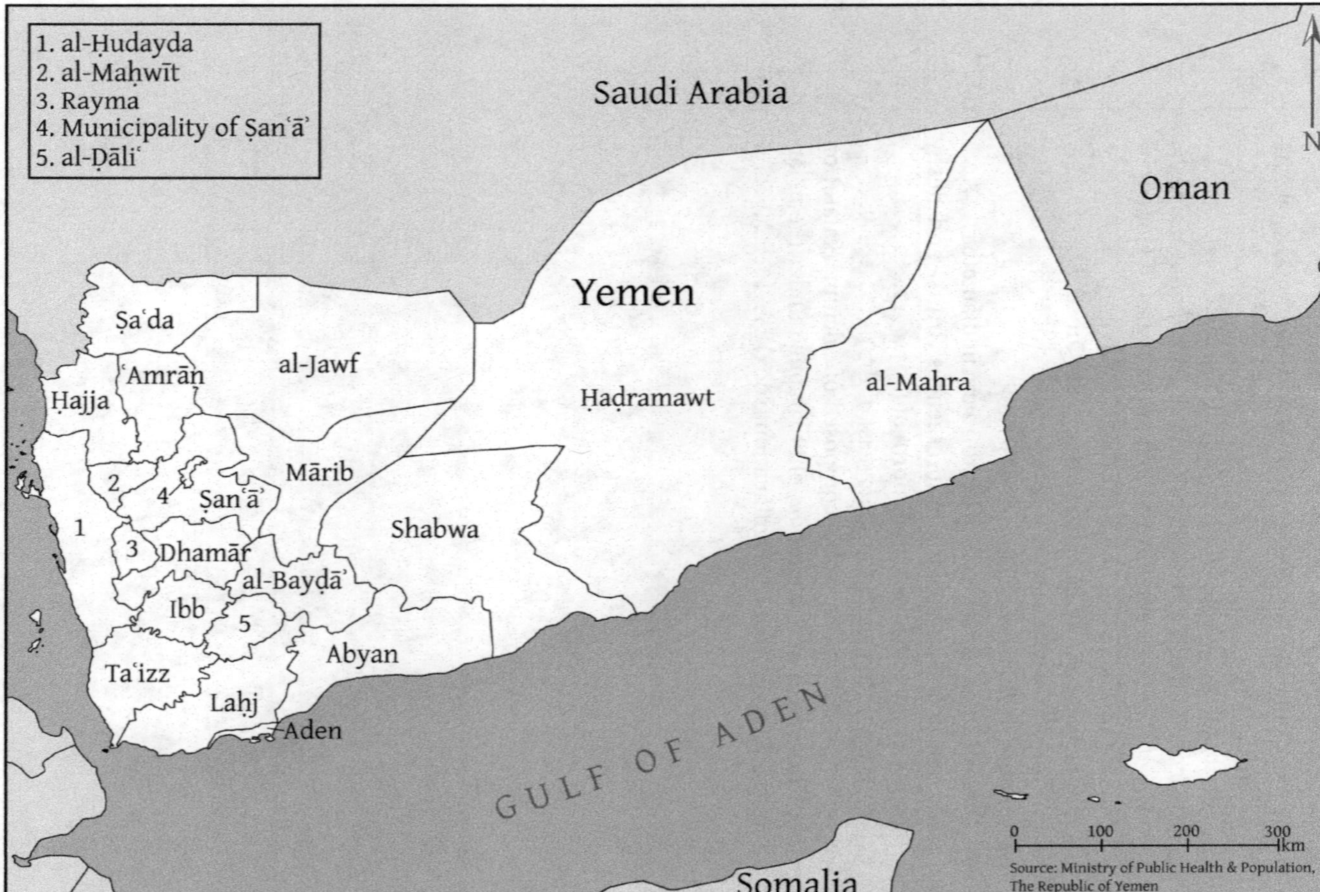

Map 1. The Governorates of Yemen (© Brandon Jacoby and Michelle Sawka)

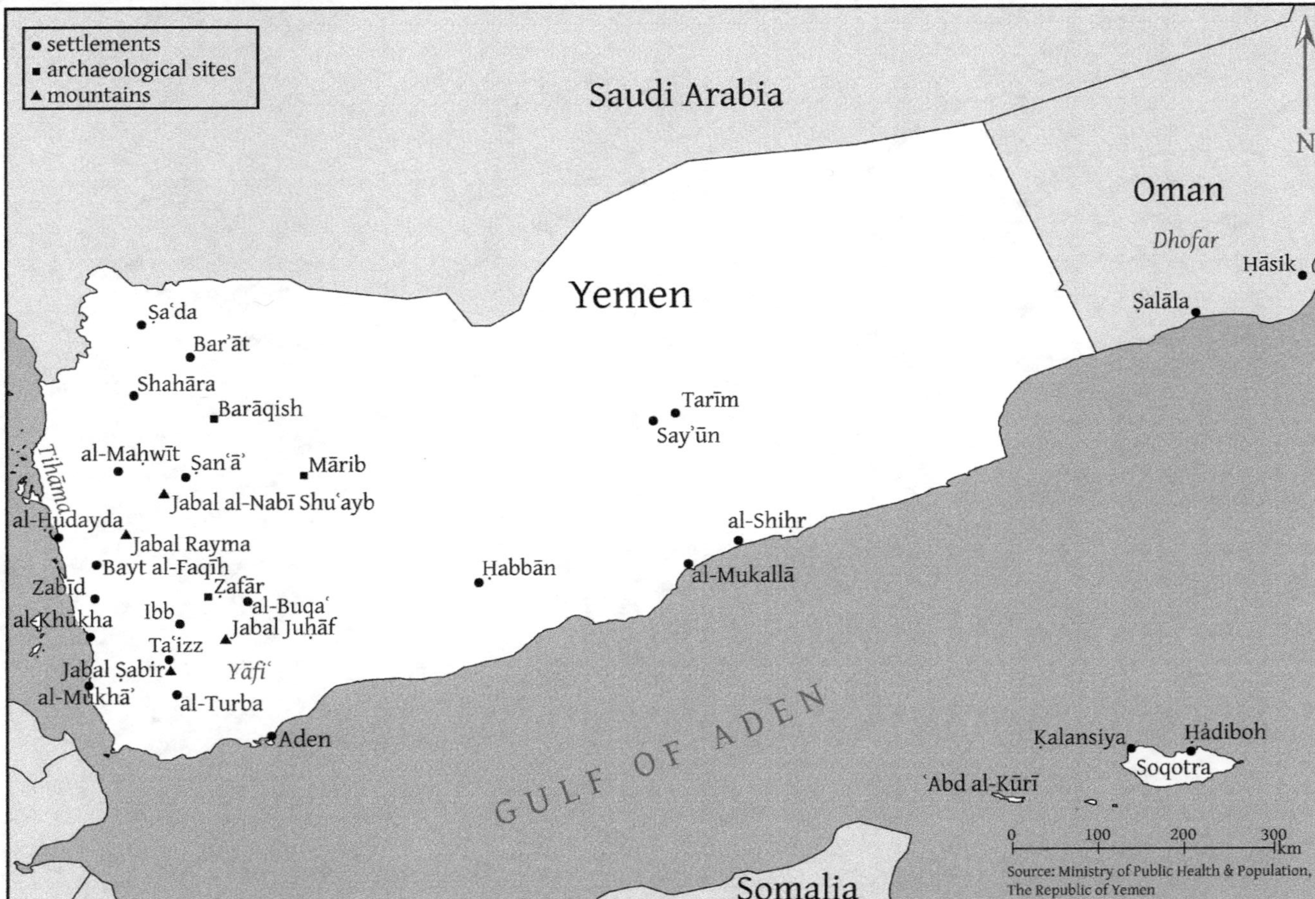

Map 2. Significant places cited (© Brandon Jacoby and Michelle Sawka)

INTRODUCTION

Hanne Schönig and Ingrid Hehmeyer

Traditional medicine in Yemen—and similarly in all other Islamic countries—is based on three main sources: classical Arabic medicine that has its foundations in Greek medical theory, the Prophet's medicine (*al-ṭibb al-nabawī*), and local pre-Islamic traditions. Its practitioners—namely druggists and healers—have studied the classical Arabic sources and the works of *al-ṭibb al-nabawī*. They have further acquired knowledge through oral transmission. Religious and magical rituals are employed side by side with *materia medica*, i.e. the substances of natural—plant, animal, or mineral—origin that are used for their medicinal properties. The different approaches to healing should not necessarily be understood as being taken independently, but rather in combination. Apart from a few drugs of animal and mineral origin, it is first and foremost Yemen's rich and diverse vegetation that has been the source of traditional remedies and that has resulted in an enormous variety of plant-based medicines.[1] Only a little plant material was imported from Iran and India. Jacques Fleurentin has determined that 54% of Yemeni medicinal plants are mentioned in the work on *materia medica* by the famous Andalusian pharmacologist and botanist Ibn al-Bayṭār (d. 1248).[2] But Fleurentin also stresses that 36% were not described by any of the classical authorities—a fact that emphasizes the originality of Yemeni herbal medicine. The specific remedies that became part and parcel of traditional Yemeni medicine result from the experience of local practitioners who had observed the remedies' effectiveness.[3] Besides the health professionals, other people with well-founded knowledge of plants—for instance farmers—acquired experience with the medical properties of herbs.[4] Apart from oral tradition, Yemeni indigenous knowledge of phytotherapy is reflected in works on *materia medica* by

---

[1] This is different in other Islamic countries, e.g. Morocco, where animal drugs are widely used.

[2] Ibn al-Bayṭār/Leclerc (trans.), *Traité*; Fleurentin, *Guérisseurs*, 109.

[3] Ibid., 110.

[4] See the chapter by Amin al-Hakimi, Anhar Ya'ni, and Frédéric Pelat in this volume.

local authors, most importantly al-Malik al-Muẓaffar (d. 1295)[5] and Shaʿbān Ibn Sālim al-Ṣanʿānī (d. 1736).[6]

In today's Yemen, synthetic medicines developed in the Western world have become widely available in the urban centres and are being used there on a large scale. Migration into cities and demographic change have contributed to this trend.[7] Also, more and more Yemenis who can afford it seek treatment abroad, in other Arab countries or in Europe. However, as in developing countries in general, traditional medicine still plays a significant role in health care in Yemen,[8] especially in rural areas and among the lower social strata. This has to do with its greater affordability and availability. In addition, as in the industrialized countries, traditional practices are very much accepted—and enjoy great popularity—as complementary or alternative medicine.

At the same time, plant resources are threatened in Yemen. The World Health Organization (WHO) adopted a strategy in 2002 to "ensure availability and affordability of TM/CAM [traditional medicine/complementary or alternative medicine], including essential herbal medicines."[9] Academic interest in the topic is also increasing. It was not until the 1980s that Western scholars began to publish on Yemeni traditional medicine. A pioneering work combining social anthropology with Arabic and Islamic studies was published by Armin Schopen in 1983 (*Traditionelle Heilmittel in Jemen*). Further, the research by Fleurentin[10] and by Anthony Miller and Miranda Morris in Soqotra[11] has to be acknowledged.[12]

In contrast to modern Western medicine, traditional medical practice—besides being to a large extent transmitted orally—includes interaction with the socio-cultural context ('Lebenswelten') of both the healer and the

---

[5] al-Malik al-Muẓaffar/al-Saqqā, *al-Muʿtamad*.

[6] al-Ṣanʿānī/Schopen and Kahl (eds. and trans., with a commentary), *Natāʾiǧ*.

[7] For a sociological analysis of these recent changes, see Muʿammar, *al-Ṭibb al-shaʿbī*.

[8] This is reflected in the numerous recent scientific publications by Yemeni authors on local medicinal plants, e.g. Alkhulaidi and Kessler, *Plants of Dhamar*; Bādhīb, *al-Nabātāt al-ṭibbiyya*; al-Dubaʿī and al-Khulaydī, *al-Nabātāt al-ṭibbiyya*; Jabalī, *al-Nabātāt al-shajariyya*; Wizārat al-Siyāḥa wa-l-bīʾa, *Nabātāt barriyya*, and the series of booklets "*Ṣaydaliyyat al-manzil al-ʿushbiyya*", each volume focusing on one or two plants, published in Ṣanʿāʾ by the Markaz ʿUbādī lil-dirāsāt wa-l-nashr, around 2000, but also articles in newspapers and journals for a wider target audience.

[9] WHO, *Essential Drugs*, [1].

[10] Fleurentin, *Guérisseurs*; Fleurentin and Pelt, 'Repertory'.

[11] Miller and Morris, *Ethnoflora*.

[12] The title of a Japanese study by Honda et al. (*Herb Drugs and Herbalists in Syria and North Yemen*) is misleading, though, because it deals mostly with Syria and refers to North Yemeni drugstores on less than five pages.

patient.[13] In particular, magico-religious rituals[14] add an additional value to "the holistic approach of indigenous knowledge systems in contrast to the reductionist approach of science."[15]

In order to do justice to the topic of this volume, *Herbal Medicine in Yemen: Traditional knowledge and practice, and their value for today's world*, a range of disciplinary approaches is required. Both the humanities and the natural sciences have an important role to play, not in competition, but in a complementary way. The aspect of interdependence of culture and nature inspires a discussion across boundaries of disciplines such as history, social anthropology, Oriental studies, biology, pharmacology, and pharmacy. Fourteen specialists on Yemen from North America, Europe, Israel, and Yemen have contributed to the book. Their research is based on textual analysis, as well as on empirical research and laboratory experiment, and covers both historical and contemporary aspects.

In her introductory contribution, pharmacist Ingrid Hehmeyer addresses the question of traditional medicine as an effective tool in issues of human health, using examples of *materia medica* and traditional practice from Yemen. She explores their historical and cultural dimensions, as well as the validity of their uses in today's society. The subsequent chapters (Lev, Schmidl) are based on textual evidence and contribute to our knowledge of medicinal herbs in earlier periods. Biologist and historian Efraim Lev, whose areas of specialization are the history of medicine and ethnopharmacology, centres upon the Yemeni medical lore found in medieval sources. He presents this information in the context of the medicinal substances found in the Cairo Genizah documents and the records of the sea trade between the eastern Mediterranean and India. Historian of science Petra G. Schmidl examines a thirteenth-century treatise on the science of the stars, the *Kitāb al-Tabṣira* by the Rasulid ruler of Yemen al-Ashraf ʿUmar (r. 1295–6), and in particular its magical and medical topics that are related to the stars in their broadest sense. The treatise explains connections between celestial events and human life on Earth with regard to prevention

---

13 Since the 1980s the effects of socio-cultural context have been claimed and studied for Western medical systems, see Sax, 'Traditional Methods', 28.

14 For research on this fascinating topic in the Islamic world, see Savage-Smith (ed.), *Magic and Divination*, especially the contribution by Dols, 'The Theory of Magic in Healing'.

15 Sillitoe, 'Local Science', 4. The holistic approach of indigenous knowledge systems has been studied within several cultures, e.g. Bodeker, 'Traditional Medical Knowledge' for Indian Ayurvedic and Chinese medicine, as well as Maass, *Cultural Context*, for a community in Guatemala.

and treatment of disease, along with the determination of the appropriate time to do so.

The subsequent chapters (Varisco, Morris, Muchawsky-Schnapper, Rodionov) take a humanities-based approach and discuss practical medical aspects of plants in contemporary Yemen. They focus on specific plants, or regions, or both. Studies on *qāt* (*Catha edulis*), be it by Western or Yemeni scholars from various disciplines, are numerous and deal primarily with its socio-economic and health-related problems. Anthropologist and historian Daniel Martin Varisco combines a study of historical sources, poetry, ethnographic accounts, and contemporary scientific analysis. He considers health impacts of *qāt* use within the ancient Greek system of humoural pathology and in Islamic legal sources, but he also claims positive effects on a person's health, and thus draws a more nuanced and objective picture of *qāt* as a drug. Miranda Morris specializes in the study of the Modern South Arabian languages and the ethnography of those who speak them. Her linguistic and ethnobotanical research on the use of aloes and frankincense in Soqotra concentrates on the more remote areas where the most valuable species flourish. Here she has discovered usages so far unknown in the Middle East, even in the towns of southern Arabia. Ethnographer Ester Muchawsky-Schnapper has studied the persistence of traditional knowledge and practice among Jews who emigrated from Yemen to Jerusalem. Secret healing knowledge has been attributed to this minority within the state of Israel. Even second-generation Yemenites still practise traditional healing methods using herbs, some of which were brought from Yemen at the time of immigration and then cultivated in a private setting. The final chapter of this section is also based on field research. Ḥaḍramawt is famous all over Yemen for its honey, and the typical bottle-shaped hives are well-known to every traveller who has visited that part of the country. Besides the medicinal qualities that are praised in the Qur'ān, specialist in Arabic studies and cultural anthropology Mikhail Rodionov has evaluated his field data and local poetry to discuss the symbolic roles and health-giving properties of honey, coffee, and tea, including the poetical rivalry and competition between the latter two.

Since the 1970s, ethnopharmacologist Jacques Fleurentin has analyzed the medicinal value of numerous plants, also taking into consideration aspects such as cultural context and magical practices. He stresses the extraordinary biodiversity of Yemen, not so much from a quantitative point of view (1750 plant species), but mainly with regard to the quality and genetic properties of certain plants, e.g. frankincense (*Boswellia sacra*), aloe

(*Aloe vera* which is the indigenous *Aloe barbadensis*), and coffee (*Coffea arabica*). With his chapter we enter the last section of the book, with three more contributions by natural scientists (Al-Duais/Jetschke, Lindequist, al-Hakimi/Ya'ni/Pelat). Plant ecologists Mohammed Al-Duais and Gottfried Jetschke, the former also a biochemist, the latter a developer of predictive models, present the example of *ḥalqa* (*Cyphostemma digitatum*), a plant that grows in Yemen's south-western highlands. Their research demonstrates that ethnobotanical knowledge can withstand the scrutiny of modern laboratory analysis. In addition, ethnobotanical work reminds us of the importance of sustainable use—instead of overexploitation—of the valuable plant resources. Pharmaceutical biologist Ulrike Lindequist enjoys well-established collaboration with Yemeni universities. Her research includes investigating the biological activity and chemical constituents of plants and fungi, and the results confirm the great potential of Yemen's natural resources for the development of new drugs. Specialist in plant breeding Amin Al-Hakimi, tropical agronomist Frédéric Pelat, and biologist Anhar Ya'ni outline the holistic setting of environment, culture and traditions in which the use of both wild and cultivated plants meets local therapeutic needs. They present numerous examples of farmers' orally transmitted knowledge, but also point out how this intangible cultural heritage is at risk of being lost to us for ever.

This volume, then, takes an interdisciplinary approach to the topic of traditional medicine in Yemen and presents it within the context of oral tradition, written sources, the socio-political and economic framework, as well as modern scientific insights. The editors are fundamentally concerned about the aspect of sustainability and the integrity of cultural property without which there would be little lasting value of this research for today's Yemen. While the focus of the book is on traditional medicine and Yemen, it is hoped that it will have much wider implications, because "[t]he discourse on the relationship between economic, ecological, and social issues in sustainable development and biodiversity conservation has gradually emphasized the re-discovery of culture [...]. In this process, indigenous knowledge as a prime part of culture has come to play an important role in international debates on development planning and conservation strategies."[16]

---

16 Maass, *Cultural Context*, 1.

Bibliography

Bādhīb, ʿAlī Sālim, *al-Nabātāt al-ṭibbiyya fī l-Yaman* (2nd edn.; Ṣanʿāʾ: Maktabat al-irshād, 1414/1993).

Bodeker, Gerard, 'Traditional Medical Knowledge and Twenty-first Century Healthcare: The Interface between Indigenous and Modern Science', in Sillitoe (ed.), *Local Science*, 23–39.

Dols, Michael W., 'The Theory of Magic in Healing', in Savage-Smith (ed.), *Magic and Divination*, 87–101.

al-Dubaʿī, ʿAbd al-Raḥmān Saʿīd, and al-Khulaydī, ʿAbd al-Walī Aḥmad, *al-Nabātāt al-ṭibbiyya wa-l-ʿiṭriyya fī l-Yaman* (2nd edn.; Ṣanʿāʾ: Markaz ʿUbādī lil-dirāsāt wa-l-nashr, 2005).

Fleurentin, Jacques, *Guérisseurs et plantes médicinales du Yémen : Au pays de l'encens, de l'aloès et du café* (Paris : Karthala, 2004).

———, and Pelt, Jean-Marie, 'Repertory of Drugs and Medicinal Plants of Yemen', *Journal of Ethnopharmacology*, 6 (1982), 85–108.

Honda, Gisho, Miki, Wataru, and Saito, Mitsuko, *Herb Drugs and Herbalists in Syria and North Yemen* (Tokyo: Institute for the Study of Languages and Cultures of Asia and Africa, 1990).

Ibn al-Bayṭār, ʿAbdallāh Ibn Aḥmad/Leclerc, Lucien (trans.), *Traité des simples par Ibn el-Beïthar* (3 vols.; Paris : Imprimerie nationale, 1877–83).

Jabalī, Saʿīd ʿAbduh, *al-Nabātāt al-shajariyya fī l-Yaman* (Aden: Jāmiʿat ʿAdan, 1993).

Al Khulaidi, Abdul-Wali A. [al-Khulaydī, ʿAbd al-Walī], and Kessler, Jan J., *Plants of Dhamar: Some Plant Species of Dhamar Montane Plains and Surrounding Areas (Yemen)* (Ṣanʿāʾ: Obadi Studies, reprint 2001 [1999]).

Maass, Petra, *The Cultural Context of Biodiversity Conservation: Seen and Unseen Dimensions of Indigenous Knowledge among Q'eqchi' Communities in Guatemala* (Göttingen: Universität sverlag, 2008).

al-Malik al-Muẓaffar Yūsuf b. ʿUmar al-Ghassānī al-Turkmānī/al-Saqqā, Muṣṭafā (ed.), *al-Muʿtamad fī l-adwiya al-mufrada* (Beirut: Dār al-qalam, 1951).

Miller, Anthony G., and Morris, Miranda, *Ethnoflora of the Soqotra Archipelago* (Edinburgh: Royal Botanic Garden, 2004).

Muʿammar, ʿAbdallāh, *al-Ṭibb al-shaʿbī wa-l-taṭawwur al-ijtimāʿī fī l-Yaman* (Cairo: Maktabat Madbūlī, 1999).

al-Ṣanʿānī, Šaʿbān Ibn Salīm/Schopen, Armin, and Kahl, Oliver (eds. and trans., with a commentary), *Die Natāʾiǧ al-fikar des Šaʿbān ibn Salīm aṣ-Ṣanʿānī: Eine jemenitische Gesundheitsfibel aus dem frühen 18. Jahrhundert* (Wiesbaden: Harrassowitz 1993).

Savage-Smith, Emilie (ed.), *Magic and Divination in Early Islam* (Aldershot: Ashgate Variorum, 2004).

Sax, Lila, 'Traditional Methods and Ethnic Choices. Prenatal Care and the Importance of Ethnicity for Health Seeking Behavior', *Cargo, Ethnologie und Medizin*, 29 (2008), 23–33.

Schopen, Armin, *Traditionelle Heilmittel in Jemen* (Wiesbaden: Steiner, 1983).

Sillitoe, Paul (ed.), *Local Science vs. Global Science: Approaches to Indigenous Knowledge in International Development* (New York: Berghahn Books, 2007).

———, 'Local Science vs. Global Science: An Overview', in id. (ed.), *Local Science*, 1–22.

Wizārat al-Siyāḥa wa-l-bīʾa [Yemen], *Nabātāt barriyya min al-Yaman* (UNDP, [s. l.] al-Āfāq lil-ṭibāʿa wa-l-nashr 2002).

Internet Sources

WHO (World Health Organization), *Essential Drugs in Brief*, 7 (July 2002) <http://www.who.int/medicines/publications/brief/en/edb07.pdf>, accessed October 2010.

THE VALIDITY OF TRADITIONAL MEDICINE AS AN EFFECTIVE TOOL IN ISSUES OF HUMAN HEALTH

Ingrid Hehmeyer

1. Preamble

The World Health Organization defines traditional medicine as "the sum total of the knowledge, skills and practices based on the theories, beliefs and experiences indigenous to different cultures, whether explicable or not, used in the maintenance of health, as well as in the prevention, diagnosis, improvement or treatment of physical and mental illness."[1] According to this definition, traditional medicine is a complex network of interaction of both ideas and practices, the study of which requires a multidisciplinary approach.

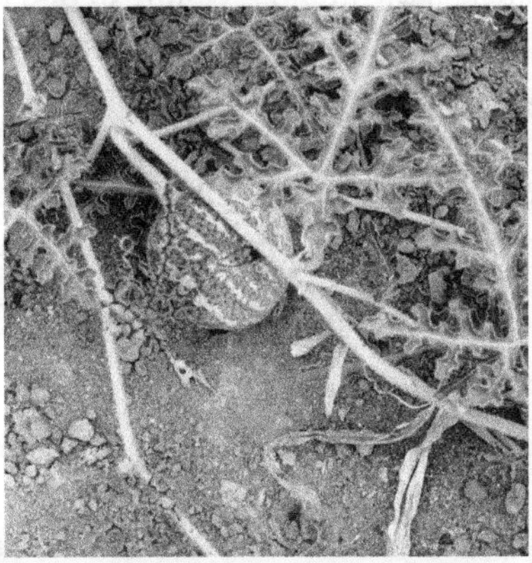

Figure 1. *Citrullus colocynthis* (Cucurbitaceae) in the Wādī Zabīd (© Ingrid Hehmeyer, 1998)

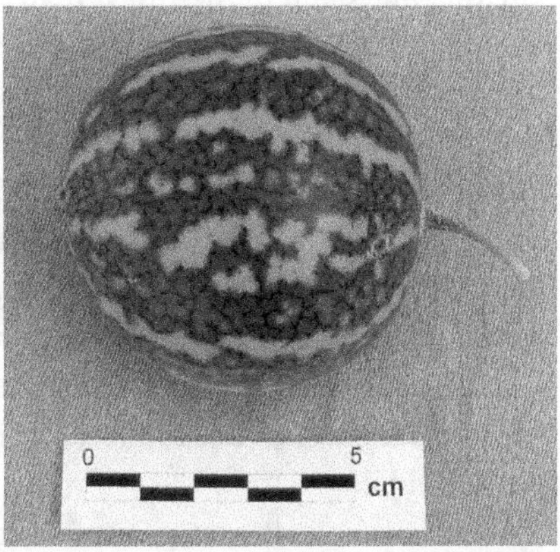

Figure 2. Fruit of *Citrullus colocynthis* (© Ingrid Hehmeyer, 2010)

This paper takes the example of a plant that grows in Yemen and explores its properties in light of the World Health Organization's definition. The anthropological fieldwork that forms the basis of the study was carried out in the city of Zabīd and its hinterland, and the plant in question is called

[1] WHO, *General Guidelines*, 1.

ḥanẓal in Arabic, colocynth in English, or colloquially bitter gourd. Its botanical name is *Citrullus colocynthis* (Cucurbitaceae) (Fig. 1). Other well-known cucurbits today are melons, cucumbers, and gourds. The colocynth is a native of arid environments in Africa and Asia. The drought-resistant perennial plant grows wild, not cultivated. Its vine-like stems spread on the ground, with deeply lobed leaves, yellow flowers, and globular fruits. Typically, these are shiny green with yellow stripes and are the size of a small apple (Fig. 2). Removal of the hard rind exposes a white spongy pulp in which numerous seeds are imbedded.

2. Evidence of the Colocynth in Ancient South Arabia

The earliest text known so far that attests to the occurrence of the colocynth in ancient South Arabia is the inscription Gl 1679 + Gl 1773 a+b = Ja 2848y, 1–10.[2] It was carved on a rock slope above the ancient dam of Mārib in boustrophedon style—that is, alternate lines are written in opposite directions, with one line from right to left and the next one from left to right, 'turning like oxen ploughing a field' which is the literal meaning of boustrophedon in Greek. Since strict right-to-left writing of Old South Arabian became standard by the seventh century BCE,[3] we may surmise that the inscription predates this time. The text talks about the fact that the god ʿAthtar, who was worshipped as a benefactor of water, finally sent rain to the region of Mārib, apparently after a period of prolonged drought. The inscription (lines 9–10) mentions in particular the "realm of Ḥanẓalān" in the Mārib oasis as having been watered by the rains. The "realm of Ḥanẓalān" is to be understood here as a designation of a proper name, referring to a specific district, but it is remarkable in so far as its literal meaning is 'colocynth field.'[4]

Seeds of the colocynth were identified in Yemen in archaeological soil samples from the excavations in Barāqish, dating to the first millennium BCE.[5] Besides the textual hint, then, there is archaeobotanical evidence that the colocynth was used in ancient South Arabia.

---

[2] See Müller, 'Dokumente', 270.
[3] Breton, *Arabia Felix*, 30.
[4] Müller, 'Dokumente', 270; Hehmeyer and Schmidt, *Wasserwirtschaft*, 57.
[5] Costantini and Costantini Biasini, 'Bioarchaeology', 362.

3. Past and Present Uses of the Colocynth in Yemen

The classical Arabic name of the colocynth, *ḥanẓal*, is clearly derived from the same root as the Old South Arabian term. Today, in the Wādī Zabīd where the plant grows wild, people immediately point out the violent purgative effect of the pulp of the fruit. It is used in case of occasional constipation, but more importantly for internal purification. In addition, the dried, pulverized pulp is manufactured into an ointment that is applied to treat rheumatic pain.[6] The active constituents are the cucurbitacins, a group of substances (chemically speaking, tetracyclic triterpenes) with exceedingly bitter taste and irritating effects that are responsible for the medicinal properties of the colocynth.

Rheumatic diseases are caused by an inflammation. The inflammation stimulates sensory nerves and this is what causes pain. If one applies a cucurbitacin-rich ointment externally to the affected area, the cucurbitacins irritate the skin, leading to an increased blood flow and stimulation of the sensory nerves in the tissue lying beneath. The result of this so-called counter-irritant effect is a weakening of the stimulation through the original inflammation and thus a lessening of the pain.[7] However, the causes of the rheumatic disorder are not treated, only the symptoms.

When applied internally, the cucurbitacins irritate the mucous membranes of the intestine and act as a hydragogue—that is, they cause a discharge of watery fluid into the intestine and thus evacuation of watery stools. Use of the colocynth is not without dangers, though. The cucurbitacins can irritate the mucous membranes to the point of causing an inflammation of the intestine accompanied by bloody diarrhoea, technically haemorrhagic colitis. If taken orally in larger quantities, the cucurbitacins are toxic.[8]

The colocynth fruit can be found in pharmacists' shops not only in Zabīd, but in all the larger cities of Yemen. In the countryside, people gather the fruits from the wild plant. Desert animals, however, avoid the plant altogether and in particular the ripe fruit that is especially rich in cucurbitacins.

---

[6] See Schopen, *Heilmittel*, 46, for further uses.

[7] Schneider, *Pharmazeutische Biologie*, 374–5; Caesar, 'Bryonia', 56–7.

[8] Al Faraj, 'Haemorrhagic Colitis', 695–6; Pfab, 'Vergiftungen', 41; Goldfain et al., 'Acute Toxic Colitis', 1412–18. Interestingly, the latter article reports three cases from Morocco that were caused by ingestion of a milk-colocynth pulp mixture taken for "ritual purposes of purification and vitalisation" (1417). The frequently cited article by Berrut et al., 'Colite pseudomembraneuse', 135–8, clearly confuses the colocynth with a different species of the cucurbits, see 136, Fig. 2.

Less tangible is a totally different kind of application of the fruit that was reported by the ethnographer Erich Brauer. In a 1934 publication entitled *Ethnography of the Yemeni Jews*, the author describes how the fruit of the colocynth was suspended in houses for protection from the evil eye (*al-ʿayn*).[9] In the Jewish community of Ṣanʿāʾ it was employed for the same purpose, as part of the wall decorations of the room where a new mother would receive well-wishers on the first or second Sabbath after the birth of a child. Until today, a new Muslim mother follows similar customs and these include the colocynth as part of the room decorations.[10] Pieces of the colocynth rind are said to be used in amulets that are worn for protection from the evil eye and are intended to ensure well-being.[11]

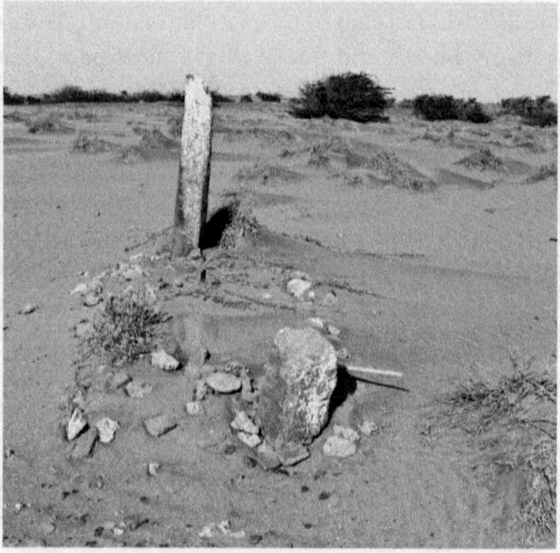

Figure 3. Grave with marker stones and colocynth plant (near al-Fazza, Tihāma) (© Elisa Fazio, 2010)

The conviction that certain people possess, by a mere glance of the eye, the power to cause misfortune, illness, and death to others, their families and their belongings, is widespread in human civilization, from ancient to modern times, and in the Middle East in particular. Whatever the nature of the connection between the glance of the eye and the inflicted evil may be, there are clearly supernatural forces involved—as there are in the ap-

9 Brauer, *Ethnologie*, 72–3.
10 See also Muchawsky-Schnapper, 'Symbolic Decorations', 69–70.
11 Schopen, *Heilmittel*, 45–6.

propriate counteraction. Defence against the potential disaster typically entails the presentation of relevant items for protection, such as objects depicting the eye, the outstretched hand, or, as in the example described here, suspension of the colocynth. Apparently, its bitter taste and poisonous qualities make it "a potent shield against evil spirits."[12] For the same reason, since early Islamic times the Bedouin of the Arabian Peninsula are reported to have named their male children Ḥanẓala.[13] In Yemen people believe that the colocynth extends its protection from evil interference even beyond death, and sowing colocynth seeds onto a burial site is part of the local mortuary practices along the Red Sea coast. Figure 3 shows two standing stones marking a grave, with a colocynth plant growing out of it. The bitterness and toxicity deter the evil spirits that may otherwise disturb the peace of the dead.

There is yet another interesting nuance regarding the colocynth, and that is a linguistic one. Brauer cites a Yemeni Arabic song in which *ḥanẓal* serves as a synonym for bitter experience in life.[14] With this connotation, *ḥanẓal* is used in Yemeni Arabic until today. In her book on *Cosmetics, Scents, and Incense*, Hanne Schönig cites the expression *amarr min al-ḥanẓal*, "more bitter than colocynth."[15] The bitterness of the colocynth is also proverbial among the Jewish community of Yemen.[16]

4. Textual Context: Non-Yemeni Sources

Regarding textual information on the colocynth, the potential dangers due to its toxicity were known even in the ancient Near East, and it is believed that the 'wild gourd' of the following story from the Hebrew Bible (II Kings 4:38–40) is the colocynth:[17]

> And Elisha came again to Gilgal: and there was a dearth in the land; and the sons of the prophets were sitting before him: and he said unto his servant, 'Set on the great pot and seethe pottage for the sons of the prophets.' And

---

12 Muchawsky-Schnapper, 'Symbolic Decorations', 69.

13 Jacob, *Beduinenleben*, 11; see Walther, *Arabische Personennamen*, 50, for examples. The same habit has been observed in the eastern Mediterranean during medieval Islamic times, see Lev and Amar, *Practical* Materia Medica, 387, and it has been documented as late as the 1970s among the Bedouin of the Negev, see Bailey and Danin, 'Bedouin Plant Utilization', 146.

14 Brauer, *Ethnologie*, 213–15.

15 Schönig, *Schminken*, 244. See also Qafisheh, *Dictionary*, 146.

16 Goitein, *Jemenica*, 65, no. 403.

17 Tristram, *Natural History*, 450–2.

> one went out into the fields to gather herbs, and found a wild vine, and gathered thereof wild gourds his lap full, and came and shred them into the pot of pottage: for they knew them not. So they poured out for the men to eat. And it came to pass, as they were eating of the pottage, that they cried out, and said, 'O thou man of God, there is death in the pot.' And they could not eat thereof.

In medieval Islamic times, the dangers of *Citrullus colocynthis* were equally understood. *Kitāb al-Sumūm* [The Book on Poisons] is attributed to the ninth-tenth-century author Ibn Waḥshiyya.[18] Reading between the lines, it is a malicious manual on the effectiveness of poisonous principles that kill humans—including lethal sounds and smells, as well as simple and compound poisons. For each of these, Ibn Waḥshiyya gives a description of the symptoms that they cause, followed by the recipe for an appropriate antidote and instructions for its administration. In the chapter on the manufacture of compound poisons that kill when eaten or drunk, the author lists the colocynth as the active ingredient in his "Description of Another Compound Poison, the Twenty-fifth". He describes the mixture as causing "sharp colic in the belly"[19] and, depending on the dose, being potentially lethal.

But the colocynth was also valued by the medieval authors for its medicinal properties. Several classical Arabic sources deal with *materia medica*, which is defined as the sum of the simple (i.e. non-compound) drugs, a 'drug' being a substance of natural (i.e. plant, animal or mineral) origin used for its medicinal properties. The most influential work on *materia medica* was composed by the thirteenth-century Andalusian pharmaceutical biologist Ibn al-Bayṭār (d. 1248). He travelled widely throughout northern Africa, the eastern Mediterranean, Asia Minor, and Italy, studying *materia medica*. His *al-Jāmiʿ li-mufradāt al-adwiya wa-l-aghdhiya* [Comprehensive Book on Simple Drugs and Foodstuffs], is an encyclopaedia of the *materia medica* known at the time, with the entries of the individual drugs organized alphabetically. The work demonstrates first of all the author's excellent knowledge of the sources compiled by his predecessors. Under the entry *ḥanẓal* Ibn al-Bayṭār cites the great authorities on *materia medica* both from the ancient past, such as Dioscorides (1st century CE) and Galen (d. after 203), and from Islamic times, among whom is Ibn Sīnā (d. 1037).[20]

---

18 See Fahd, 'Ibn Waḥshiyya', 963b–965b, for the controversy over his identity.
19 Levey, *Toxicology*, 65.
20 Ibn al-Bayṭār/Leclerc (trans.), *Traité*, 1, 461–4.

In the introduction to his *Kitāb al-Ṣaydana fī l-ṭibb* [Book on Pharmacy] which was completed in the 1040s, al-Bīrūnī, one of the great scholars and innovative thinkers of medieval Islam, points out that good knowledge of *materia medica* forms the basis of pharmacy.[21] In the chapter on the colocynth, which is unfortunately not cited by Ibn al-Bayṭār, al-Bīrūnī describes the medicinal value of the plant, in particular as a purgative, while also warning against its potential dangers.[22] Specifically, if a plant bears only one fruit, it should be avoided since its effect is too powerful. The author gives the following explanation: "the root's power is transferred in toto to the flower"[23]—that is, the active constituents are transported from the root, the location of their synthesis, to the fruit. This, of course, is pure speculation on the part of the author and, in fact, botanically incorrect. The cucurbitacins are not transported within the plant, but are synthesized *in situ* within those plant organs where they are typically found.[24]

The great authority on the preparation and application of compound drugs was the ninth-century physician and pharmacist Sābūr Ibn Sahl (d. 869). His *al-Aqrābādhīn al-ṣaghīr* [Small Dispensatory] comprises 408 recipes. For each of these, the author lists the ingredients with their doses, instructions for manufacture, and directions for application. Sābūr had 299 simple drugs of plant origin at his disposal.[25] The colocynth is specified as an ingredient in twenty-three recipes.[26]

The classical Arabic texts also refer to a different use of the colocynth that people today in the Middle East tend to keep silent about. Like other purgatives that have a violent effect on the lower intestines, the colocynth can be used to cause an abortion, i.e. as an abortifacient. ʿArīb Ibn Saʿd al-Kātib al-Qurṭubī (d. *c.*980) was a physician from the western part of the Islamic world, al-Andalus, who wrote a treatise *Kitāb Khalq al-janīn wa-tadbīr al-ḥabālā wa-l-mawlūd* [On the Development of the Fetus, the Treatment of Pregnant Women, and the Newborn Baby]. It is clear from the title of the work that the author's main concern was in healthy pregnancies

---

21 al-Bīrūnī/Said (ed. and trans.), *Pharmacy*, 1–2 and 6. See Hehmeyer, 'Pharmaceutical Utensils', 237 and n. 3, for further details.

22 al-Bīrūnī/Said (ed. and trans.), *Pharmacy*, 131–2.

23 Ibid., 132.

24 Frohne and Pfänder, *Giftpflanzen*, 148.

25 This equals 79.1% of the total *materia medica*, see Kahl (trans.), *Dispensatory*, 14–16. Animal substances make up 10.6% and substances of mineral origin 10.3%.

26 Sābūr's work was edited by Kahl in 1994 (*Dispensatorium*) and a translation was submitted by the same author in 2003 (*Dispensatory*).—For further references on the colocynth, see Lev and Amar, *Practical* Materia Medica, 385–7.

and deliveries. But in this context he also identified cases where an abortion was called for. The *materia medica* that he recommended for that purpose includes the colocynth.[27] May one suggest that Sābūr Ibn Sahl's recipe no. 69—which contains a substantial quantity of colocynth pulp, and that he describes as making "the menstrual blood flow that stopped untimely"—points in a similar direction?[28] This particular concoction would have had an exceedingly violent effect because colocynth pulp was combined with aloe and cassia, both of which are strong laxatives as well, in addition to some other ingredients that are known for their abortive effects, such as cinnamon and parsley.[29] In today's Middle East women still take colocynth pulp to induce an abortion, despite its toxicity, and the medical literature reports cases of women who have died as a result.[30]

5. Yemeni Sources

The colocynth is also mentioned in a thirteenth-century Yemeni treatise on *materia medica*, *al-Muʿtamad fī l-adwiya al-mufrada* [The Reliable Source on Simple Medicines], most probably composed by the third Rasulid sultan of Yemen, al-Ashraf ʿUmar (d. 1296).[31] Al-Ashraf ʿUmar is well-known as a scholar who wrote a number of scientific works, several of which focus on medical topics.[32] The authorship of *al-Muʿtamad* has been contested, though. Daniel Varisco states in his book *Medieval Agriculture and Islamic Science* that the "text is usually assigned to the [...] father, al-Malik al-Muẓaffar," the second Rasulid ruler (d. 1295), and that "there is no evidence that this important and widely circulated herbal should not be attributed to al-Malik al-Muẓaffar."[33] The confusion is well reflected in the

---

[27] ʿArîb Ibn Saʿîd [*sic*] Al-Kâtib Al-Qûrtûbi [*sic*]/Makaci (trans.), *Génération*, 86. For the correct name of the author, see Pellat, "Arīb', 628a–b.

[28] Sābūr Ibn Sahl/Kahl (trans.), *Dispensatory*, 69–70. Recipes nos. 114 and 115 are simply recommended to "make the menstrual blood flow" (84–5).

[29] Wichtl, *Teedrogen*, 154, 433, 435–6. As for parsley, it is the fruits and the root that are used until today to induce abortions. Sābūr's text, though, does not specify the organ of the plant that should be added to the recipe, see Sābūr Ibn Sahl/Kahl (ed.), *Dispensatorium*, 82, line 12.

[30] Qédan, 'Volksmedizin', 70; Venzlaff, *Drogenhändler*, 64; Bellakhdar, *Pharmacopée*, 262–3; Akhmisse, *Médecine*, 113.

[31] Brockelmann, *GAL* I, 650 (494) and S I, 901.

[32] Varisco, *Almanac*, 14–16.

[33] Ibid., 16. Varisco's book is a critical edition, English translation, and detailed analysis of an agricultural almanac that was compiled by the same al-Ashraf ʿUmar as one of fifty

edition that is used by the present writer (Hehmeyer): while the father's name is given on the title page, the editor states that the author is "al-Malik al-Muẓaffar al-Ashraf"—and thus gets the honorific titles of father and son mixed up.[34] The problem was apparently caused by a mistake in the manuscript that was used as the basis for one of the edited and printed versions of the text and that—it seems wrongly—attributed the work to al-Ashraf 'Umar's father, while the real author was al-Ashraf 'Umar himself.[35] Both had excellent knowledge of medicine, as is acknowledged by the official court historian of the Rasulids, al-Khazrajī (d. 1410), who was intimately acquainted with the individuals. Reading between the lines of a report about a medical crisis one gets the impression that in the 1270s the son had already surpassed his father in the mastery of medical science.[36]

Varisco has pointed out that *al-Muʿtamad* "is in fact largely derivative from previous Arabic herbals and offers little information specific to Yemen."[37] This is entirely correct, and at the beginning of *al-Muʿtamad* the author even cites the great authorities on *materia medica* whom he employs as sources. Ibn al-Bayṭār is among them.[38] Nevertheless, the work does make a valuable contribution insofar as it reflects a deliberate choice of the material that the author included—or, conversely, decided not to include—in his text, first of all because he selected *materia medica* with which he was familiar from his native country of Yemen.

Like his predecessors, he organized the entries alphabetically. For the colocynth, the author lists, among others, the following uses: as a purgative, as a treatment of rheumatic pain, and as an agent of abortion (abortifacient). At the same time, he warns about the dangers of the drug and its potentially lethal properties.[39]

---

chapters comprising his major work on astronomy, *al-Tabṣira fī ʿilm al-nujūm* [Enlightenment on the Science of the Stars] (see Petra Schmidl's chapter in this volume).

34 Ibn Rasūl/Muhannā (ed.), *al-Muʿtamad*, 9.

35 See al-Ziriklī, *al-Aʿlām*, 5, 69 and n. 3. I am indebted to Jābir ʿAbduh ʿAlī ʿAbdallāh, M.A., Department of History, University of al-Ḥudayda, Yemen, for having drawn my attention to this discrepancy and to the reference.

36 al-Khazrajī/Redhouse (trans.) and ʿAsal (ed.), *Pearl-strings*, 1, 233 (English translation), and 4, 277–8 (Arabic text). See Bosworth, 'al-K͟hazrad͟jī', 1188b, for general information on the author.

37 Varisco, *Almanac*, 16.

38 Incidentally, Ibn al-Bayṭār's own chapter on the colocynth is equally a compilation of information gathered by his predecessors and does not constitute his original research.

39 Ibn Rasūl/Muhannā (ed.), *al-Muʿtamad*, 103–5.

6. Conclusion

At this point it is clear that the medicinal properties of the colocynth provide a well-founded basis for its administration to treat certain physical conditions. Even though until quite recently chemical analysis to identify the active constituents—the cucurbitacins in the case of *Citrullus colocynthis*—was not available, experience showed that the drug worked: people could observe the evidence. It is therefore not surprising that the colocynth has formed part of the Yemeni *materia medica* for a long period of time, both in terms of its practical application and its description in the medical manuals.

Use of the colocynth for protection from the evil eye and as an amulet reflects a different principle.[40] It calls upon supernatural forces and, instead of treating a physical symptom, it targets the mind. In classical Islamic medicine, a clear understanding prevails of the human being as an entity of body and mind. The physician al-Rāzī (d. *c.*925), one of the great independent medical thinkers and practitioners, addressed both aspects in his works. While being a meticulous clinical observer of physical illnesses and their symptoms, it is mostly in his alchemical writings that he openly admits that there are unexplained phenomena in nature.[41]

In their 1982 article "Repertory of Drugs and Medicinal Plants of Yemen," Jacques Fleurentin and Jean-Marie Pelt have pointed out that traditional medical practices include those that are *materia medica*-based, and those that are not of an explicable nature.[42] But the authors have hinted at the fact that this straight-forward categorization may be an oversimplification. For example, a purgative may be administered in order to eliminate evil spirits, and while there will be an explicable and observable medical effect, the reason for the prescription is not constipation, but the belief that the patient is suffering from a condition induced by evil spirits who have to be expelled.[43] In traditional medicine, the causes of illness can also be of supernatural origin. This has been one of the most basic principles of human health concerns since ancient times and the evidence can be found beginning with the earliest medical texts from the ancient Near East.

---

[40] See Claisse-Dauchy, *Médecine traditionnelle*, 98–9, for two hypothetical explanations of the magical associations of the colocynth that may provide the reason for the plant's use in magic-medicinal practices in today's Morocco.

[41] See Goodman, 'al-Rāzī', 474b–475a.

[42] Fleurentin and Pelt, 'Repertory', 87.

[43] Ibid., 105.

An example was observed by the present writer in Zabīd in the year 2007. Figure 4 shows Sharīf Qāsim ʿAbdallāh al-Ahdal, a local healer (second from left) and his young patient (second from right) who was suffering from a serious skin disease. Of course, even in modern medicine skin diseases are notorious for being difficult to diagnose, and equally difficult to treat. After seeing a local doctor whose prescription of various Western medicines did not ease the boy's condition, his father took him to a specialist in the capital city of Ṣanʿāʾ, again to no avail. Following their return to Zabīd, the father decided to try a local healer as a last resort. Sharīf Qāsim ʿAbdallāh al-Ahdal came to the house every other day to treat his patient, rubbing on a preparation whose recipe he did not wish to reveal. Each treatment started and ended with the healer taking a sip of water and spitting three times onto the skin lesions—and by doing this he was, in effect, spitting at the evil spirits causing the disease. The boy's condition improved considerably, at least over the next weeks.

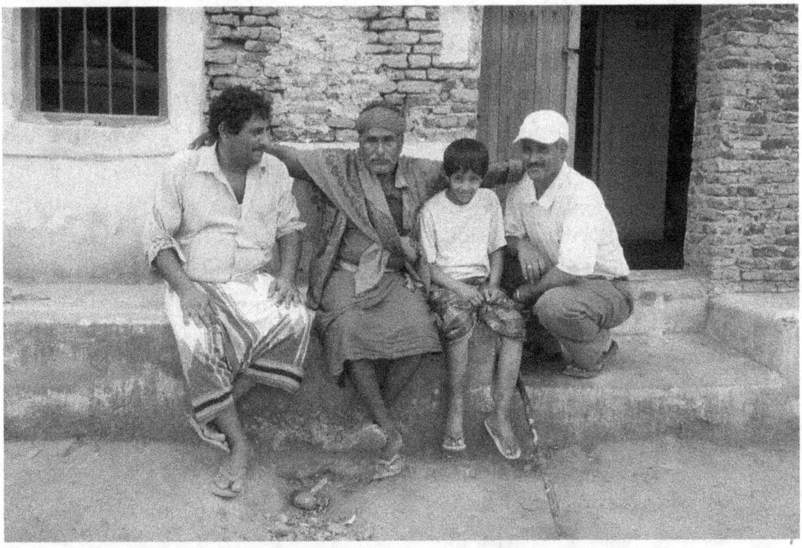

Figure 4. Sharīf Qāsim ʿAbdallāh al-Ahdal, a local healer in Zabīd (second from left) with his young patient (second from right) (© Ingrid Hehmeyer, 2007)

One may easily be critical here and judge that such irrational practices do not deserve to be called 'medical.' In a 2002 article in the *Annals of Internal Medicine*, Daniel Moerman and Wayne Jonas have pointed out the significance of what they termed "meaningfulness" in our understanding of the physiologic or psychological response of a patient to treatment.[44] The practitioner's manner, the authority that transpires from him or her, or the performance of certain procedures and rituals, are all meaningful for the therapeutic outcome. For the patient, the 'meaning response' can be an important component within the complex healing process, and the practitioner has to be aware of the fact that there is more involved in successful therapy than simply applying a drug with medicinally active constituents. To underline their position, the authors give an example from the history of medicine, from the *Dialogues of Plato*, that attribute the following to Socrates:

> [The cure for the headache] was a kind of leaf, which required to be accompanied by a charm, and if a person would repeat the charm at the same time that he used the cure, he would be made whole; but that without the charm the leaf would be of no avail.[45]

Western physicians trained in a rational, science-based approach to diagnosis and treatment have observed in Yemen with admiration the wholehearted commitment that a traditional healer offers to his patient. His practices regularly include magico-religious rituals.[46] In traditional medicine—as for most human beings—there is no strict separation between the rational and the supernatural, which is why the WHO's definition specifically includes "knowledge, skills and practices [...], whether explicable or not."[47] May one suggest that in order to enhance the success of modern Western medical procedures a combination with certain traditional treatment options might also have beneficial effects? After all, Western medicine can neither explain what causes many diseases, nor offer a cure for them. Under any circumstance, maximising the 'meaning response' should be a priority.

Bibliography

Akhmisse, Mustapha, *Médecine, Magie et Sorcellerie au Maroc ou L'Art traditionnel de guérir* , (Casablanca : Eddar El Beida [1985]).

Al Faraj, S., 'Haemorrhagic Colitis Induced by *Citrullus*', *Annals of Tropical Medicine and Parasitology*, 89 (1995), 695–6.

44 Moerman and Jonas, 'Meaning Response', 472–5.

45 Ibid., 471; a literal translation from Plato's dialogue *Charmides* 155e.

46 Middendorp. 'Eingeborenenmedizin', 10. The present writer has made similar observations.

47 WHO, *General Guidelines*, 1.

'Arîb Ibn Sa'îd [*sic*] Al-Kâtib Al-Qûrtûbi [*sic*]/Makaci, Mustapha (trans.), *Le livre de la génération du fœtus et le traitement des femmes enceintes et des nouveau-nés* ([Algiers :] Anep, 2002).

Bailey, Clinton, and Danin, Avinoam, 'Bedouin Plant Utilization in Sinai and the Negev', *Economic Botany*, 35 (1981), 145–62.

Bellakhdar, Jamal, *La pharmacopée marocaine traditionnelle : Médecine arabe ancienne et savoirs populaires* (Paris : Ibis, 1997).

Berrut, C., Bisetti, A., Widgren, S., Tissot, J.-D., and Loizeau, E., 'Colite pseudomembraneuse causée par l'ingestion de coloquinte', *Schweizerische Medizinische Wochenschrift*, 117 (1987), 135–8.

The Holy Bible/Authorised King James Version (London: The Crusaders' Union [c.1950]).

al-Bīrūnī, Abū l-Rayḥān Muḥammad Ibn Aḥmad/Said, Hakim Mohammed (ed. and trans.), *Kitāb al-Ṣaydana fī l-ṭibb/al-Biruni's Book on Pharmacy and* Materia Medica (1. vol; Karachi: Hamdard National Foundation, 1973).

Bosworth, Clifford E., 'al-Khazradjī', *EI*², IV (1978), 1188b.

Brauer, Erich, *Ethnologie der jemenitischen Juden* (Kulturgeschichtliche Bibliothek, 1. Reihe: Ethnologische Bibliothek, 7; Heidelberg: Winter, 1934).

Breton, Jean-François, *Arabia Felix from the Time of the Queen of Sheba: Eighth Century B.C. to First Century A.D.* (Notre Dame/IN: University of Notre Dame Press, 1999).

Brockelmann, Carl, *Geschichte der arabischen Litteratur* (2 vols., 3 suppls.; 2nd edn.; Leiden: Brill, 1943–9).

Caesar, Wolfgang, 'Zaunrübe—Bryonia: Ein Homöopathikum bei stechenden Schmerzen', *PTA Heute*, 9 (2008), 56–7.

Claisse-Dauchy, Renée, *Médecine traditionnelle du Maghreb : Rituels d'envoûtement et de guérison au Maroc* (Paris : L'Harmattan; Montréal/Canada : L'Harmattan INC, 1996).

Costantini, Lorenzo, and Costantini Biasini, Loredana, 'Laboratory of Bioarchaeology', *East and West*, 36/4 (1986), 354–65.

*EI*² = *The Encyclopaedia of Islam* (New Edition) (12 vols., and suppl.; Leiden: Brill, 1960–2005).

Fahd, Toufic, 'Ibn Waḥshiyya', *EI*², III (1971), 963b–965b.

Fleurentin, Jacques, and Pelt, Jean-Marie, 'Repertory of Drugs and Medicinal Plants of Yemen', *Journal of Ethnopharmacology*, 6 (1982), 85–108.

Frohne, Dietrich, and Pfänder, Hans Jürgen, *Giftpflanzen: Ein Handbuch für Apotheker, Ärzte, Toxikologen und Biologen* (5th edn.; Stuttgart: Wissenschaftliche Verlagsgesellschaft, 2004).

Goitein, Solomon D. F., *Jemenica: Sprichwörter und Redensarten aus Zentral-Jemen* (reprint Leiden: Brill, 1970).

Goldfain, D., Lavergne, A., Galian, A., Chauveinc, L., and Prudhomme, F., 'Peculiar Acute Toxic Colitis after Ingestion of Colocynth: A Clinicopathological Study of Three Cases', *Gut*, 30 (1989), 1412–18.

Goodman, L. E., 'al-Rāzī', *EI*², VIII (1995), 474a–477b.

Hehmeyer, Ingrid, 'Pharmaceutical Utensils from the Islamic Period and Their Practical Use', *Bulletin of the Canadian Society for Mesopotamian Studies*, 36 (2001), 235–42.

———, and Schmidt, Jürgen, *Antike Technologie: Die Sabäische Wasserwirtschaft von Mārib* (Archäologische Berichte aus dem Yemen, 5; Mainz: Zabern, 1991).

Ibn al-Bayṭār, 'Abdallāh Ibn Aḥmad/Leclerc, Lucien (trans.), *Traité des simples par Ibn el-Beïthar* (3 vols.; Paris : Imprimerie nationale, 1877–83).

Ibn Rasūl, Yūsuf Ibn 'Umar Ibn 'Alī/Muhannā, Muḥammad Riḍwān (ed.), *al-Mu'tamad fī l-adwiya al-mufrada* (al-Manṣūra: Maktabat jazīrat al-ward, 2004).

Jacob, Georg, *Altarabisches Beduinenleben* (Berlin: Mayer & Müller, 1897).

al-Khazrajī, 'Alī Ibn al-Ḥasan/Redhouse, James W. (trans.), and 'Asal, Muḥammad (ed.), *The Pearl-strings: A History of the Resúliyy Dynasty of Yemen, by 'Aliyyu 'bnu 'l-Hasan 'el-Khazrejiyy* (E. J. W. Gibb Memorial Series, 3, 5 vols.; Leiden: Brill; London: Luzac, 1906–18).

Lev, Efraim, and Amar, Zohar, *Practical* Materia Medica *of the Medieval Eastern Mediterranean According to the Cairo Genizah* (Sir Henry Wellcome Asian Series, 7; Leiden: Brill, 2008).

Levey, Martin, *Medieval Arabic Toxicology: The Book on Poisons of Ibn Waḥshīya and Its Relation to Early Indian and Greek Texts* (Transactions of the American Philosophical Society, New Series, 56, part 7; Philadelphia: The American Philosophical Society, 1966).

al-Malik al-Muẓaffar, see Ibn Rasūl.

Middendorp, U. G., 'Beobachtungen zur Eingeborenenmedizin in Nord-Yemen', *Acta Tropica*, 26/1 (1969), 1–14.

Moerman, Daniel E., and Jonas, Wayne B., 'Deconstructing the Placebo Effect and Finding the Meaning Response', *Annals of Internal Medicine*, 136/6 (2002), 471–6.

Muchawsky-Schnapper, Ester, 'Symbolic Decorations for a Woman after Childbirth in San'a', *The Israel Museum Journal*, 7 (Spring 1988), 61–74.

Müller, Walter W., 'Altsüdarabische Dokumente', in Otto Kaiser (ed.), *Texte aus der Umwelt des Alten Testaments*, 1/3 (Gütersloh: Mohn, 1983), 268–82.

Pellat, Charles, "Arīb b. Sa'd al-Kātib al-Ḳurṭubī', *EI*², I (1960), 628a–b.

Pfab, Rudi, 'Vergiftungen mit der Koloquinthe (Sodomsapfel): Eine bei uns unbekannte, in Reiseländern häufige Giftpflanze', *MMW Fortschritte der Medizin*, 141/31–2 (1999), 41–2.

Qafisheh, Hamdi A., *NTC's Yemeni Arabic-English Dictionary* (Lincolnwood (Chicago)/IL: NTC, 2000).

Qédan, Saleh, 'Heimische Arzneipflanzen der arabischen Volksmedizin', *Planta medica*, 26 (1974), 65–74.

Sābūr Ibn Sahl/Kahl, Oliver (ed.), *Dispensatorium Parvum* (*al-Aqrābādhīn al-ṣaghīr*) (Islamic Philosophy, Theology and Science: Texts and Studies, 16; Leiden: Brill, 1994).

——— (trans.), *The Small Dispensatory* (Islamic Philosophy, Theology and Science: Texts and Studies, 53; Leiden: Brill, 2003).

Schneider, Georg, *Pharmazeutische Biologie* (2nd edn.; Mannheim: Bibliographisches Institut-Wissenschaftsverlag, 1985).

Schönig, Hanne, *Schminken, Düfte und Räucherwerk der Jemenitinnen: Lexikon der Substanzen, Utensilien und Techniken* (Beiruter Texte und Studien, 91; Würzburg: Ergon, 2002).

Schopen, Armin, *Traditionelle Heilmittel in Jemen* (Wiesbaden: Steiner, 1983).

Tristram, Henry B., *The Natural History of the Bible: Being a Review of the Physical Geography, Geology and Meteorology of the Holy Land; With a Description of Every Animal and Plant Mentioned in the Holy Scripture* (9th edn.; London: Society for Promoting Christian Knowledge, 1898).

Varisco, Daniel Martin, *Medieval Agriculture and Islamic Science: The Almanac of a Yemeni Sultan* (Publications on the Near East, 6; Seattle: University of Washington Press, 1994).

Venzlaff, Helga, *Der marokkanische Drogenhändler und seine Ware: Ein Beitrag zu Terminologie und volkstümlichem Gebrauch traditioneller arabischer Materia medica* (Akademie der Wissenschaften und der Literatur, Veröffentlichungen der orientalischen Kommission, 31; Wiesbaden: Steiner, 1977).

Walther, Wiebke, *Untersuchungen zu vor- und frühislamischen arabischen Personennamen* (unpublished PhD thesis, University of Halle/Saale, 1966).

Wichtl, Max (ed.), *Teedrogen und Phytopharmaka* (3rd edn.; Stuttgart: Wissenschaftliche Verlagsgesellschaft, 1997).

al-Ziriklī, Khayr al-Dīn, *al-A'lām: Qāmūs tarājim li-ashhar al-rijāl wa-l-nisā' min al-'arab wa-l-musta'ribīn wa-l-mustashriqīn* (5; 4th edn.; Beirut: Dār al-'ilm lil-malāyīn, 1979).

Internet sources

WHO (World Health Organization), *General Guidelines for Methodologies on Research and Evaluation of Traditional Medicine* (2000) <http://whqlibdoc.who.int/hq/2000/WHO_EDM_TRM_2000.1.pdf>, accessed 13 September 2009.

EASTERN MEDITERRANEAN PHARMACOLOGY AND INDIA TRADE AS A BACKGROUND FOR YEMENI MEDIEVAL MEDICINAL PLANTS[1]

Efraim Lev

There is still a lot to be learned about medicinal substances of vegetal origin that were used in medieval Yemen. The aim of this chapter is to enlarge our knowledge by employing as yet unexploited historical sources. The focus is on extracting data from two main groups of documents: firstly, the reconstructed inventory of medicinal substances from the eastern Mediterranean (based on practical medical fragments found in the Cairo Genizah); and secondly various documents (traders' letters and documents dealing with tax) that relate to the sea trade that passed (mostly) through the Red Sea between India and Egypt. In addition, a number of literary sources will be evaluated.

The chapter opens with a short introduction to the Genizah and its importance to the history of medicine and pharmacology. This is followed by the classification of documents and their significance to the research. The contribution of each group of Genizah fragments to the knowledge relating to the use of medicinal plants and the reconstruction of the inventory of practical medicinal plants is dealt with later. The main part of the work presents some of the research studies regarding trade in the Red Sea and Yemeni ports. These sources shed light on medicinal plants that were traded in the sea routes through Yemen. Examination of certain historical sources related to agriculture in medieval Yemen provides evidence of the kinds of medicinal plants that were cultivated there as well as information regarding the local Yemeni names of medicinal plants in that period (I presume that non-indigenous plants would have had a Yemeni Arabic name especially if they had local applications).

---

[1] The chapter is partly based on Lev, 'Drugs'. This research would not have taken place without a generous grant from St. John's College, Cambridge, which hosted the author as an Overseas Visiting Scholar (2003–4). The author would like to express his deepest thanks to Prof. Zohar Amar, Bar-Ilan University, Israel for his helpful remarks. Special thanks go to my colleagues at the Taylor-Schechter Genizah Research Unit at the Cambridge University Library who shared with me their vast knowledge and experience and supported me with helpful comments: Dr. Ben Outhwaite (head), Prof. Stefan Reif (former head), and Dr. Avihai Shivtiel.

The chapter ends by presenting a table that collates all the collected data, followed by a short discussion. This will enable the reader to make a comparison between the plants that were used in medicine in the medieval Mediterranean and those that were recorded for the purpose of trade (and, I will suggest, therefore made use of) in Yemen.

My first assumption is that medicinal plants and their different parts and products that were traded in the sea routes and passed through Yemeni seaports were used medicinally by the Yemeni population, especially in the port cities and their vicinity. The second assumption is that the reconstructed inventory of practical medicinal plants of the medieval eastern Mediterranean—as recorded in the practical medical Genizah fragments—is comparable to the Yemeni one of the same period. According to previous research that included the study of inventories of traditional medicine around the Middle East, the core of any historical or present day inventory of medicinal substances is similar. However, the wild species that augment it differ according to the local climate, geography, and phytogeographical zones of the country.[2] Therefore, the differences between the medieval eastern Mediterranean and the Yemeni inventories of medicinal plants are mainly the local wild plants, in addition to locally cultivated species; the wild plants were not traded and were thus not recorded in regular commercial documents. In this context I should mention the important work done recently by Daniel Martin Varisco on medieval Yemeni agriculture that supplies us with data regarding locally cultivated plants, including those that had medicinal applications.[3]

1. The Cairo Genizah and Its Contribution

European scholars have known since the early nineteenth century of the hoard of documents that was found in the Genizah of the Ben Ezra synagogue of the Palestinian Jews of al-Fuṣṭāṭ (Old Cairo). The extraordinary circumstance of its preservation for such a long period, from about the tenth to the nineteenth century, against the ravages of time and decay was due to the exceptionally dry climate of Egypt. By the end of the nineteenth century the 'spell was broken,' and these manuscripts were bought from

[2] Lev, 'Ethno-diversity', 7.

[3] Mainly Varisco, 'Agriculture in al-Hamdānī's Yemen'; id., *Almanac*, 165–202. In the future I hope to establish a research group in order to study medieval medical literary (Arabic as well as Hebrew) sources that mention wild and cultivated medicinal plants in Yemen in order to improve our knowledge and help us reconstruct this inventory.

the synagogue officials and guards. The fragments slowly reached the hands of collectors and came to the attention of European scholars; different academic institutes and libraries purchased manuscripts and assembled their own collections.[4] Solomon Schechter (d. 1915) and Charles Taylor (d. 1908) were responsible for recovering the majority of the Ben Ezra Genizah manuscripts from Cairo in 1896 so that the Taylor-Schechter (T-S) Genizah collection at Cambridge University Library is the largest in the world, holding more than 150,000 fragments (three times more than all the others combined). The importance of the Genizah texts that supply information on almost every aspect of life in the medieval Mediterranean communities, was demonstrated by, among others, Shlomo Dov Goitein, Moshe Gil, Menachem Ben-Sasson.[5] An early study by Albert Dietrich of medicinal materials in Muslim Egypt was based on one manuscript rich with information on the trade in drugs.[6] A number of other scholars have since dealt with this subject-matter, mainly Goitein, Colin F. Baker, Paul Fenton, Mark R. Cohen, Esti Dvorjetsky, and especially Haskell D. Isaacs.[7]

The medical profession has been studied in works on the Genizah documents in general and on the life of the Jewish communities and societies in the Mediterranean.[8] Medicine, as a subject in its own right, has been given due attention only in the last few years with the publication of a catalogue of 1616 medical fragments and para-medical manuscripts in the Cambridge T-S collection by Isaacs with the assistance of Baker.[9] Further research on the Cambridge T-S collection has provided information on more than 160 fragments referring to medicine in general and to *materia medica* in particular.[10]

Many medieval Egyptian Jews practised medicine. To date, a systematic examination of Genizah fragments, as part of an ongoing long-term project, has yielded the names of more than fifty physicians.[11] The fact that a large number of Jews were engaged in the medical profession in Egypt and other Muslim territories emerges from other historical sources, but

---

[4] Reif, *A Jewish Archive*, 1–22; Richler, *Guide to Hebrew*, 60–4.

[5] Goitein, *A Mediterranean Society*; Gil, *Palestine*; id., *Kingdom*; Ben-Sasson, *Jews*.

[6] Dietrich, *Drogenhandel*.

[7] Goitein, *A Mediterranean Society*, 1, 153–4, 209–24; 2, 240–72; Baker, 'Islamic and Jewish Medicine'; Fenton, 'Importance'; Cohen, 'The Burdensome Life'; Isaacs, 'Impact of Western Medicine'; Dvorjetski, 'The Contribution of the Genizah'; Isaacs, 'Medical Certificate'.

[8] Goitein, 'The Medical Profession'.

[9] Isaacs, *Medical and Para-Medical Manuscripts*.

[10] Niessen and Lev, 'Addenda'.

[11] Lev, 'Work in Progress'.

mainly from books by medieval biographers and historians of medicine such as Ibn Abī Uṣaybiʿa (d. 1270)[12] who mentions more than fifteen Jewish practitioners in Cairo whom he met or knew of in his or earlier times.

The majority of the fifty Jewish physicians documented to date in the Genizah fragments lived and practised medicine in Cairo, with a few in Alexandria and in other smaller towns in Egypt between the eleventh and the thirteenth centuries. For some of them we even have information on their specialization: doctors of the eye, a specialist in wounds, and a physician who worked in a hospital.

2. Medicinal Substances Extracted from Plants and Used in Medicine

The literature on medicine in medieval Muslim countries in general,[13] and in Egypt in particular,[14] is vast. However, it mainly discusses theory and not practice. Studying and analyzing medical fragments from the Cairo Genizah has led to the development of a method for distinguishing the different kinds of data provided by them.[15] A crucial step was to differentiate between theoretical and practical medical knowledge.

Theoretical medical knowledge is mainly contained in general medical books. To date 1550 fragments of medical books have been identified in the Cambridge T-S collection, and dozens in each of the other collections mentioned above.[16]

Practical medical knowledge is commonly found in prescriptions, lists of drugs, and letters.[17] The bulk of the fragments in this group are the prescriptions, of which 140 unique original examples have been found in the Cambridge T-S collection.[18] Seventy lists of *materia medica* are known so far.[19]

The main sources on which we relied to reconstruct the bulk of medicinal plants that were in use from the tenth to the thirteenth century by

[12] Ibn Abī Uṣaybiʿa/Müller, *ʿUyūn al-anbāʾ*.

[13] Ullmann, *Islamic Medicine*; Levey, *Pharmacology*; Savage-Smith, 'Medicine'; ead., 'Ṭibb'; Pormann and Savage-Smith, *Medieval Islamic Medicine*.

[14] Ibn Riḍwān/Dols (trans.) and Gamal (ed.), *Medieval Islamic Medicine*.

[15] For more information about the method, see Lev and Amar, 'Practice Versus Theory'.

[16] Lev, 'Work in Progress', 46–9.

[17] Id. and Amar, 'Practice Versus Theory'.

[18] Eid., *Practical* Materia Medica, 43–8; Lev, 'Medieval Egyptian Judaeo-Arabic Prescriptions'.

[19] Id., 'Drugs'.

the members of the Jewish community in medieval Cairo were, therefore, lists of *materia medica* and practical prescriptions from the Cambridge T-S collection.[20] The inventory of practical *materia medica* comprises 278 substances of which 220 (79.5%) are of vegetal origin.[21] The number and proportion are entirely comparable with the size range of medicinal plants in other practical inventories[22] and with the proportions found in different sources and practices, from classical medical books to present-day traditional medicine.[23] The most frequently mentioned plants and plant products were:[24] myrobalan (79), rose (71), almond (41), pepper, endive, galingal and saffron (34 each), nard and licorice (32 each), lentisk and sugar cane (31 each), basil and borage (24 each), gum arabic, aloe, sesame (21 each), lemon and camphor (20 each).

2.1. *Lists of* materia medica

One hundred and sixty-eight plants and plant products were recorded in lists of *materia medica*, 84.2% of the total number of substances of vegetal origin. The most frequently mentioned plants and plant products, and hence, we suggest, most frequently employed were: myrobalan, pepper, and saffron. Twenty-nine plants and plant products appear only in lists of *materia medica* and, so far, have not been found in any prescriptions:[25] acacia, agrimony, ajava, anemone, arar tree, azerole tree, banana, betel pepper, bitter vetch, broad-leaved pepperwort, bryony, cedar, coconut palm, cornelian cherry, dragon's blood, elecampane, Jew's mallow, juniper, manna, mulberry, Nile papyrus, Oriental plane tree, orpine, sea holly, stonecrop, polypody, struthium, sumac, and thyme. These drugs were available to the patients in the Jewish pharmacies.

They may have been mentioned also in prescriptions that did not survive, or they may have been used by members of the Jewish community in Cairo without being prescribed, for instance in traditional medicine.[26]

---

20 Lev and Amar, '"Fossils"'.

21 Eid., 'Practice Versus Theory'; eid., *Practical* Materia Medica, 521–49. On the problems and methodology of identification and systematic categorization of *materia medica* in the Genizah, see ibid., 29–34.

22 Eid., 'Reconstruction'.

23 Lev, 'Reconstructed *materia medica*', id., 'Medicinal Substances'; id. and Amar, 'Ethnopharmacological Survey'.

24 See tables below.

25 See tables below.

26 Lev, 'Drugs'.

2.2. *Practical Prescriptions*

Evidence of 195 substances of vegetal origin (88.2% of the total number) was found in prescriptions in the Genizah collection. The most frequently mentioned plants and plant products and therefore, we suggest, most commonly used were: almond, myrobalan, rose, and sugar. Fifty-four plants and plant products were mentioned only in prescriptions and have not been found in any list of *materia medica*:[27] apricot, asafoetida, asparagus, barley, basil, bean, beet, ben tree, bitumen trefoil, cabbage, calamus, centaury, chamomile, chickpea, common caper, cypress tree, dill, dodder of thyme, Egyptian clover, Egyptian marjoram, fumitory, gum ammoniac, hellebore, horehound, hyssop, jasmine, leek, lemongrass, lentil, lettuce, linseed, lovage, malabathrum, meadow saffron, melon, mint, mustard, opopanax, pear, pellitory of Spain, stone pine (nuts), red behen, savory, sea squill, service tree, spinach, stavesacre, sweet clover, tamarisk, tar, wallflower, white behen, wild nard, and willow. This may be due to the relatively large number of prescriptions (140), compared to lists of *materia medica* (70), that have survived and been discovered in the Genizah collections.[28]

3. Plants Traded between Egypt and South East Asia

Merchants' letters found in the Genizah contain information on other aspects of medieval trade. They mention names of drugs and their origins and provide information about routes and other aspects of the drug trade of that era. A large proportion of the substances referred to in merchants' letters also served members of this medieval society as foodstuffs, spices, condiments, and cosmetics, and they were used for industrial purposes as well (tanning, dyeing, etc.). The reconstructed inventory of practical medicinal plants corresponds directly to our knowledge of the trade. Historical works on trade in the medieval Mediterranean have been published by Eliyahu Ashtor, Goitein, Gil, Ben-Sasson, Dietrich, Norman A. Stillman, David Jacoby, Lev, Zohar Amar and Lev;[29] and in the Red Sea and Indian

[27] See tables below.

[28] Id. and Amar, 'Reconstruction'.

[29] Ashtor, 'Spice Prices', 'The Crusader', 'Levantine Sugar Industry', 'Il regno dei crociati', 'European Trade'; id. and Cervidalli, 'Levantine Alkali Ashes'; Goitein, *A Mediterranean Society*, 1, 153–4, 209–22; Gil, *Palestine*; Ben-Sasson, *Jews*; Dietrich, *Drogenhandel*; Stillman, 'Merchant House'; Jacoby, *Trade*, id., *Commercial Exchange*; Lev, 'Trade'; id. and Amar, 'Practice Versus Theory'; Amar and Lev, 'The Significance'.

Ocean by Eleni Roxani Margariti, and Goitein and Mordechai Akiva Friedman.[30]

The trade between Egypt and South Asia during the medieval period was vast, and numerous Genizah documents provide many data on the topic.[31] Most of the sixty plants and products originating from plants that are explicitly mentioned in the historical sources had medicinal uses. The list of plants and plant products consists both of general names, such as aromatic plants, spices, gums, chewing gums; and named species of plants that scholars have been able to identify.[32] Since the Yemeni ports were crucial stopovers for the ships on their routes between India and Egypt, we can assume that these plants were available to the Yemeni traders and therefore to Yemeni customers, at least on a small scale.[33]

From recent research focusing on the Yemeni sea port of Aden we learn that, according to the Genizah documents dealing with taxes at this port, various plants were traded, the vast majority of which had medicinal applications. Among them we should mention some plants that were exported to Egypt, such as aromatic substances and aromatic woods, brazilwood, cinnamon, date, and rhubarb. The sources also mention that cardamom and pepper were imported from India into Yemen.[34]

A further source of information regarding the maritime trade and commerce in Ayyubid Aden that deals mainly with trade practices and taxes is the book of the thirteenth-century 'Easterner' Abū Bakr b. Muḥammad b. Masʿūd b. ʿAlī b. Aḥmad Ibn al-Mujāwir named *Tārīkh al-Mustabṣir*.[35] The author mentions the various taxes that were levied on many commodities, of which half were of a medicinal nature, such as: camphor, cardamom, clove, flax, indigo, iron, lac, madder, pepper, perfumed cherry bark, saffron, 'sugar' of bamboo, and tamarind. Other commodities are listed that were medicinal, but on which no tax was levied: date, dried fruits/nuts, flax oil, frankincense, honey, olive oil, preserved fruits (myrobalan), sesame, sugar, soap, saltwort, syrup,[36] and aloeswood.[37]

Evidence of a few other medicinal substances coming from India and going to Egypt can be found among the commodities mentioned in documents that were found in al-Quṣayr, a site on the shores of the Red Sea

---

30 Margariti, *Aden*; Goitein and Friedman, *India Traders*.
31 Ibid.
32 Ibid., see table below.
33 See column F in the table below.
34 Margariti, *Aden*. See column M in the table below.
35 Smith, 'Have You Anything to Declare?'. See column S in the table below.
36 Smith, 'Have You Anything to Declare?'.
37 Id., 'More on the Port Practices'. See column S in the table below.

between the Mediterranean Sea and the Indian Ocean. These include food and drinks that were also employed in medical practice such as: apple, barley, bean, butter, carrot, chickpea, date, eggplant, grape vine, Jew's mallow, lemon, lentil, liquor, nut, onion, pepper, sugar, syrup, watermelon, wheat, in addition to other medicinal plants and products such as: henna, perfumed cherry, perfume, rose water, saffron, and soap.[38] The data extracted from the sources mentioned above are presented below in the table alongside the reconstructed inventory of practical medicinal plants in the medieval Mediterranean according to the Cairo Genizah.

Further information regarding medieval Yemeni medicinal plants may in future be gained from a study of Rasulid tax archives. Some such documents have been edited and published recently by Muḥammad Jāzim.[39]

4. More Sources—Plants Cultivated and Employed Medicinally in Medieval Yemen

A few manuscripts of the Yemeni medieval literature dealing with agriculture and science have been studied by Varisco, for example those written by al-Hamdānī (d. *c.*947). These works supply us with data regarding plants that were cultivated in Yemen, many of which are known to have been put to medicinal uses.[40]

Other sources might be medical books written by medieval Yemeni authors, though this is a different category. The most important book on the topic is probably *al-Muʿtamad fī l-adwiya al-mufrada* by al-Malik al-Muẓaffar Yūsuf.[41] There is no doubt that the author relies extensively on prior medical authorities. However, one part at the end of the book—the glossary of local Yemeni names of the medicinal substances mentioned in the book—might be of relevance to us. The existence of trade in the commodities mentioned above is, in my opinion, circumstantial evidence for the medical application of these substances in Yemen, and I would strongly suggest a thorough investigation of these sources, but that is beyond the scope of the current publication.

38 Guo, *Commerce*, 67–9. See column G in the table below.

39 Jāzim and Arbach (eds.), *al-Fāṣil*; Jāzim (ed.), *Irtifāʿ al-dawla*.

40 For example Varisco and Smith, *Manuscript*; Varisco, *Medieval Folk Astronomy*, id., *Almanac*, 165–202, id., 'Agriculture in al-Hamdānī's Yemen'. See column V in the table below.

41 al-Malik al-Muẓaffar/al-Saqqā, *al-Muʿtamad*. See Ingrid Hehmeyer's chapter in this volume for the suggestion that the author of the work was, in fact, al-Malik al-Muẓaffar's son, al-Ashraf ʿUmar.

5. Comparison and Analysis of the Practical vs. Commercial Data

The data regarding medicinal plants extracted from the various sources dealing with international trade and commerce in medieval Yemen are compared here with the list of practical medicinal plants employed in the medieval Mediterranean basin according to the Cairo Genizah documents. Data from studies focusing on medicinal uses of local plants in that period were added to the table in order to allow a comparison to be made between the products that were taxed when imported from outside Yemen and the products that were actually employed within the country. Moreover, the indigenous Yemeni names of medicinal plants of that period were also included here on the assumption that if foreign medicinal plants had a local name, they probably had local employment.

The sources relied upon here are described in detail above: L – Genizah practical fragments,[42] F – Genizah trade,[43] S – Aden,[44] M – Aden,[45] G – al-Quṣayr,[46] and V – Yemeni medieval agriculture.[47] Analysis and discussion of the data are presented below.

Table. Medicinal plants between Yemen and Egypt – practical *vs.* commercial sources

Scientific name and botanical family	Common name	L	F	S	M	G	V
Acacia nilotica (Leguminosae)	gum arabic tree	X	X				
Acacia spp. (Leguminosae)	acacia	X					
Acorus calamus (Araceae)	calamus	X					
Adiantum capillus-veneris (Pteridophyta)	maidenhair	X					
Agaricus spp. (Agaricaceae)	agaric	X					
Agrimonia eupatoria (Rosaceae)	agrimony	X					
Alhagi maurorum (Leguminosae)	manna	X					
Allium cepa (Alliaceae)	onion	X				X	X
Allium porrum (Alliaceae)	leek	X					

[42] Lev and Amar, *Practical* Materia Medica.

[43] Goitein and Friedman, *India Traders*.

[44] Smith, 'Have you anything to declare?', id., 'More on the Port Practices'.

[45] Margariti, *Aden*.

[46] Guo, *Commerce*.

[47] Varisco, *Almanac*, 165–202, id., 'Agriculture in al-Hamdānī's Yemen'. The English names are from Varisco.

Table. Continued.

Scientific name and botanical family	Common name	L	F	S	M	G	V
Allium sativum (Alliaceae)	garlic	X	X				X
Aloe spp. (Aloaceae)	aloe	X	X				
Alpinia galanga (Zingiberaceae)	galingal	X	X				
Althaea officinalis (Malvaceae)	marshmallow	X					
Ammi copticum (Umbelliferae)	ajwain, ajava	X					
Amomum spp. (Zingiberaceae)	amomum	X					
Amygdalus communis (Rosaceae)	almond	X	X				X
Anacyclus (*Anthemis*) *pyrethrum* (Compositae)	pellitory of Spain	X					
Anchusa italica and *A. officinalis* (Boraginaceae)	borage	X					
Andropogon schoenanthus (Gramineae)	lemongrass	X					
Anemone coronaria (Ranunculaceae)	anemone	X					X
Anethum graveolens (Umbelliferae)	dill, anet	X					X
Apium graveolens (Umbelliferae)	celery	X					X
Aquilaria agallocha (Thymelaeaceae)	aloeswood	X	X	X			
Areca catechu (Arecaceae)	betel palm	X	X				X
Aristolochia spp. (Aristolochiaceae)	birthwort	X					
Artemisia spp. (Compositae)	wormwood	X					X
Asarum europaeum (Aristolochiaceae)	wild nard	X					
Asparagus officinalis (Liliaceae)	asparagus	X					X
Asphodelus aestivus (Asphodelaceae)	asphodel	X					
Asplenium onoperis (Pteridophyta)	black spleenwort	X					
Astragalus gummifera (Leguminosae)	tragacanth	X					
Astragalus sarcocolla (Leguminosae)	sarcocolla	X					
Bambusa vulgaris (Gramineae)	bamboo	X	X		X		
Berberis cretica (Berberidaceae)	berberry	X					
Beta vulgaris (Chenopodiaceae)	beet	X					
Bituminaria bituminosa (Leguminosae)	bitumen trefoil	X					
Boswellia sacra (Burseraceae)	frankincense	X	X	X			
Brassica oleracea (Brassicaceae)	cabbage	X					X
Bryonia cretica (Cucurbitaceae)	bryony	X					
Buxus sempervirens (Buxaceae)	box	X					

Table. Continued.

Scientific name and botanical family	Common name	L	F	S	M	G	V
Caesalpinia sappan (Leguminosae)	brazilwood		X		X		
Cannabis sativa var. *indica* (Cannabaceae)	cannabis	X					
Capparis spinosa (Capparaceae)	common caper	X					
Carthamus tinctorius (Compositae)	safflower	X	X				X
Carum carvi (Umbelliferae)	caraway	X					
Cassia acutifolia (Leguminosae)	cassia, senna	X	X				
Cassia fistula (Caesalpiniaceae)	purging cassia	X					X
Cedrus libani (Pinaceae)	cedar of lebanon	X					
Centaurea spp. (Compositae)	centaury	X					
Centaurea behen (Compositae)	white behen	X					
Ceratonia siliqua (Leguminosae)	carob	X					X
Cercis siliquastrum (Leguminosae)	Judas tree	X					
Chelidonium majus (Papaveraceae)	celandine	X	X				
Cicer arietinum (Leguminosae)	chickpea	X				X	X
Cichorium intybus, also *C. endivia, C. pumilum* (Compositae)	chicory, endive	X					X
Cinnamomum camphora (Lauraceae)	camphor	X			X	X	
Cinnamomum aromaticum (Lauraceae)	malabathrum	X					
Cinnamomum verum (Lauraceae)	cinnamon	X	X		X		
Cistus ladanifer (Cistaceae)	ladanum (= labdanum)	X	X				
Citrullus colocynthis (Cucurbitaceae)	colocynth	X					
Citrullus vulgaris (Cucurbitaceae)	watermelon	X				X	X
Citrus limon (Rutaceae)	lemon	X	X			X	X
Citrus medica (Rutaceae)	citron	X					X
Cocos nucifera (Arecaceae)	coconut palm	X	X				X
Colchicum autumnale (Liliaceae)	meadow saffron	X					
Commiphora gileadensis (Burseraceae)	balsam of Mecca	X					X
Commiphora wightii (Burseraceae)	bdellium	X					
Commiphora myrrha (Burseraceae)	myrrh	X	X				
Convolvulus scammonia (Convolvulaceae)	scammony	X	X				
Corchorus olitorius (Malvaceae)	Jew's mallow	X				X	
Cordia myxa (Boraginaceae)	sebesten	X					

Table. Continued.

Scientific name and botanical family	Common name	L	F	S	M	G	V
Coriandrum sativum (Umbelliferae)	coriander	X					X
Cornus mas (Cornaceae)	cornelian cherry	X					
Corylus avellana (Corylaceae)	hazelnut	X					
Costus speciosus (Zingiberaceae)	costus	X	X				
Crataegus azarolus (Rosaceae)	azerole tree	X					
Crocus sativus (Iridaceae)	saffron	X	X	X	X	X	
Cucumis melo (Cucurbitaceae)	melon	X					X
Cucumis melo var. *chate* (Cucurbitaceae)	chate melon	X					
Cucumis sativus (Cucurbitaceae)	cucumber	X					X
Cuminum cyminum (Umbelliferae)	cumin	X	X				X
Cupressus sempervirens (Cupressaceae)	cypress tree	X					
Curcuma longa (Zingiberaceae)	turmeric	X	X				X
Cuscuta spp. (Cuscutaceae)	dodder	X					
Cuscuta epithymum (Cuscutaceae)	dodder of thyme	X					
Cydonia oblonga (Rosaceae)	quince	X					X
Cyperus longus (Cyperaceae)	sedge	X					
Cyperus papyrus (Cyperaceae)	papyrus, Nile papyrus	X					
Cytinus hypocistis (Rafflesiaceae)	hypocist	X					
Daucus carota (Umbelliferae)	carrot	X				X	X
Delphinium staphisagria (Ranunculaceae)	stavesacre	X					
Dorema ammoniacum (Umbelliferae)	ammoniacum	X					
Doronicum orientale (Compositae)	leopard's bane	X					
Dracaena draco, D. cinnabari (Dracaenaceae)	dragon's blood	X					
Drimia maritima (Asparagaceae)	sea squill	X					
Elettaria cardamomum (Zingiberaceae)	cardamom	X	X	X	X		
Eruca sativa (Brassicaceae)	garden rocket	X					
Eryngium spp. (Umbelliferae)	sea holly	X					
Erysimum cheiri = *Cheiranthus cheiri* (Brassicaceae)	wallflower	X					
Eugenia caryophyllata (Myrtaceae)	clove	X	X	X			
Euphorbia spp. (Euphorbiaceae)	spurge	X					

Table. Continued.

Scientific name and botanical family	Common name	L	F	S	M	G	V
Ferula assa-foetida (Umbelliferae)	asafoetida	X		X			
Ferula galbaniflua (Umbelliferae)	galbanum	X					
Ferula persica (Umbelliferae)	sagapenum	X					
Foeniculum vulgare (Umbelliferae)	fennel	X					X
Fraxinus excelsior or *F. syriaca* (Oleaceae)	ash tree	X					
Fumaria officinalis (Fumariaceae)	fumitory	X					X
Glaucium corniculatum (Papaveraceae)	horned poppy	X					
Glycyrrhiza glabra (Leguminosae)	licorice	X					
Gossypium herbaceum (Malvaceae)	cotton	X					X
Gypsophila struthium (Caryophyllaceae)	struthium	X					
Helleborus niger (Liliaceae) or *Veratrum album* (Ranunculaceae)	hellebore	X					
Hordeum spp. (Gramineae)	barley	X				X	X
Hyoscyamus albus (Solanaceae)	henbane	X					
Hyssopus officinalis (Labiatae)	hyssop	X					
Indigofera tinctoria (Leguminosae)	indigo	X	X	X			X
Inula helenium (Compositae)	elecampane	X					
Ipomoea turpethum (Convolvulaceae)	turpeth	X					
Iris florentina or *I. mesopotamica* (Iridaceae)	iris	X					
Jasminum spp. (Oleaceae)	jasmine	X					X
Juglans regia (Juglandaceae)	walnut	X					X
Juniperus spp. (Cupressaceae)	juniper	X					
Lactuca sativa (Compositae)	lettuce	X					X
Lagenaria vulgaris (Cucurbitaceae)	bottle gourd	X					X
Lathyrus sativus (Leguminosae)	chickling vetch	X					
Laurus nobilis (Lauraceae)	laurel	X					
Lavandula officinalis (Labiatae)	lavender	X					
Lawsonia inermis (Lythraceae)	henna	X				X	X
Lens esculenta (Leguminosae)	lentil	X				X	X
Lepidium latifolium (Brassicaceae)	broad-leaved pepperwort	X					
Lepidium sativum (Brassicaceae)	garden cress	X					X
Levisticum officinale (Umbelliferae)	lovage	X					

Table. Continued.

Scientific name and botanical family	Common name	L	F	S	M	G	V
Linum usitatissimum (Linaceae)	linseed, flax	X	X	X			X
Liquidambar orientalis (Altingiaceae)	storax		X				
Lycium afrum (Solanaceae)	box thorn	X	X				
Mandragora autumnalis (Solanaceae)	mandrake	X					
Marrubium vulgare (Labiatae)	horehound	X					
Matricaria aurea (Compositae)	chamomile	X					
Melilotus albus (Leguminosae)	sweet clover	X					
Melissa officinalis (Labiatae)	balm	X					
Mentha sativa (Labiatae)	mint	X					X
Moringa peregrina (Moringaceae)	ben tree	X	X				X
Morus nigra (Moraceae)	mulberry	X					X
Musa paradisiaca (Musaceae)	banana	X					X
Myristica fragrans (Myristicaceae)	nutmeg	X	X				
Myrtus communis (Myrtaceae)	myrtle	X					X
Nardostachys jatamansi (Valerianaceae)	(spike)nard	X	X				
Nigella sativa (Ranunculaceae)	black cumin	X					X
Nymphaea spp.; *Nuphar* spp. (Nymphaeaceae)	lotus	X					
Ocimum basilicum (Labiatae)	(sweet) basil	X	X				
Ocimum basilicum var. *pilosum* (Labiatae)	basil	X					
Olea europaea (Oleaceae) (oil)	olive tree	X	X	X			X
Opopanax chironium (Umbelliferae)	opopanax	X					
Orchis spp. (Orchidaceae)	salep	X					
Origanum majorana (Labiatae)	sweet marjoram	X					
Origanum vulgare (Labiatae)	wild marjoram	X					X
Origanum maru (Labiatae)	Egyptian marjoram	X					
Paeonia spp. (Paeoniaceae)	peony	X					
Papaver somniferum (Papaveraceae)	opium poppy	X					
Pastinaca sativa (Umbelliferae)	parsnip	X					
Peganum harmala (Nitrariaceae)	wild rue	X					
Phoenix dactylifera (Arecaceae)	date palm	X	X	X	X	X	X
Phragmites communis (Gramineae)	common reed	X					
Pimpinella anisum (Umbelliferae)	anise	X					X

Table. Continued.

Scientific name and botanical family	Common name	L	F	S	M	G	V
Pinus spp. and *Cedrus* spp. (Pinaceae), *Cupressus* spp. (Cupressaceae) (tar)	pine, cypress, cedar	X					
Pinus pinea (Pinaceae) (nuts)	stone pine	X					
Piper betel (Piperaceae)	betel pepper	X					
Piper cubeba (Piperaceae)	cubeb pepper	X	X				
Piper longum (Piperaceae)	long pepper	X					
Piper nigrum (Piperaceae)	pepper	X	X	X	X	X	
Pistacia atlantica (Anacardiaceae)	Atlantic pistachio	X					
Pistacia lentiscus (Anacardiaceae)	lentisk	X					
Pistacia vera (Anacardiaceae)	pistachio	X	X				X
Plantago afra (Plantaginaceae)	plantain	X					
Platanus orientalis (Platanaceae)	Oriental plane tree	X					
Polypodium vulgare (Pteridophyta)	polypody	X					
Portulaca oleracea (Portulacaceae)	purslane	X					X
Prunus armeniaca (Rosaceae)	apricot	X					X
Prunus cerasia (sweet cherry), *P. cerasus* (sour cherry) (Rosaceae)	cherry	X					
Prunus domestica (Rosaceae)	plum	X					X
Prunus mahaleb (Rosaceae)	perfumed cherry	X		X		X	
Punica granatum (Punicaceae)	pomegranate	X					X
Pyrus communis (Rosaceae)	pear	X					X
Pyrus malus (Rosaceae)	apple	X				X	X
Quercus spp. (Fagaceae) (gall)	oak	X	X				
Raphanus sativus (Brassicaceae)	radish	X	X				X
Rheum spp. (Polygonaceae)	rhubarb	X	X		X		
Rhus coriaria (Anacardiaceae)	sumac	X					
Ricinus communis (Euphorbiaceae)	castor oil	X					
Rosa canina (Rosaceae)	dog rose	X				X	X
Rosmarinus officinalis (Labiatae)	rosemary	X					
Rubia tinctorum (Rubiaceae)	madder	X		X			X
Rumex spp. (Polygonaceae)	sorrel, dock	X					
Ruta chalepensis and *R. graveolens* (Rutaceae)	fringed rue, common rue	X					X

Table. Continued.

Scientific name and botanical family	Common name	L	F	S	M	G	V
Saccharum officinarum (Gramineae)	sugar cane	X	X	X		X	X
Salix spp. (Salicaceae)	willow	X					
Santalum album (Santalaceae)	sandalwood	X					
Satureja spp. (Labiatae)	savory	X					
Sedum spp. (Crassulaceae)	orpine, stonecrop	X					
Sesamum indicum (Pedaliaceae)	sesame	X					X
Sinapis alba (Brassicaceae)	mustard	X					X
Solanum melongena (Solanaceae)	eggplant	X				X	X
Sorbus domestica = *Pyrus sorbus* (Rosaceae)	service tree	X					
Spinacia oleracea (Chenopodiaceae)	spinach	X					X
Statice limonium (Plumbaginaceae)	red behen	X					
Tamarindus indica (Leguminosae)	tamarind	X		X			X
Tamarix gallica, T. orientalis (Tamaricaceae)	tamarisk	X					
Taxus baccata (Taxaceae)	yew	X					
Terminalia spp. (Combretaceae)	myrobalan	X	X	X			
Tetraclinis articulata (Cupressaceae)	arar tree	X					
Teucrium capitatum (Labiatae)	thyme	X	X				X
Trifolium alexandrinum (Leguminosae)	Egyptian clover	X					X
Trigonella foenum-graecum (Leguminosae)	fenugreek	X					X
Triticum vulgare (Gramineae)	wheat	X				X	X
Usnea spp. (Parmeliaceae)	lichen	X	X				
Vicia ervilia (Leguminosae)	bitter vetch	X					
Vicia faba (Leguminosae)	broad bean	X				X	X
Viola odorata (Violaceae)	sweet violet	X					
Vitis vinifera (Vitaceae)	grape vine	X	X			X	X
Zingiber officinale (Zingiberaceae)	ginger	X	X				X
Zingiber zerumbet (Zingiberaceae)	wild ginger		X				
Ziziphus spina-christi (Rhamnaceae)	Christ's thorn	X					X
Ziziphus jujuba (Rhamnaceae)	jujube	X					

5.1. *Discussion*

Analysis of the data presented in the table reveals that sixty-six medicinal plants were identified in the commercial sources (columns F, S, M, G).[48] These include only three plants that were not part of the Genizah inventory of practical medicinal plants (brazilwood, wild ginger, and storax), therefore, the vast majority found practical application for medical purposes in the eastern Mediterranean according to the Genizah documents (column L).

It appears that the Yemeni people, during the Middle Ages, were doubly fortunate: on the one hand they had access to the local medicinal plants of the various and diverse geo-botanical zones of Yemen, and on the other hand they benefited from the intensive Indian Ocean trade, especially between Egypt and the South Asian ports. Therefore, we can assume that in the larger cities of medieval Yemen, physicians and pharmacists had at their disposal hundreds of medicinal substances, mainly medicinal plants. The inventory of medicinal plants of the Jewish community of Cairo, mentioned above and reconstructed from the Genizah documents, may give us an indication of the likely size and content. This assumption is based on the fact that these inventories tend to be similar in numbers and content, as is for instance also the case with the one of the medieval Levant that has been reconstructed from different historical sources.[49]

When the list of plants (39) of the reconstructed core inventory of Middle Eastern medicinal substances[50] was compared to the table above, twenty-one plants from this list were identified among the sixty-six found in the commercial sources (columns F, S, M, G in the table). These were mainly spices of Indian origin such as: cardamom, cinnamon, clove, galingal, ginger, nutmeg, pepper, tamarind, turmeric, and other commodities of diverse geographical origin: cassia (senna), cumin, frankincense, henna, linseed, olive, perfumed cherry, rose, saffron, and sugar cane. Additionally, eighteen plants were not identified from among the sixty-six plants. However, they were identified in the list of medicinal plants of the practical inventory of the Genizah (column L in the table); these were mainly wild and cultivated medicinal plants such as: anise, black cumin, coriander, fennel, fenugreek, garden cress, licorice, lentisk, pine, rosemary, rue, and sumac. Interestingly enough, many of these plants (black cumin, coriander,

48 In addition to general names such as aromatic plants, soap, spices, gums, chewing gum, or perfume.

49 Lev, 'Reconstructed *materia medica*', id., 'Medicinal Substances'.

50 Id., 'Ethno-diversity'.

fennel, fenugreek, mint, rue, and wormwood) were recorded by Varisco as cultivated in medieval Yemen,[51] and some are easy to grow in gardens (rosemary, chamomile).

It is worth mentioning that Varisco records thirty-three plants that were cultivated or taxed in medieval Yemen. Among them, nineteen are known as having been put to medicinal use in the past: anemone, broad bean, colcasia, earth almond, faba bean, fig, gillyflower, gourd, lily, lupine, marigold, mung bean, narcissus, orange, parsley, poppy, screwpine, snake cucumber, and watercress.[52]

An attempt was made to support the assumption that medicinal plants that were transported through Yemeni ports (i.e. mentioned in the tax lists) were also known and available to the inhabitants of the Yemeni city ports, at least on a small scale. I compared the list of medicinal plants mentioned in the traders' letters and tax documents with two different sources telling us about their actual exploitation or cultivation in medieval Yemen. It turns out that out of the sixty-six medicinal plants mentioned by these sources, thirty-two were recorded by Varisco[53] from sources dealing with medieval Yemeni agriculture and were known and used by the Yemenis. Out of the thirty-four plants that were not recorded by Varisco, ten (aloe, asafoetida, bamboo, cassia, cinnamon, Jew's mallow, lichen, perfumed cherry, saffron, and wild ginger) were clearly identified in the unique glossary of local Yemeni names at the end of al-Malik al-Muẓaffar Yūsuf's book.[54] I suggest that if a substance has a medieval Yemeni name, it saw practical use in the country by its inhabitants. When the list of the remaining plants was studied it turned out that the vast majority of them were clearly identified as mentioned and described in the book itself (aloeswood, basil, box thorn, brazilwood, camphor, cardamom, celandine, clove, costus, galingal, gum arabic, labdanum, myrobalan, myrrh, nutmeg, oak gall, pepper, rhubarb, scammony, spikenard, and storax).[55] It should be mentioned that many of these plants that were well known and widely employed in the medieval period, remain so today in the traditional medicine of Yemen and of many Arab and Asian countries and cultures.

---

51 Varisco, 'Agriculture in al-Hamdānī's Yemen', id., *Almanac*, 165–202.

52 Ibid.

53 Ibid.

54 al-Malik al-Muẓaffar/al-Saqqā, *al-Muʿtamad*, 558–72.

55 Ibid.

6. Conclusion

As has been clearly demonstrated from the Genizah trading documents, most of the medicinal plants from South Asia were available in Yemen due to its geographical location as well as its maritime and overland trading activities. Both the medicinal plants and plant products that arrived through trade and the ones that originate from Yemen contribute to the complex nature of the Yemeni *materia medica*, and can be considered as Yemen's possible contribution, as an entrepôt, to Cairene medicine and pharmacology. The trade in several of the above-mentioned medicinal plants and other substances was in the hands of members of the Jewish community of medieval Cairo who traded with India, Sicily, Syria, North Africa, and other ports and cities.[56]

Bibliography

Amar, Zohar, and Lev, Efraim, 'The Significance of the Genizah's Medical Documents for the Study of Medieval Mediterranean Trade', *Journal of the Economic and Social History of the Orient*, 50/4 (2007), 524–41.

Ashtor, Eliyahu, 'Spice Prices in the Near East in the 15th Century', *Journal of the Royal Asiatic Society*, 1 (1976), 26–41.

———, 'The Crusader Kingdom and Trade in the Levant', in Benjamin Z. Kedar (ed.), *The Crusaders in Their Kingdom* [Hebrew] (Jerusalem: Yad Yitshak Ben Zvi, 1978), 30–54.

———, 'Levantine Sugar Industry in the Late Middle Ages', in Abraham L. Udovitch (ed.), *The Islamic Middle East, 700–1900: Studies in Economic and Social History* (Princeton: Darwin Press, 1981), 91–132.

———, 'Il regno dei crociati e il commercio di Levante', in Gabriella Airaldi and Benjamin Z. Kedar (eds.), *I Comuni Italiani nel Regno Crociato di Gerusalemme. Atti del Colloquio* (*The Italian Communes in the Crusader Kingdom of Jerusalem*) (Genoa: Università di Genova, 1986), 5–56.

———, 'European Trade in the Late Medieval Land of Israel', in Benjamin Z. Kedar, Trude Dothan, and Samuel Safrai (eds.), *Commerce in Palestine Throughout the Ages* [Hebrew] (Jerusalem: Yad Yitshak Ben Zvi, 1990), 280–99.

———, and Cervidalli, G., 'Levantine Alkali Ashes and European Industries', *The Journal of European Economic History*, 12 (1983), 493–500.

Baker, Colin F., 'Islamic and Jewish Medicine in the Medieval Mediterranean World: The Genizah Evidence', *Journal of the Royal Society of Medicine*, 89 (1996), 577–80.

Ben-Sasson, Menachem, *The Jews of Sicily 825–1068* [Hebrew] (Jerusalem: Yad Izhak Ben Zvi, 1991).

Cohen, Mark R., 'The Burdensome Life of a Jewish Physician and Communal Leader: A Genizah Fragment from the Alliance Israélite Universelle Collection', *Jerusalem Studies in Arabic and Islam*, 16 (1993), 125–36.

Dietrich, Albert, *Zum Drogenhandel im islamischen Ägypten* (Heidelberg: Winter, 1954).

[56] Goitein, *A Mediterranean Society*, 1, 148–56, 209–24; Isaacs, *Medical and Para-Medical Manuscripts*, xi; Dietrich, *Drogenhandel*.

Dvorjetski, Esti, 'The Contribution of the Genizah to the Study of the Medicinal Hot Springs in Eretz-Israel', in Ron Margolin (ed.), *Proceedings of the Twelfth World Congress of Jewish Studies* (2; Jerusalem: World Congress of Jewish Studies, 1990), 85–93.

Fenton, P., 'The Importance of the Cairo Genizah for the History of Medicine', *Medical History*, 24 (1980), 347–8.

Gil, Moshe, *Palestine During the First Muslim Period (643–1099)* [Hebrew] (Tel-Aviv: Tel Aviv University and the Ministry of Defence Publishing House, 1983). English short edition (Cambridge: Cambridge University Press, 1992).

———, *In the Kingdom of Ishmael* [Hebrew] (4 vols.; Tel-Aviv: Tel Aviv University and Ministry of Defence Publishing House; Jerusalem: The Bialik Institute, 1997).

Goitein, S. Dov, 'The Medical Profession in the Light of the Cairo Genizah Documents', *Hebrew Union College Annual*, 34 (1963), 177–94.

———, *A Mediterranean Society* (5 vols.; Berkeley: University of California Press, 1967–88).

———, and Friedman, Mordechai Akiva, *India Traders of the Middle Ages: Documents from the Cairo Geniza ('India Book')* (Jerusalem: The Ben-Zvi Institute; Leiden: Brill, 2008).

Guo, Li, *Commerce, Culture, and Community in a Red Sea Port in the Thirteenth Century: The Arabic Documents from Quseir* (Islamic History and Civilization, Studies and Texts, 52; Leiden: Brill, 2004).

Ibn Abī Uṣaybi'a/Müller, August (ed.): Ibn Abi Useibia, *'Uyūn al-anbā' fī ṭabaqāt al-aṭibbā'* (Farnborough: Gregg International Publishers, 1972).

Ibn Riḍwān, 'Alī/Dols, W. Michael (trans.), Gamal, S. Adil (ed.), *Medieval Islamic Medicine: Ibn Riḍwān's Treatise 'On the Prevention of Bodily Ills in Egypt'* (Berkeley: University of California Press, 1984).

Isaacs, Haskell D., 'The Impact of Western Medicine on Muslim Physicians and Their Writing in the 17th Century', *Bulletin of the British Association of Orientalists*, 11 (1979–80), 52–7.

———, 'A Medieval Arab Medical Certificate', *Medical History*, 35 (1991), 250–7.

———, (with the assistance of C.F. Baker), *Medical and Para-Medical Manuscripts in the Cambridge Genizah Collections* (Cambridge: Cambridge University Press, 1994).

Jacoby, David, *Trade, Commodities and Shipping in the Medieval Mediterranean* (Variorum Collected Studies Series; Aldershot: Ashgate, 1997).

———, *Commercial Exchange across the Mediterranean: Byzantium, the Crusader Levant, Egypt and Italy* (Hampshire: Ashgate/Variorum Aldershot, 2005).

Jāzim, Muḥammad 'Abd al-Raḥīm (ed.), *Irtifā' al-dawla al-Mu'ayyadiyya: Jibāyat bilād al-Yaman fī 'ahd al-sulṭān al-Malik al-Mu'ayyad Dā'ūd b. Yūsuf al-Rasūlī (al-mutawaffā sanat 721 h/1321 m) / Le Livre des Revenus du sultan rasûlide al-Malik al-Mu'ayyad Dâwûd b. Yûsuf (m. 721/1321)* (La bibliothèque yéménite / al-Maktaba al-Yamaniyya / Die Jemenitische Bibliothek, 2; Ṣan'ā': al-Ma'had al-faransī lil-āthār wa-l-'ulūm al-ijtimā'iyya bi-Ṣan'ā', al-Ma'had al-almānī lil-āthār, Ṣan'ā' /Centre Français d'Archéologie et de Sciences Sociales, Deutsches Archäologisches Institut, Ṣan'ā' Branch, 2008).

———, and Arbach, Mounir (eds.), *al-Fāṣil bayn al-ḥaqq wa-l-bāṭil: Min mafākhir abnā' Qaḥṭān wa-l-Yaman li-mu'allif majhūl (Les mérites véritables de Qaḥṭân et du Yémen)* (La bibliothèque yéménite, 3; Ṣan'ā': CEFAS, 2009).

Lev, Efraim, 'Reconstructed *materia medica* of the Medieval and Ottoman al-Sham', *Journal of Ethnopharmacology*, 80 (2002), 167–79.

———, *Medicinal Substances of the Medieval Levant* [Hebrew] (Tel-Aviv: Eretz & Tel Aviv University Press, 2002).

———, 'Trade of Medical Substances in the Medieval and Ottoman Levant (Bilad Al-Sham)', in Yaacov Lev (ed.), *Towns and Material Culture in the Medieval Middle East* (Leiden: Brill, 2002), 159–83.

———, 'Work in Progress: The Research of Medical Knowledge in the Cairo Genizah: Past, Present and Future', in Shulie Reif (ed.), *The Written Word Remains: The Archive and the*

Achievement. Articles in Honour of Professor Stefan C. Reif (Cambridge: Taylor-Schechter Genizah Research Unit at Cambridge University Library, 2004), 37–51.

———, 'Ethno-diversity within Current Ethno-pharmacology as Part of Israeli Traditional Medicine: A Review', *Journal of Ethnobiology and Ethnomedicine*, 2/4 (2006), 1–12.

———, 'Drugs Held and Sold by Pharmacists of the Jewish Community of Medieval (11th–14th Centuries) Cairo According to Lists of *materia medica* Found at the Taylor-Schechter Genizah Collection, Cambridge', *Journal of Ethnopharmacology*, 110 (2007), 275–93.

———, 'Medieval Egyptian Judaeo-Arabic Prescriptions (and the Edition of Three Medical Prescriptions)', *Journal of the Royal Asiatic Society* 18/4 (2008), 449–64.

———, and Amar, Zohar, 'Ethnopharmacological Survey of Traditional Drugs Sold in Israel at the End of the 20th Century', *Journal of Ethnopharmacology*, 72 (2000), 191–205.

———, and Amar, Zohar, 'Reconstruction of the Inventory of *Materia Medica* Used by Members of the Jewish Community of Medieval Cairo According to Prescriptions Found in the Taylor-Schechter Genizah Collection, Cambridge', *Journal of Ethnopharmacology*, 108 (2006), 428–44.

———, and Amar, Zohar, 'Practice versus Theory: Medieval *Materia Medica* According to the Cairo Genizah', *Medical History*, 51/4 (2007), 507–26.

———, and Amar, Zohar, *Practical* Materia Medica *of the Medieval Eastern Mediterranean According to the Cairo Genizah* (Sir Henry Wellcome Asian Series, 7; Leiden: Brill, 2008).

———, and Amar, Zohar, '"Fossils" of Practical Medical Knowledge from Medieval Cairo', *Journal of Ethnopharmacology*, 119/1 (2008), 24–40.

Levey, Martin, *Early Arabic Pharmacology: An Introduction Based on Ancient and Medieval Sources* (Leiden: Brill, 1973).

al-Malik al-Muẓaffar Yūsuf b. 'Umar al-Ghassānī al-Turkmānī/al-Saqqā, Muṣṭafā (ed.), *al-Mu'tamad fī l-adwiya al-mufrada* (Beirut: Dār al-ma'rifa, 1975).

Margariti, Eleni Roxani, *Aden & the Indian Ocean Trade. 150 Years in the Life of a Medieval Arabian Port* (Chapel Hill: University of North Carolina Press, 2007).

Niessen, Friedrich, and Lev, Efraim, 'Addenda to Isaacs *Catalogue of the Medical and Paramedical Manuscripts in the Cambridge Genizah Collection* Together with the Edition of Two Medical Documents T-S 12.33 and T-S NS 297.56', *Hebrew Union College Annual*, 77 (2006), 131–65.

Pormann, Peter E., and Savage-Smith, Emilie, *Medieval Islamic Medicine* (Cairo: The American University in Cairo Press, 2007).

Reif, Stefan C., *A Jewish Archive from Old Cairo* (Richmond/Surrey: Curzon Press, 2000).

Richler, Benjamin, *Guide to Hebrew Manuscript Collections* (Jerusalem: The Israel Academy of Sciences and Humanities, 1994).

Savage-Smith, Emilie, 'Medicine', in Roshdi Rashed (ed.), *Encyclopedia of the History of Arabic Science* (London: Routledge, 1996), 3, 903–62.

———, 'Ṭibb', *The Encyclopaedia of Islam* (New Edition) (X; Leiden: Brill, 1999), 452a–461a.

Smith, G. Rex, 'Have You Anything to Declare? Maritime Trade and Commerce in Ayyubid Aden: Practices and Taxes', *Proceedings of the Seminar for Arabian Studies*, 15 (1995), 127–40.

———, 'More on the Port Practices and Taxes of Mediaeval Aden, *New Arabian Studies*, 3 (1996), 208–18.

Stillman, Norman A., 'The Eleventh Century Merchant House of Ibn 'Awkal (a Geniza Study)', *Journal of the Economic and Social History of the Orient*, 16 (1973), 15–87.

Ullmann, Manfred, *Islamic Medicine* (Edinburgh: Edinburgh University Press, 1978).

Varisco, Daniel M., *Medieval Agriculture and Islamic Science: The Almanac of a Yemeni Sultan* (Publications on the Near East, 6; Seattle: University of Washington Press, 1994).

———, *Medieval Folk Astronomy and Agriculture in Arabia and the Yemen* (Variorum Collected Studies Series; Aldershot: Ashgate, 1997).

———, 'Agriculture in al-Hamdānī's Yemen: A Survey from Early Islamic Geographical Texts', *Journal of the Economic and Social History of the Orient*, 52/3 (2009), 382–412.
———, and Smith, G. Rex (eds.), *The Manuscript of al-Malik al-Afḍal al-ʿAbbās b. ʿAlī b. Dāʾūd b. Yūsuf b. ʿUmar b. ʿAlī Ibn Rasūl (d. 778/1377): A Medieval Arabic Anthology from the Yemen.* Edited with an Introduction (Warminster: Aris & Phillips for the Gibb Memorial Trust, 1998).

MAGIC AND MEDICINE IN A THIRTEENTH-CENTURY TREATISE ON THE SCIENCE OF THE STARS[1]

Petra G. Schmidl

At the end of the thirteenth century the Rasulid sultan al-Ashraf ʿUmar wrote a treatise on the science of the stars, *Kitāb al-Tabṣira fī ʿilm al-nujūm* [Enlightenment on the Science of the Stars] that claims to be an introduction to or a textbook of this discipline. It also contains magical and medical subjects scattered throughout the text. A closer look at the author, his text, and the magical and medical topics he deals with will reveal possible reasons to include magic and medicine in a treatise on the science of the stars.

1. The Author

al-Ashraf ʿUmar, the third of the Rasulid sultans and the author of the *Tabṣira*, ruled over Yemen for less than two years before he died in 1296.[2] By writing a number of scientific treatises concerning diverse topics he made a "considerable contribution to science."[3] His treatises deal with genealogy, agriculture, hippiatry, medicine, and magic, although it appears his treatise on oneiromancy, *Ishāra fī l-ʿibāra fī ʿilm taʿbīr al-ruʾya*

---

[1] This chapter—and the talk on which it is based—is a spin-off of a research project called "The Sultan and the Stars" generously supported by the Fritz Thyssen Stiftung, Düsseldorf, during 2008–9. I am very grateful for the grant that enabled me to spend an interesting time conducting research on the *Kitāb al-Tabṣira* of al-Ashraf ʿUmar. The work is intended to lead to an edition and translation of the introduction and the table of contents, accompanied by a commentary. This research will take into account the specific role of al-Ashraf ʿUmar. I wish to thank all my colleagues who helped me in preparing this paper, in particular Rainer Brömer, David A. King, Zeina Matar, Armin Schopen, and Daniel M. Varisco, as well as Gillian Grant and the staff at the Bodleian Library in Oxford for their kind permission to reproduce clips from *Kitāb al-Tabṣira* and for their help and patience. Although carefully proofread, all remaining mistakes are the author's responsibility.

[2] On the Rasulids *e.g.* Smith, 'Rasūlids'; Schmidl, *Volkstümliche Astronomie*, 1, 33–5; also Ibn Ḥātim/Smith (ed. and trans.), *Kitāb al-Simṭ*, 2, 83–90; al-Khazrajī/Redhouse (trans.) and ʿAsal (ed.), *Pearl-strings, passim*. On al-Ashraf ʿUmar, see Schmidl, 'al-Ashraf ʿUmar'; King, *MAY*, 27–9; al-Khazrajī/Redhouse (trans.) and ʿAsal (ed.), *Pearl-strings*, 1, 236–46 (English translation), and 4, 284–98 (Arabic text); also Suter, *'Mathematiker und Astronomen'*, 160–1; *id.*, *'Nachträge'*, 177.

[3] Schmidl, 'al-Ashraf ʿUmar', 66.

[Explanative Instruction (?) on the Science of Interpreting Dreams] is not preserved.[4] Concerning the science of the stars, al-Ashraf 'Umar wrote an instrument book comprising instructions for the construction of astrolabes, sundials, water clocks, and a magnetic compass for finding the direction to Mecca, the *qibla*. In addition, two *ijāzāt* ('statements of approval') by al-Ashraf 'Umar's teachers attached to his instrument book attest that the sultan himself made astrolabes "skillfully and accurately;"[5] it is one of the great windfalls of the history of science that one of these astrolabes is still preserved (IIC #0109 = #3549).[6] The resemblances of the scales and features shown in the schemes of the manuscript and on the instrument itself are striking. Most interesting are the symbols used for the planets on the back of the astrolabe (see below).[7] Apart from the instrument book and the astrolabe, the sultan's third contribution to the science of the stars is the *Tabṣira,* introduced below in detail.

Although none of al-Ashraf 'Umar's predecessors and successors was as enthusiastic and as creative as the third Rasulid sultan himself, all of them were interested in the sciences and the arts. This interest is reflected in the architecture and the artefacts preserved from the Rasulid period and also in texts, in particular those on agriculture and on astronomy.[8] Several astronomical treatises were closely related to the sultans, some of them written by the sultans themselves, some of them patronized by the rulers or their attendants and covering different topics of astronomy and astrology.[9] For instance, al-Fārisī (d. 1278/9), a scholar with varied interests, dedicated his *al-Zīj al-mumtaḥan al-Muẓaffarī*, an astronomical handbook

---

[4] For an overview of al-Ashraf 'Umar's treatises, see Varisco, *Almanac*, 14–16. See also Ingrid Hehmeyer's chapter in this volume.

[5] King, *SATMI* 2, XIVa, 645. Id., *SATMI* 2, XIVa, 632–46, including a translation of both *ijāzāt*; also id., *MAY*, 28–9. The chapter on the magnetic compass and its use as a *qibla* indicator is edited, translated, and commented on in Schmidl, 'Magnetic Compass'; also King, *World-Maps*, 109–11, and the figure in id., 'Astronomie im Jemen', 279, with the beginning of the chapter on the compass bowl and its scheme (taken from the manuscript Cairo, *Taymūr riyāḍā*, 105; also the description in id., *Cairo Survey*, 132). A reconstruction of the compass bowl is to be found in the Institute for the History of Arabic-Islamic Science, Frankfurt (Sezgin and Neubauer, *Wissenschaft und Technik*, 2, 58; also Sezgin, *Science and Technology*, 46).

[6] King, *SATMI* 2, XIVa, 623–32.

[7] See ibid., 625–6 (figs. 2.1, 2.2; front and back of the astrolabe itself), 634–5 (figs. 3.1, 3.2; schemes of the front and back taken from his instrument book); see also id., 'Astronomie im Jemen', 280–1 (front of the astrolabe itself).

[8] E.g. Smith, 'Rasūlids', 456b–457a; Finster, 'Architektur der Rasūliden'; King, 'Astronomie im Jemen'; Porter, 'Kunst der Rasuliden'; Varisco, 'Rasūlidische Landwirtschaft'; on patronage in general also Brentjes, 'Patronage'.

[9] King, *MAY*, esp. 11–15; id., *Cairo Survey*, 131–4.

with tables, to al-Muẓaffar Yūsuf, the second of the Rasulid sultans and al-Ashraf 'Umar's father, and wrote his *Nihāyat al-idrāk fī asrār 'ulūm al-aflāk*, an astrological treatise for the sultan's treasury.[10]

2. The Text

In these inspiring surroundings al-Ashraf 'Umar made his instruments and wrote his scientific treatises, one of them a text on the science of the stars—the *Tabṣira*. The treatise is preserved only in an undated and unsigned manuscript in Oxford (Bodleian Library, Huntington 233), abbreviated as "H" in this chapter.[11] David King suggested that the manuscript was copied around 1400, and Daniel Varisco identified several Yemeni characteristics of the handwriting.[12]

The title, *Kitāb al-Tabṣira fī 'ilm al-nujūm* [Enlightenment on the Science of the Stars], is written at the top of the title page (H,3a), followed by the name of the author *al-Malik al-Ashraf Mumahhid al-Dunyā wa-l-Dīn Abū l-Fatḥ 'Umar b. Mawlānā l-Sulṭān al-Malik al-Muẓaffar Yūsuf b. 'Umar b. 'Alī b. Rasūl.* A close inspection of the manuscript in Oxford in May 2009 revealed that the title page is a compound of several layers of paper due to the production, restoration and/or conservation process. The layer that is most likely the oldest bears two pentagrams in the lower right corner of the page (see below). The layer with the title and the name of the author appears to be later than the one with the five-pointed stars. It is uncertain if the layers were put together by the copyist or somebody else, and therefore it is also not clear whether the title and the name of the author originally belonged on the title page. Because of these uncertainties it appears appropriate to search for evidence in the manuscript itself.

Concerning the authorship, al-Ashraf 'Umar himself is not mentioned in the *Tabṣira*. But there are numerous indications scattered throughout the text pointing towards its compilation in Yemen probably at the end of the thirteenth century. First, the author of the *Tabṣira* is familiar with

---

[10] On al-Fārisī and his œuvre Schmidl, 'al-Fārisī'; ead., *Volkstümliche Astronomie*, 1, 18–23; King, *SATMI* 1, *passim*; Ihsanoğlu and Rosenfeld, *Mathematicians*, 219; King, *MAY*, 23–6; Brockelmann, *GAL* I, 625 (474), and S I, 866–7 (mixing up al-Fārisī with al-Kawāshī); al-Khazrajī/Redhouse (trans.) and 'Asal (ed.), *Pearl-strings*, 4, 204 (Arabic text); Suter, 'Mathematiker und Astronomen', 139 and 218 (n. 72); id., 'Nachträge', 175; on his *zīj* also King and Samsó, *Zīj Report*, 52, Kennedy, *Survey*, 10; Lee, 'Astronomical Tables of Al Farsi'; a table of contents in Pingree, *Gregory Chioniades*, 1, 9–16.

[11] See *Catalogue Oxford*, 1, 196b–197a (no. CMV).

[12] King, *SATMI* 1, III, 487; Varisco, *Almanac*, 16.

the œuvre of al-Fārisī, the scholar who worked at the court of al-Muẓaffar Yūsuf, al-Ashraf ʿUmar's father (see above). He is mentioned in chapter xiv of the *Tabṣira* dealing with the use of magic squares (H,28b,18; see also below). In addition, one of the three *qibla* schemes presented at the end of al-Fārisī's folk astronomical treatise bears close resemblance to the *qibla* scheme in chapter xxxvii of the *Tabṣira*.[13] Second, the astronomical parameters used in the *Tabṣira* are calculated for Yemen, most probably for Ṣanʿāʾ by using φ = 14;30° for its geographical latitude, a common medieval value.[14] Chapter xlvii contains a geographical table, accompanied by a short explanation of how to determine the geographical latitude of a location by means of the solar altitude at noon. This explanation seems to be using the example of Ṣanʿāʾ because it employs the geographical latitude of φ = 14;30°. In the table, however, Taʿizz is emphasized by adding *al-maḥrūs* ('[may it be] protected'; H,153b). In addition, that city's geographical latitude is given with the most precise value in the whole table, φ = 13;43° (H,153b). In 1255 al-Muẓaffar Yūsuf had made Taʿizz the Rasulid capital,[15] possibly a reason for the emphasis.

Concerning the title, *Kitāb al-Tabṣira fī ʿilm al-nujūm* [Enlightenment on the Science of the Stars], a slightly different phrase is found in the introduction. Here al-Ashraf ʿUmar characterizes his treatise as "*hādhā l-majmūʿ*" ('this collection [of texts]'; H,3b,8) being a "*tabṣira lil-mubtadiʾ fī ʿilm al-nujūm*" ('an enlightenment for the beginner in the science of the stars'; H,3b,5).

Following the introduction, a detailed table of contents reflects what al-Ashraf ʿUmar thought to be important for the beginner (Table 1).

A large portion at the beginning—chapters i to xix, except for chapter xiv that contains the use of magic squares (see below) and the reference to al-Fārisī (see above)—deals with descriptive astrology, i.e. astrological methods distinguished from mathematical astrology that is mainly concerned with the computation of horoscopes.[16] Likewise, chapters xxxix

13 Schmidl, *Volkstümliche Astronomie*, 2, 666–7; figures of al-Fārisī's schemes in King, 'Makka 4. As the Centre of the World' (fig. 4); id., *World-Maps*, 53; id., 'Astronomie im Jemen', 276.

14 For examples, see the data in chapters xxvii, xxviii, and xxxiii; also King, *SATMI* 1, I, 80–1 and 91, III, 487-8, VIa, 697; on the geographical latitude of Ṣanʿāʾ, see Kennedy and Kennedy, *Geographical Coordinates*, 300–1.

15 E.g. Smith, 'Taʿizz', 117a.

16 See Ullmann, *Natur- und Geheimwissenschaften*, 273: "In Laienkreisen wurde vor allem die nicht-horoskopische Astrologie gepflegt, jener Zweig, der ohne Kenntnis der Mathematik und der komplizierten astrologischen Systematik praktiziert werden konnte."

Table 1. The contents of the *Tabṣira*

H	Chapter	Contents
6a–27a	i–xiii	descriptive astrology
27a–31b	xiv	magic
31b–35a	xv	descriptive astrology
35a–43a	xvi–xvii	elections
43a–45a	xviii–xix	descriptive astrology
45a–50a	xx–xxiii	Sun and Moon
50a–52b	xxiv	fixed stars
52b–56a	xxv	elections
56a–63a	xxvi	calendars
63b–94a	xxvii–xxx	timekeeping
94b–96b	xxxi	descriptive astrology
96b–109a	xxxii	almanac
109a–116a	xxxiii–xxxvi	*anwāʾ* and *azmina*
116a–117a	xxxvii	*qibla*
117b–119a	xxxviii	calendars
119b–135b	xxxix–xl	elections
135b–139b'[a]	xli	magic
139b'[a]–146b	xlii–xliv	descriptive astrology
146b–153a	xlv–xlvi	instruments
153b–154a	xlvii	geography
154a–160b	xlviii	elections
160b–165b	xlix–l	symbols, ciphers

[a] There is at least one folio missing, because the end of chapter xli and the beginning of chapter xlii are omitted.

to xliv provide similar topics—except for chapter xli that is comprised of magical techniques (see below). Together with chapters xxv, xxxi, and xlviii, descriptive astrology is dealt with in more than half of the chapters. A second larger group, chapters xxxii to xxxviii, concerns information usually found in *anwāʾ* and *azmina* books, apart from the determination of the *qibla* in chapter xxxvii. Distinguishing between *anwāʾ* and *azmina* books is not an easy task. Usually, both explain the *anwāʾ* system, in which the heliacal risings[17] and acronychal settings[18] of specific stars and groups of stars subdivide the solar year and help foresee the weather. They

[17] I.e. the rising of a celestial body just before sunrise when it becomes first visible in the eastern dawn sky.

[18] I.e. the setting of a celestial body shortly after sunset when it is last visible in the western dusk sky.

provide information on times and seasons, list the lunar mansions, and explain the winds and the rains, accompanied by proverbs, poems, and commentaries.[19] The arrangement of the other chapters of the *Tabṣira* seems to be more or less random.

The survey of the contents of the *Tabṣira* shows a very individual composition with several striking points in its arrangement and topics. While the basic information on descriptive astrology at the beginning is well-situated, the placement of the final two chapters, xlix and l, appears rather peculiar. They contain a description of the Indian numbers and their use, although al-Ashraf ʿUmar takes it for granted that the reader of the *Tabṣira* is familiar with them from some of the forty-eight chapters dealt with before. The only two chapters on instruments, xlv and xlvi, seem to be of no great value. Covering the described range of topics in one treatise also appears unusual. A generation before al-Ashraf ʿUmar compiled the *Tabṣira*, al-Aṣbaḥī (d. *c.*1260/1), a Yemeni scholar trained in religious law and grammar, wrote a book on the determination of prayer times, the *Kitāb al-Yawāqīt*.[20] In one chapter he writes a rejection of profane astronomy and astrology. He says:

> This introduction prohibits determining prayer times by means of the calculations of the scientists of the stars (*al-munajjimūn*) and the philosophers (*al-falāsifa*), as well as (by means) of geometry. Know that it is not allowed to determine prayer times by means of the degrees of an astrolabe or by the calculations belonging to the science of the stars. [...] The scientists of the stars take their knowledge from Euclid, the *Sindhind*, Aristotle, and other philosophers. They are all infidels [...].[21]

Later in this chapter al-Aṣbaḥī even compares the science of the stars with divination and fortune telling. His rejection of Greek and Indian methods may be interpreted as a general refusal of mathematical or scientific astronomy—one of the two astronomical traditions usually distinguished in modern research on pre-modern astronomy in Islamic societies, the other being folk astronomy.[22] It is not surprising, then, that in order to determine prayer times al-Aṣbaḥī relies in his treatise solely on the methods of the latter.

---

19 For an introduction, see Pellat, 'Anwā'', also Schmidl, *Volkstümliche Astronomie*, 1, 86–91.

20 Ibid., 5–7; King, *SATMI* 1, III, 484–5; Ihsanoğlu and Rosenfeld, *Mathematicians*, 323 ("London (Sup. 110)" has to be read "Cambridge (Sup. 110)"); King, *MAY*, 22.

21 See Schmidl, *Volkstümliche Astronomie*, 1, 132–3.

22 Ibid., 78–92; King, 'Mathematical Astronomy'; Varisco, 'Islamic Folk Astronomy'.

The author of the *Tabṣira* had a different attitude towards these issues. The work contains not only subjects al-Aṣbaḥī rejects, but presents them together with other topics of which he approves. al-Ashraf ʿUmar puts astrology and problems related to profane astronomy next to sacred astronomy in the service of Islam.[23] Methods of mathematical or scientific astronomy al-Aṣbaḥī rejects, and folk astronomical methods he approves can be found side by side.[24]

3. Magic and Medicine

Only the headings of chapter xli and chapter xiv point towards magical topics. While chapter xli comprises three subjects—palmomancy,[25] onomatomancy,[26] and seating arrangements in court—chapter xiv focuses on making talismans and amulets, also a major concern in chapter xxv dealing with lunar elections (see below). al-Ashraf ʿUmar describes the purpose of these pieces endowed with magic power as "*muttaṣil bi-l-suʿūd barīʾ min al-nuḥūs*" ('connected with fortune, [and] free of misfortune'; H,29b,18).[27]

3.1. *Planetary Symbols*

While introducing al-Ashraf ʿUmar, his scientific œuvre, and his contributions to the science of the stars, two examples of possible magical

---

23 Schmidl, *Volkstümliche Astronomie* 1, 92–103; King, 'Astronomie im Dienste des Islam'; id., *Astronomy in the Service of Islam*.

24 For instance, in chapter xxxvii al-Ashraf ʿUmar describes a *qibla* scheme that can be used for finding the direction to Mecca (e.g. King, 'Makka 4. As the Centre of the World'). Previous to this, in chapter xxxi he deals with the knowledge of the lords of the hours, and slightly later, in chapter xlii, with the twelve houses, as well as in chapters xlv and xlvi with astronomical instruments. He arranges astrological topics and profane astronomy around a problem of sacred astronomy. In addition, the geographical table in chapter xlvii can also be used for finding the direction to Mecca by calculating the angle between the meridian of any locality and the great circle that goes through that locality and Mecca (*inḥirāf al-qibla*, e.g. King, *World-Maps*, 56–7). This method belongs to the mathematical tradition, while the same problem is solved in the *qibla* scheme in chapter xxxvii by folk astronomical methods that are completely different and much simpler. Further investigations have to be conducted to decide whether dealing with profane astronomy and astrology side by side with sacred astronomy, and the use of mathematical methods parallel to folk astronomical methods, are as unusual as they appear at the moment.

25 A divinatory practice that interprets the convulsions occurring in all parts of the human body.

26 A divinatory practice that makes use of the numerical value of letters.

27 For an introduction, see Ruska and Carra de Vaux (Bosworth), 'Tilsam'; Savage-Smith, 'Introduction', in ead. (ed.), *Magic and Divination*, xxii–xxv.

significance were mentioned—the planetary symbols on the back of his astrolabe, and the two pentagrams on the title page of the *Tabṣira* (see above).

Table 2. The planetary symbols used by al-Ashraf ʿUmar (columns 2–5 with kind permission from King, *SATMI* 2, 626 and 635; column 6 courtesy of the Bodleian Library, Oxford)

Names of the planets	*Instrument Book*, line 1 of table	*Instrument Book*, line 2 of table	*Instrument Book*, line 3 of table	Back of astrolabe	*Tabṣira* (H,22a)
Saturn					
Jupiter					
Mars					
Sun					
Venus					
Mercury					
Moon					

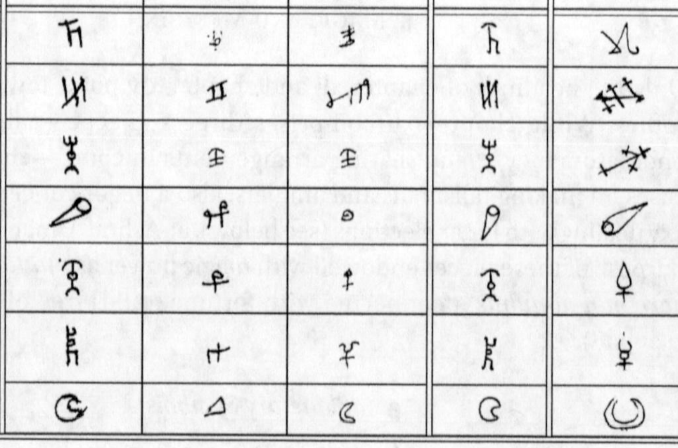

The planetary symbols appear in a diagram that consists of three circular astrological scales and is found both on the back of the astrolabe (i.e. on the instrument itself), and in the instrument book. The first scale is inscribed with the 'terms' (*ḥudūd, fines*, i.e. five areas of unequal size for each zodiacal sign), the second one with the 'faces' (*al-wujūh, facies*, i.e. three equal parts of ten degrees for each zodiacal sign), and the third one with the lord of the day, of the night, and the companion of the corresponding triplicity of a sign.[28] In addition, below the diagram in the instrument book there is a table that depicts three different versions of each planetary symbol (see Table 2). The first version (line 1 of the table) is identical with the planetary symbols found in the diagram of the back of the astrolabe in the instrument book. In the *Tabṣira,* chapter viii deals with the astrological characteristics, natures, and associations of the planets and also presents planetary symbols. The chapter includes a table that gives the Arabic, the

[28] King, *SATMI* 2, XIVa, 631; for pictures of the astrolabe <http://www.metmuseum.org/Collections/search-the-collections/140001577>, accessed 14 November 2011; on the astrological scales Hartner, 'Astrolabe', 2548–9.

Persian, and the Greek names of each planet, supplemented by the associated symbol and the final-letter-abbreviation of the planet's name (H,22a; Table 3).[29] The latter is commonly used in astronomy and astrology as an alternative symbol for the respective planet.[30]

Table 3. The planets, their names in different languages, and their symbols (H,22a; column 4 courtesy of the Bodleian Library, Oxford; column 6 by PGS)

Names of the planets	In Persian	In Greek	Their symbols	Their signs in astronomy	English names
Zuḥal	*Kaywān*	*Q-rūn-s* "without dots"[31]		*l*	Saturn
al-Mushtarī	*Barjīs*[32]	*Ṭ* (?)-*ʾūs*	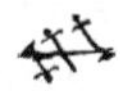	*y*	Jupiter
al-Mirrīkh	*Bahzām*[33]	*ʾ-rās*	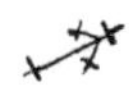	*kh*	Mars
al-Shams	"not found in Persian"	*al-Yūl-s*	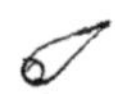	*s*	Sun
al-Zuhra	*Anāhīd* "without dots"[34]	*ʾ-f-rūd* (?)-*ṭī*		*h*	Venus
ʿUṭārid	"its name not found"	*H-r-m-s*	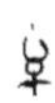	*d*	Mercury
al-Qamar	"its name not found"	*Sālū* (?)-*nī*	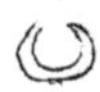	*r*	Moon

[29] al-Bīrūnī/Sachau (ed. and trans.), *Chronology*, 192/172, gives a table listing the Arabic, Greek, Persian, Syriac, Hebrew, Sanskrit, and Khwārizm names of the seven planets.

[30] King, *SATMI* 2, XIIIc, 515. There are several astrolabes combining planetary symbols with final-letter-abbreviations, e.g., on the back of the astrolabes made by al-Khujandī in 984/5 (IIC #0111; King, *SATMI* 2, XIIIc, 503–17, esp. 507 (fig. 9b), 514–15); by Ḥāmid b. ʿAlī al-Wāsiṭī in the ninth/tenth centuries (IIC #3713; King, *SATMI* 2, XIIIc, 500–3, esp. 501–2 (fig. 8.2b)); by Badr, *mawlā* of Hibat Allāh al-Aṣṭurlābī in 1130/1 (IIC #2557; King, *SATMI* 2, X, 54 (fig. 4.7.3)); by Ḥāmid b. Maḥmūd al-Iṣfahānī in 1152/3 (IIC #0004; King, *SATMI* 2, X, 48–9 (fig. 4.5.2), and Gunther, *Astrolabes*, 1, 117 (pl. XXIV)); and by Muḥammad b. Jaʿfar b. ʿUmar al-Aṣṭurlābī, also called al-Jalāl, in 1393/4 (IIC #2710; King, *SATMI* 2, XIVd, 771–4, esp. 773 (fig. 4b)). But none of these instruments is of Yemeni provenance.

[31] The *addendum* "without dots" given in the *Tabṣira* makes clear that al-Ashraf ʿUmar copied a source written in Arabic letters.

[32] al-Bīrūnī/Sachau (ed. and trans.), *Chronology*, 192/172, gives *Hurmuzd* as the Persian name of Jupiter; *Barjīs* seems to be not the Persian, but another Arabic name (see Hartner, 'al-Mushtarī', 680a, referring to *Lisān al-ʿArab*, vii, 323).

[33] al-Bīrūnī/Sachau (ed. and trans.), *Chronology*, 192/172, gives *Bahrām* as the Persian name of Mars.

[34] Ibid., *Nāhīd* is given as the Persian name of Venus; on the *addendum*, see above n. 31.

The symbols given in the *Tabṣira* are slightly different from the versions found on the astrolabe and in the instrument book (see Table 2). They serve purely astrological, not magical purposes, although they bring to mind the seven seals or signs (*al-khawātim al-sabʿa* or *al-ashkāl al-sabʿa*).[35]

3.2. *The Pentagrams*

The two pentagrams on the title page stand on their own without information regarding their purpose, or who was responsible for drawing them. A talismanic protection might be envisaged. Both five-pointed stars are inscribed in a circle, and Indian numbers are written in the resulting sections. The sum of opposite numbers is constant. The first pentagram (Fig. 1) comprises the numbers 1 to 10, with 11 as its sum in the middle. The second version (Fig. 2) has the numbers 1 to 5 and 10 to 14 written in the sections, but without 15 (the sum) in its centre.[36]

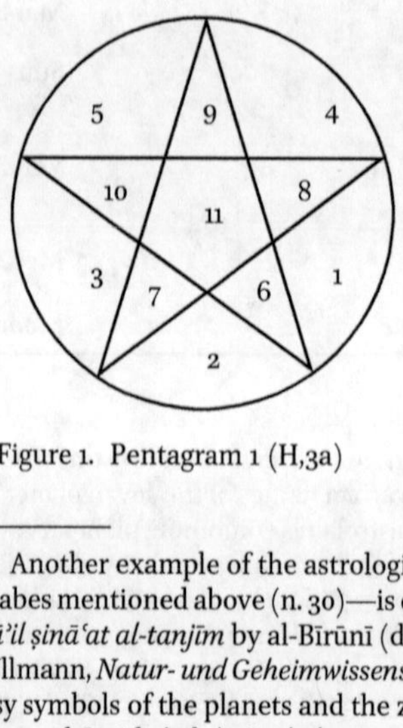

Figure 1. Pentagram 1 (H,3a)

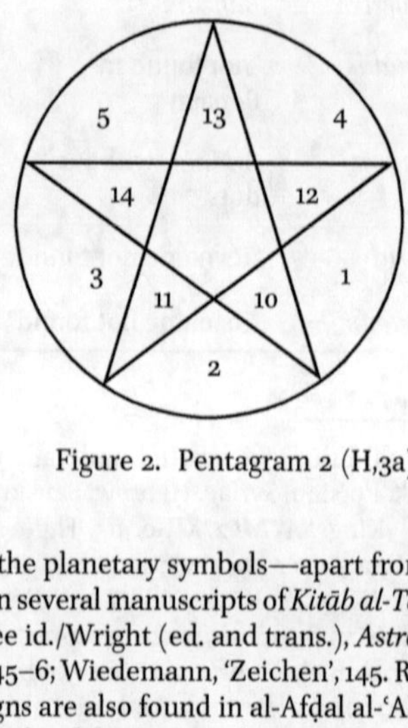

Figure 2. Pentagram 2 (H,3a)

[35] Another example of the astrological use of the planetary symbols—apart from the astrolabes mentioned above (n. 30)—is displayed in several manuscripts of *Kitāb al-Tafhīm li-awāʾil ṣināʿat al-tanjīm* by al-Bīrūnī (d. *c.*1050), see id./Wright (ed. and trans.), *Astrology*, 199; Ullmann, *Natur- und Geheimwissenschaften*, 345–6; Wiedemann, 'Zeichen', 145. Rather clumsy symbols of the planets and the zodiacal signs are also found in al-Afḍal al-ʿAbbās/Varisco and Smith (eds.), *Anthology*, 248. An example of their magical use is given in the *Picatrix* by Pseudo-Maslama al-Majrīṭī (d. *c.*1007) at the beginning of chapter 2:10 (Arabic text in Ritter (ed.), *Pseudo-Mağrīṭī*, 106–7; German translation in Ritter and Plessner (trans.), *"Picatrix"*, 113–14; Latin version in Pingree (ed.), *Latin Version*, 64–5). For an overview of the planetary symbols used in Europe since the Renaissance, see Gettings, *Dictionary of Occult, Hermetic, and Alchemical Sigils, passim.* Examples of the seven signs and their magical use are given, for instance, in *Shams al-maʿārif al-kubrā* by al-Būnī (d. 1225 (?)), ed. (1) and (2), esp. 1, 86; also Winkler, *Siegel*, 68–70, 114–19; Hehmeyer, 'Water and Sign Magic', 85–92; Porter, 'Seals', 189–90, (fig. 8.10); Canaan, 'Decipherment', 168–70.

[36] Winkler, *Siegel*, 119–27, lists examples of pentagrams and hexagrams and emphasizes their interchangeability. Doutté, *Magie et religion*, 251, presents four hexagrams with letters inscribed in their points.

3.3. *Magic Squares*

This sort of arithmetical gadget calls to mind the magic squares, in Arabic *al-wafq* or *wafq al-ʿadad*, literally 'the harmonious (arrangement)' or 'the harmonious (arrangement) of the numbers'.[37] In such squares each number only appears once. Numbers in each line, column, and diagonal add up to the same numerical value. In chapter xiv of the *Tabṣira* al-Ashraf ʿUmar presents eight of them, using Indian numbers. Each square is associated either with one of the seven planets of pre-modern astronomy, or with the zodiac (Figs. 3 to 10).

Generally speaking, at first sight it appears not to matter whether one starts with the innermost planet of pre-modern astronomy, the Moon, and associates it with the square of order 3, or whether one begins with the outermost planet, Saturn, and relates it to the smallest square.[38] But over

4	3	8
9	5	1
2	7	6

Figure 3. The square of order 3 for the Moon (H,27a)[39]

4	14	15	1
9	7	6	12
5	11	10	8
16	2	3	13

Figure 4. The square of order 4 for Mercury (H,28b)[40]

[37] For an introduction to their compilation Sésiano, 'Wafḳ'; to their history Sésiano, *Carrés magiques*, 1–19; to their magical significance Macdonald, 'Budūḥ'; Savage-Smith, 'Introduction', in ead. (ed.), *Magic and Divination*, xxv–xxvii.

[38] Ahrens, 'Studien', 199–200, and id., 'Planetenamulette', 466–8, mentions two examples with a square of order 3 for the Moon: *Maqāla fī wujūd ʿillat al-ʿadād al-mutaḥābba*, a treatise on arithmetics, amicable numbers, and related subjects, by Abū l-Walīd Ismāʿīl b. ʿAlī b. al-Ḥasan b. Abī Naṣr al-Mālaqī (Ahlwardt, *Handschriften-Verzeichnisse*, 9/3, 505–6 (no. 4115 = Mq. 98), the manuscript is dated *c.* 1450); and *Practica Arithmeticae* by Hieronymus Cardanus (d. 1576), this example without associating the square of order 10 with the zodiac.

[39] Similar to Sésiano, *Carrés Magiques*, 5 (fig. 15), and Ahrens, *'Studien'*, 190 (fig. 9), both displaying all eight possibilities to arrange a simple square of order 3. In the *Tabṣira* the completely filled-in square of order 3 is followed by a square that only presents the odd numbers in the form of a cross (H,27b). This special feature is also described in Ahrens, *'Studien'*, 239–40; also Canaan, *'Decipherment'*, 147–8. The possibility of writing only the even numbers in the corners is missing in the *Tabṣira*. This variety coined the name of these magic devices, *budūḥ*, by writing the even numbers 2, 4, 6, and 8 in *abjad*-notation, ب د و ح.

[40] Provided the direction of writing was not adjusted to Latin custom, the square of order 4 is similar to the one in Cammann, *'Islamic and Indian Magic Squares'*, 1, 191 (fig. b).

11	9	2	25	18
19	12	10	3	21
22	20	13	6	4
5	23	16	14	7
8	1	24	17	15

Figure 5. The square of order 5 for Venus (H,29a)

6	12	34	35	23	1
7	11	27	28	8	30
24	25	16	15	18	13
33	14	22	21	17	4
5	29	9	10	26	32
36	20	3	2	19	31

Figure 6. The square of order 6 for the Sun (H,29b)

time the second association became more common.[41] It is reflected in the following explanation: the numerical value of Saturn (زحل) is 45 (7 + 8 + 30 = 45), three times the number of the lines, columns, and diagonals in a square of order 3 (15 × 3 = 45), and 15 is the so-called 'number of Saturn.'[42]

al-Ashraf ʿUmar uses the first arrangement described above, and attributes the Moon to the square of order 3. He concentrates on the astrological dependencies and the magical applications of these squares. Among other things, he gives information on the exaltations and the domiciles of the planets, the metals and incenses that are associated with them (Table 4),[43] as well as the appropriate times to prepare these

He relies on an edition of the *Rasāʾil* of the Ikhwān al-Ṣafāʾ (printed in Cairo in 1928) that used a Cairo manuscript (also in Sésiano, *Carrés Magiques*, 255 (fig. 413)); Hermelink, '*Älteste Quadrate*', 207; Dieterici, *Propädeutik*, 43. On the Cairo manuscript, see also King, *Cairo Survey*, 44–5. On the compilation of a square of order 4, see below n. 46.

[41] This was pointed out by Anne Regourd during the workshop in Halle; also Macdonald, 'Budūḥ', 153b; Bergsträsser, 'Magische Quadrate', 231; Cammann, 'Islamic and Indian Magic Squares', 2, 292–4.

[42] Ahrens, 'Studien', 198–201; id., 'Planetenamulette', 467; also Wiedemann, 'Auszüge', 453; Cammann, 'Islamic and Indian Magic Squares', 1, 208; Gettings, *Dictionary of Astrology*, 190: "[...] 15, which is the number of Saturn." These 'planetary numbers' were used for a variety of magical practices.

[43] For similar information on the association of the planets, with more details, see chapter viii of the *Tabṣira*. For the metals used for making talismanic squares, see e.g. Ahrens, 'Planetenamulette', 468–75; Sésiano, *Carrés magiques*, 254–63, including information on the substances used for their fumigation; and also al-Bīrūnī/Wright (ed. and trans.), *Astrology*, 243 (§ 409–11); Strunz, *Astrologie*, 36–40. For further examples of magic squares used as talismans, see e.g. Porter, 'Seals' (fig. 8.6); Doutté, *Magie et religion*, 191–4, 234, and 251.

22	19	9	6	45	42	32
33	23	20	10	7	46	36
37	34	24	21	11	1	47
48	38	35	25	15	12	2
3	49	39	29	26	16	13
14	4	43	40	30	27	17
18	8	5	44	41	31	28

Figure 7. The square of order 7 for Mars (H,30a)

8	58	59	5	4	62	63	1
49	15	14	52	53	11	10	56
41	23	22	44	45	19	18	48
32	34	35	29	28	38	39	25
40	26	27	37	36	30	31	33
17	47	46	20	21	43	42	24
9	55	54	12	13	51	50	16
64	2	3	61	60	6	7	57

Figure 8a. The square of order 8 for Jupiter (H,30b)[44]

8			5	4			1
	15	14			11	10	
	23[a]	22			19	18	
32			29	28			25
40			37	36			33
	47	46			43	42	
	55	54			51	50	
64			61	60			57

Figure 8b. The incomplete square of order 8 (H,30b)[45]

[a] corr., 33 in H.

44 Similar to Ahrens, *'Planetenamulette'*, 473 (fig. 12), but attributed to Mercury, and also in Bischoff, *Mystik und Magie*, 75.

45 This incompletely filled-in square reflects most probably the first step of compiling a square of order 8. First, divide the square of order 8 into four squares of order 4 and mark the cells of the main diagonals in all four squares (grey cells in Fig. 8b). Start filling the cells from the top right, i.e. 1 is written in that cell. Keep counting while following the cells horizontally from right to left and write the respective number—i.e. 4—in the next marked cell, then 5 in the next, and so on until the cell in the bottom left is reached with the number 64. This is the (intermediate) stage displayed in the *Tabṣira*. Second, start counting anew with the bottom left cell, this time from left to right. Fill in the number 2 in the first still empty cell, then 3 in the next one (non-shaded cells in fig. 8b), and so on until the top right is reached. (Sésiano, 'Wafḳ', 29b). The square of order 4 of the *Tabṣira* was compiled in the same way.

37	33	20	16	3	80	67	63	50
51	38	34	21	17	4	81	68	55
56	52	39	35	22	18	5	73	69
70	57	53	40	36	23	10	6	74
75	71	58	54	41	28	24	11	7
8	76	72	59	46	42	29	25	12
13	9	77	64	60	47	43	30	26
27	14	1	78	65	61	48	44	31
32	19	15	2	79	66	62	49	45

Figure 9. The square of order 9 for Saturn (H,31a)

10	9	93	94	5	96	97	98	2	1
11	19	18	84	85	86	87[a]	13	12	90
71	22	28	27	75	76	24	23	79	80
61	62	33	37	36	35	34	68	69	70
50	52	53	44	46	45	57	58	59	41
60	49	43	54	56	55	47	48	42	51
40	32	63	67	66	65	64	38	39	31
21	72	78	77	26	25[b]	74	73	29[c]	30
81	89	88	17	15	16	14	83	82	20
100	99	8	4	95[d]	6	7	3[e]	92	91

Figure 10. The square of order 10 for the zodiac (H,31b). It includes corrections of the following (obvious) mistakes in the manuscript:
[a] corr., 97 in H. [b] corr., 75 in H. [c] corr., 39 in H. [d] corr., 45 in H. [e] corr., 93 in H.
The magic squares were not mirrored to adjust the writing direction to Latin custom, i.e. the number in the top right cell is in the same place as in the manuscript.

Table 4. The associations of the magic squares with the planets, metals, and incenses (H,27a–31b)

Magic square	Planet	Metal	Incense(s)
of order 3	Moon	silver	styrax, musk, camphor
of order 4	Mercury	quicksilver	ambergris
of order 5	Venus	brass/copper (?) (*al-nuḥās al-aṣfar*)	saffron
of order 6	Sun	gold	ambergris
of order 7	Mars	iron	mukul
of order 8	Jupiter	tin (*al-qazdīr*)	costus, camphor, sandalwood
of order 9	Saturn	lead (*al-usrub* or *al-raṣāṣ al-aswad*)	agarwood, ambergris, and musk
of order 10	zodiac	"all of the seven metals"	ambergris, musk, agarwood

talismanic squares, usually defined by the aspects, the positions of the planets with respect to each other and with respect to the zodiac.[46]

3.4. *Lunar Elections*

The problem of choosing the appropriate time to make talismans is also reflected in chapter xxv dealing with lunar elections. Elections, electing, choosing, or beginning acts at the appropriate time, *ikhtiyārāt* or *ibtidāʾāt* in Arabic, are a standard concept in astrology—since at least Greek antiquity. For a given time, specific activities are declared to be either auspicious or inauspicious. In chapter xxv that deals with determining the appropriate time al-Ashraf ʿUmar makes use of the lunar mansions. The lunar mansions subdivide the ecliptic, the apparent path of the Sun around the Earth, into twenty-eight parts, in the same way as the zodiac subdivides this path into twelve equal parts, the twelve zodiacal signs. The Moon moves through these twenty-eight lunar mansions approximately over the course of one lunar month, entering a new mansion each day. al-Ashraf ʿUmar organizes his chapter in a similar way by discussing one lunar mansion per paragraph. The protasis 'when the Moon enters the lunar mansion (of ...)' is followed by the apodosis 'then do ... or do not ...' ("*idhā anzala al-qamar fīhi fa-aʿmil ... wa-lā ...*"), listing activities related to several topics—including politics, agriculture, health, and magic—that are

46 See e.g. Wiedemann, 'Zu den magischen Quadraten', 96: "Man behauptet, daß diese Figuren [die magischen Quadrate] besondere Eigenschaften haben, wenn sie zu bestimmten Zeiten aufgezeichnet (angewandt) werden."

declared to be either auspicious or inauspicious at that time. The advice concerning magic recommends or disapproves of making talismans, amulets, and other magical devices at the specified time, while the advice concerning medicine recommends or disapproves of applying medicine, or treating the ill.[47]

3.5. *Bloodletting*

Chapter xxxix of the *Tabṣira* involves another example of a medical treatment that depends on the appropriate time as determined by the Moon. The first part informs about the seasons, their natures and their conditions, and also includes advice related to diet. In the second part follows a list that gives advice on bloodletting for each day of the lunar month.[48] When the Moon is waxing, bloodletting apparently encourages certain diseases, while, when waning, it cures them (Table 5).[49]

Table 5. H,120b-121a. Because most of the Arabic terms for diseases do not refer to properly defined symptoms, their translation is not always completely clear.[50]

H	Arabic text	English translation
120b,1	معرفة أوقات تنفيس الدم في أيّام الشهور العربي ومايكرمها ويحمد فيها (؟)	Information on the times for bloodletting in the Arabic months
2	اليوم الأوّل من أخرج فيه الدم أورثه صداع الرأس	First day (of the lunar month)—bloodletting causes headaches.
3	اليوم الثاني من أخرج فيه الدم أورثه الكلف	Second day (of the lunar month)—bloodletting causes freckles.
4	اليوم الثالث من أخرج فيه الدم أورثه الأوضاح	Third day (of the lunar month)—bloodletting causes vitiligo (*al-awḍāḥ*).

47 Chapter xxv is translated with a comment in Varisco, 'Magical Significance'; see also Schmidl, 'Lunar Elections'.

48 Ibn al-Ṣalt/Klein-Franke (ed.), *Iatromathematics*, 69–71, reports that Ibn Buṭlān (d. 1066) discussed the dependency of bloodletting on the phases of the Moon.

49 This was pointed out by Armin Schopen in a personal written communication (December 2010). I tend to agree with him now, although initially I assumed that when the Moon is waxing, an easing—not a worsening—of the disease is implied in the *Tabṣira*.

50 E.g. al-Ṣanʿānī/Schopen and Kahl (eds. and trans., with a commentary), *Natāʾiǧ*, 229. The translation is mainly based on the aforementioned personal written communication by Schopen (see above n. 49) and supplemented by al-Ṣanʿānī/Schopen and Kahl (eds. and trans., with a commentary), *Natāʾiǧ, passim*; Schopen, *Heilmittel, passim*; Ullmann, *Medizin im Islam, passim*; id., *Islamic Medicine, passim*.

Table 5. Continued.

H	Arabic text	English translation
5	اليوم الرابع من أخرج فيه الدم أورثه الرمد الشديد	Fourth day (of the lunar month)—bloodletting causes severe inflammation of the eyes.
6	اليوم الخامس من أخرج فيه الدم أورثه النمش في الوجه	Fifth day (of the lunar month)—bloodletting causes chloasma.
7	اليوم السادس من أخرج فيه الدم أورثه الرعاف	Sixth day (of the lunar month)—bloodletting causes nosebleeds.
8	اليوم السابع من أخرج فيه الدم أورثه السعال	Seventh day (of the lunar month)—bloodletting causes coughs.
9	اليوم الثامن من أخرج فيه الدم أورثه ضيق النفس	Eighth day (of the lunar month)—bloodletting causes dyspnoea.
10	اليوم التاسع من أخرج فيه الدم أورثه اللقوة	Ninth day (of the lunar month)—bloodletting causes facial paralysis.
11	اليوم العاشر من أخرج فيه الدم أورثه الجرب	Tenth day (of the lunar month)—bloodletting causes scabies.
12	إليوم الحادي عشر من أخرج فيه الدم أورثه الحصب	Eleventh day (of the lunar month)—bloodletting causes measles/smallpox.
13	إليوم الثاني عشر من أخرج فيه الدم أورثه الخناق	Twelfth day (of the lunar month)—bloodletting causes diphtheria/pharyngitis.
14	إليوم الثالث عشر من أخرج فيه الدم أورثه الجذام	Thirteenth day (of the lunar month)—bloodletting causes leprosy (*al-judhām*).
15	إليوم الرابع عشر من أخرج فيه الدم أورثه البرص	Fourteenth day (of the lunar month)—bloodletting causes leukoderma (*al-baraṣ*).
16	إليوم الخامس عشر من أخرج فيه الدم أورثه سائر الأعلال	Fifteenth day (of the lunar month)—bloodletting causes all other diseases (?).
17	اليوم السادس عشر من أخرج فيه الدم نقعه من الصداع	Sixteenth day (of the lunar month)—bloodletting stops headaches.

Table 5. Continued.

H	Arabic text	English translation
H,121a,1	اليوم السابع عشر من أخرج فيه الدم نقعه من الكلف	Seventeenth day (of the lunar month)—bloodletting stops freckles.
2	اليوم الثامن عشر من أخرج فيه الدم نقعه من الوضح	Eighteenth day (of the lunar month)—bloodletting stops vitiligo (*al-waḍaḥ*).
3	اليوم التاسع عشر من أخرج فيه الدم نقعه من الرمد	Nineteenth day (of the lunar month)—bloodletting stops inflammation of the eyes.
4	اليوم العشرون من أخرج فيه الدم نقعه من النمش في الوجه	Twentieth day (of the lunar month)—bloodletting stops chloasma.
5	اليوم الحادي والعشرون من أخرج فيه الدم نقعه من الرعاف	Twenty-first day (of the lunar month)—bloodletting stops nosebleeds.
6	اليوم الثاني والعشرون من أخرج فيه الدم نقعه من السعال	Twenty-second day (of the lunar month)—bloodletting stops coughs.
7	اليوم الثالث والعشرون من أخرج فيه الدم نقعه من ضيق النفس	Twenty-third day (of the lunar month)—bloodletting stops dyspnoea.
8	اليوم الرابع والعشرون من أخرج فيه الدم نقعه من اللقوة	Twenty-fourth day (of the lunar month)—bloodletting stops facial paralysis.
9	اليوم الخامس والعشرون من أخرج فيه الدم نقعه من الجرب	Twenty-fifth day (of the lunar month)—bloodletting stops scabies.
10	اليوم السادس والعشرون من أخرج فيه الدم نقعه من الحصب	Twenty-sixth day (of the lunar month)—bloodletting stops measles/smallpox.
11	اليوم السابع والعشرون من أخرج فيه الدم نقعه من الخناق	Twenty-seventh day (of the lunar month)—bloodletting stops diphtheria/pharyngitis.
12	اليوم الثامن والعشرون من أخرج فيه الدم نقعه من الجذام	Twenty-eighth day (of the lunar month)—bloodletting stops leprosy (*al-judhām*).
13	اليوم التاسع والعشرون من أخرج فيه الدم نقعه من البرص	Twenty-ninth day (of the lunar month)—bloodletting stops leukoderma (*al-baraṣ*).
14	اليوم الثلاثون من أخرج فيه الدم نقعه من سائر الأعلال	Thirtieth day (of the lunar month)—bloodletting stops all other diseases (?).

3.6. *Appearance and Disappearance of Diseases*

Additional general information on diseases—their appearance and disappearance, but without mentioning specific treatments—is found in chapter xxxii of the almanac. However, instead of the Moon, it is the Sun that determines when medicine should be taken, or when diseases (tend to) appear or disappear (Table 6).

Table 6. Medical information in chapter xxxii of the *Tabṣira* (according to Varisco, *Almanac, passim*)

Day of the year	Medical information
Tishrīn II, 13	Infectious diseases lifted from people.
Kānūn I, 28	There are fewer illnesses.
Ādhār, 14	Time for taking medicine.
Ādhār, 20	Pestilential diseases are common.
Nīsān, 10	Head colds and eye diseases are common.
Ḥazīrān, 27	Start of Hippocrates' prohibition on (taking) medicine.
Tammūz, 8	Pestilential diseases go away.
Tammūz, 11	Eye diseases are common.
Āb, 10	Last of Hippocrates' prohibition on taking medicine.
Aylūl, 9	Onstart of infectious diseases in people.

3.7. *The Four Seasons, the Zodiacal Signs, and the Planets*

The almanac is also one of the chapters of the *Tabṣira* where the four seasons are associated with the four humours (Table 7)—phlegm, blood, yellow and black bile—a correlation based on Galenic traditions.[51] Each humour possesses a pair of qualities (or natures, characteristics, virtues),

[51] Another example showing the association of the seasons and the humours can be found at the beginning of chapter xxxix of the *Tabṣira*. It also contains the bloodletting list (see above Table 5). For a general introduction to medieval Yemeni medicine, see Varisco, 'Arzneikunde', 306–7. On the Galenic tradition, see e.g. id., *Almanac*, 202–5; Schmidt (ed. and trans.), *Ps.-Galeni liber de humoribus*, 78: "[...] denn das Blut und die Luft und schließlich auch der Frühling (sind) feucht und warm, [...]; (es sind) aber von den Gallen(säften) der gelbe und der Sommer und das Feuer warm und trocken; der schwarze (Gallensaft) aber und die Erde und der Herbst (sind) trocken und kalt; der Schleim aber und das Wasser, aber auch der Winter (sind) kalt und feucht" (see also the Greek text ibid., 2). Another example is described in *Kitāb al-Azmina* by Ibn Māsawayh (d. *c.*857): "Le printemps [...]. C'est une période chaude et humide, durant laquelle le sang est en mouvement. [...] L'été [...]. C'est une période chaude et sèche, durant laquelle la bile jaune est en mouvement. [...] L'automne [...]. C'est une période froide et sèche, durant laquelle l'atrabile est en mouvement. [...]. L'hiver [...]. C'est une période froide et humide, durant laquelle la pituite est en mouvement. [...]." (Ibn Māsawayh/Troupeau (trans.), *'Livre des temps'*, 115–17).

i.e. two of the following: heat, cold, dryness, and moistness. Phlegm is moist and cold, blood moist and hot, yellow bile dry and hot, and black bile dry and cold.[52]

Table 7. Association of the four seasons and the four humours in chapter xxxii of the *Tabṣira* (according to Varisco, *Almanac, passim*)

Day of the year	Seasons and humours
Kānūn I, 14	Entry of the Sun into Capricornus, beginning of winter.
Kānūn I, 16	The humour of phlegm is active.
Ādhār, 13	Entry of the Sun into Aries, beginning of spring.
Ādhār, 14	The humour of blood is active.
Ḥazīrān, 14	Entry of the Sun into Cancer (beginning of summer).
Ḥazīrān, 15	The humour of yellow bile is active.
Aylūl, 15	Entry of the Sun into Libra (beginning of autumn).
Aylūl, 16	The humour of black bile is active.

Clearly, the qualities of the humours and the seasons are interrelated, apart from influencing human health and the treatment of diseases.[53] In a similar way the twelve zodiacal signs are associated with the humours, and accordingly with their qualities.[54] In addition, and mainly by resemblance and analogy, each of the twelve zodiacal signs is correlated with certain creatures, animals, birds, plants, herbs, trees, metals, jewels, stones, colours, incenses, as well as with parts of the human body. There are similar associations for the planets.[55] The influence of both, the zodiacal signs and the planets, depends on their position in relation to the local horizon and to each other. If they are in an auspicious position they strengthen acts performed.[56] al-Ashraf ʿUmar lists these associations in detail in the chapters at the beginning of the *Tabṣira* concerned with descriptive astrology—the zodiacal signs in chapter i, the planets in chapter viii (also including the planetary symbols; see above)—and, with less detail and for another purpose, in chapter xiv (introducing the magic squares; see above).

---

52 On the four humours and their qualities see, for instance, Hankinson, 'Philosophy of Nature', 218–20.

53 See Daniel Martin Varisco's chapter in this volume.

54 On the humours of the signs see, for instance, al-Bīrūnī/Wright (ed. and trans.), *Astrology*, 210 (§ 347).

55 E.g. on the natures, qualities, and associations of the signs, ibid., 211–24 (§ 348-72); and of the planets, ibid., 230–55 (§ 379–437).

56 E.g. Ibn al-Ṣalt/Klein-Franke (ed.), *Iatromathematics*, 65.

Altogether there is a symphony of connections between the macrocosm and the microcosm, the fundamental principle of the astrological *Weltbild*.[57] There are strong indications that celestial events have influence on human life and health. They have to be taken into consideration in the maintenance of health and in the treatment of diseases. This close relationship may be one of the main reasons for including magical and medical topics in the *Tabṣira*. Another reason could be the importance of choosing the appropriate time for performing specific acts—for example making talismans or treating diseases. After all, timekeeping is one of the major problems dealt with in pre-modern astronomy in Islamic societies.[58]

4. Conclusion

The great variety of subjects concerning magic and medicine scattered throughout the *Tabṣira* support the statement in the introduction that it is intended to be "a collection of texts" (H,3b,9), and its basic contents allows it to be "an enlightenment for the beginner in the science of the stars" (H,3b,5). This concept reflects that al-Ashraf ʿUmar was "a teachable pupil and a versatile scholar,"[59] familiar with much more than only astronomy and astrology. His treatise on the science of the stars, the *Tabṣira*, allows one to catch a unique glimpse of what a thirteenth-century Yemeni sultan thought was important for a beginner to learn about the science of the stars. This includes magical and medical topics that are related to the stars in their broadest sense.

Bibliography

al-Afḍal al-ʿAbbās/Varisco, Daniel Martin, and Smith, G. Rex (eds.), *The Manuscript of al-Malik al-Afḍal al-ʿAbbās b. ʿAlī b. Dāʾūd b. Yūsuf b. ʿUmar b. ʿAlī Ibn Rasūl (d. 778/1377): A Medieval Arabic Anthology from the Yemen* (E.J.W. Gibb Memorial Trust; Warminster: Aris & Phillips, 1998).

Ahlwardt, Wilhelm Theodor, *Die Handschriften-Verzeichnisse der königlichen Bibliothek zu Berlin. 9: Verzeichnis der arabischen Handschriften* (3; Berlin: Asher, 1891).

Ahrens, Wilhelm Ernst Martin Georg, 'Studien über die "magischen Quadrate" der Araber', *Der Islam,* 7 (1917), 186–250.

———, 'Die "magischen Quadrate" al-Būnī's', *Der Islam,* 12 (1912), 157–77.

---

57 E.g. Akasoy, Burnett, and Yoeli-Tlalim (eds.), *Astro-Medicine*, ix; Schmidt (ed. and trans.), *Ps.-Galeni liber de humoribus*, 31.

58 E.g. the substantial evidence in King, *SATMI* 1, *passim*.

59 Schmidl, 'al-Ashraf ʿUmar', 67a.

———, '"Magische Quadrate" und Planetenamulette', *Naturwissenschaftliche Wochenschrift*, 35 (1920), 465–75.

Akasoy, Anna, Burnett, Charles, and Yoeli-Tlalim, Ronit (eds.), *Astro-Medicine. Astrology and Medicine, East and West* (Florence: SISMEL, 2008).

BEA = Hockey, *Biographical Encyclopedia of Astronomers*.

Bergsträsser, G., 'Zu den magischen Quadraten', *Der Islam*, 13 (1923), 227–35.

Bibliothecae Bodleianae codicum manuscriptorum orientalium catalogus. Pars 1. Joannes Uri. (Oxonii: Typographeus Clarendonianus, 1787).

al-Bīrūnī/Sachau, C. Edward (ed. and trans.), *The Chronology of Ancient Nations: An English Version of the Arabic Text of the Athâr-ul-Bâkiya of Albîrûnî, or "Vestiges of the Past"* (London: Allen & Co., 1879). Repr. Frankfurt: Minerva, 1969, and in *IMA*, 31.

al-Bīrūnī/Wright, R. Ramsey (ed. and trans.), *The Book of Instruction in the Art of Astrology of al-Bīrūnī* (i.e. *Kitāb al-Tafhīm li-awā'il ṣinā'at al-tanjīm*) (London: Luzac, 1934). Repr. in *IMA*, 29.

Bischoff, Erich, *Mystik und Magie der Zahlen* (Berlin: Barsdorf, 1920). Repr. Schwarzenburg: Ansata, 1977, and Wiesbaden: Fourier, 1992. (The edition used in this chapter).

Blois, F. C. de, 'Ta'rīkh I. Dates and Eras in the Islamic World 1. In the Sense of "Date, Dating", etc.', *EI²*, X (2000), 257b–264b.

Brentjes, Sonja, 'Courtly Patronage of the Ancient Sciences in Post-Classical Islamic Societies', *al-Qanṭara*, 29 (2008), 403–36.

Brockelmann, Carl, *Geschichte der arabischen Litteratur* (2 vols., 3 suppls.; 2nd edn.; Leiden: Brill, 1943–9).

al-Būnī, Aḥmad b. 'Alī, *Shams al-ma'ārif al-kubrā* ([n.p.: unknown publisher], 1318/1900–1, the edition labelled (1) in this chapter).

al-Būnī, Aḥmad b. 'Alī, *Shams al-ma'ārif al-kubrā* (Cairo: [unknown publisher, n.d.], the edition labelled (2) in this chapter).

Cammann, Schuyler, 'Islamic and Indian Magic Squares', Part 1: *History of Religions*, 8/3 (1969), 181–209; Part 2: *History of Religions*, 8/4 (1969), 271–99.

Canaan, Tewfik, 'The Decipherment of Arabic Talismans', *Berytus*, 4 (1937), 69–110, and 5 (1938), 141–51. Repr. in Emily Savage-Smith (ed.), *Magic and Divination*, 125–77.

Catalogue Oxford = *Bibliothecae Bodleianae catalogus*.

Daum, Werner (ed.), *Jemen. 3000 Jahre Kunst und Kultur des Glücklichen Arabien* (Innsbruck: Pinguin, Frankfurt/Main: Umschau, 1987).

Dieterici, Friedrich, *Die Philosophie bei den Arabern im X. Jahrhundert n. Chr.: Gesamtdarstellung und Quellenwerke III. Die Propädeutik der Araber im zehnten Jahrhundert* (Berlin: Mittler & Sohn, 1865). Repr. Hildesheim: Olms, 1969 (the edition used in this chapter), and in the series *Islamic Philosophy*, 22 (Frankfurt: Institut für Geschichte der Arabisch-Islamischen Wissenschaften, 1999).

Doutté, Edmond, *Magie et religion dans l'Afrique du Nord* (Alger : Jourdan, 1908). Repr. Paris : Maisonneuve/Geuthner, 1984 (the edition used in this chapter).

EI² = *The Encyclopaedia of Islam* (New Edition) (12 vols., and suppl.; Leiden: Brill, 1960–2005).

Finster, Barbara, 'Die Architektur der Rasūliden', in Daum (ed.), *Jemen*, 237–55.

Gettings, Fred, *Dictionary of Astrology* (London: Routledge & Kegan Paul, 1985).

———, *Dictionary of Occult, Hermetic, and Alchemical Sigils* (London: Routledge & Kegan Paul, 1981).

Gingerich, Owen, and King, David A., 'Some Astronomical Observations from Thirteenth-Century Egypt', *Journal for the History of Astronomy*, 13 (1982), 121–8. Repr. in David A. King, *Islamic Mathematical Astronomy* (London: Variorum, 1986), VII.

Gunther, Robert T., *The Astrolabes of the World* (2 vols.; Oxford: Oxford University Press, 1932). Repr. in one volume, London: The Holland Press, 1976.

Hankinson, Robert J., 'Philosophy of Nature', in id. (ed.), *The Cambridge Companion to Galen* (Cambridge: Cambridge University Press, 2008), 210–41.

Hartner, Willy, 'The Principle and Use of the Astrolabe', in Arthur Upham Pope (ed.), *Survey of Persian Art: From Prehistoric Times to the Present* 3 (London: Oxford University Press, 1939), 2530–54, 12 figs. Repr. in Günther Kerstein et al. (eds.), *Oriens-Occidens: Ausgewählte Schriften zur Wissenschafts- und Kulturgeschichte. Festschrift zum 60. Geburtstag* (Hildesheim: Olms, 1968), 287–311 (the edition used in this chapter). Also repr. in *Astrolabica*, 1 (1978), and in *IMA*, 94, 338–75.

———, 'al-Mus͟htarī', *EI*², VII (1993), 680a–b.

Hehmeyer, Ingrid, 'Water and Sign Magic in al-Jabin, Yemen', *The American Journal of Islamic Social Sciences*, 25/3 (2008), 82–96.

Hermelink, Heinrich, 'Die ältesten magischen Quadrate höherer Ordnung und ihre Bildungsweise', *Sudhoffs Archiv*, 42 (1958), 199–217.

———, 'Arabische magische Quadrate mit 25 Zellen', *Sudhoffs Archiv*, 43 (1959), 351–4.

Hockey, Thomas, et al. (eds.), *Biographical Encyclopedia of Astronomers* (New York: Springer, 2007).

Ibn Ḥātim/Smith, G. R[ex] (ed. and trans.), *The Ayyūbids and Early Rasūlids in the Yemen (567–694/1173–1295)* (London: Luzac, 1974/8).

Ibn Māsawayh/Troupeau, Gérard (trans.), 'Le *livre des temps* de Jean Ibn Māsawayh', *Arabica*, 15 (1968), 113–42.

Ibn al-Ṣalt/Klein-Franke, Felix (ed.), *Iatromathematics in Islam: A Study on Yuhanna Ibn aṣ-Ṣalt's Book on Astrological Medicine* (Texte und Studien zur Orientalistik, 3; Hildesheim: Olms, 1984).

Ihsanoğlu, Ekmeleddin, and Rosenfeld, Boris A., *Mathematicians, Astronomers and Other Scholars of Islamic Civilization and Their Works (7th–19th c.)* (Series of Studies and Sources on History of Science, 11; Istanbul: IRCICA, 2003).

IIC = International Instrument Checklist (instruments #0001 to #0336: Gunther, *Astrolabes*. Following numbers, although not consecutively numbered: Price et al., *Checklist*. Instruments #4000 onwards: King, *Frankfurt Catalogue*).

IMA = *Islamic Mathematics and Astronomy* Series (vols. 28–99; Frankfurt: Institut für Geschichte der Arabisch-Islamischen Wissenschaften, 1998).

Kennedy, E.S., *A Survey of Islamic Astronomical Tables* (Transactions of the American Philosophical Society, New Series, 46/2; Philadelphia: American Philosophical Society, 1956; 2nd edn. Philadelphia: American Philosophical Society, 1989; references in this chapter are given according to the 2nd edn.).

———, and Kennedy, Mary H., *Geographical Coordinates of Localities from Islamic Sources* (Frankfurt: Institut für Geschichte der Arabisch-Islamischen Wissenschaften, 1987).

al-Khazrajī, ʿAlī Ibn al-Ḥasan/Redhouse, James W. (trans.), and ʿAsal, Muḥammad (ed.), *The Pearl-strings: A History of the Resúliyy Dynasty of Yemen, by ʿAliyyu ʾbnu ʾl-Hasan ʾel-Khazrejiyy* (E.J.W. Gibb Memorial Series, 3, 5 vols.; Leiden: Brill; London: Luzac, 1906–18).

King, *Cairo Survey* = King, *Survey of Scientific Manuscripts*.

———, *MAY* = King, *Mathematical Astronomy in Medieval Yemen*.

———, *SATMI* 1 = King, *In Synchrony with the Heavens* 1.

———, *SATMI* 2 = King, *In Synchrony with the Heavens* 2.

King and Samsó, *Zīj Report* = King and Samsó, 'Astronomical Handbooks'.

King, David A., *Mathematical Astronomy in Medieval Yemen: A Biobibliographical Survey* (American Research Center in Egypt; Malibu: Udena Publications, 1983).

———, 'Makka 4. As the Centre of the World', *EI*², VI (1991), 180b–187a.

———, 'The Medieval Yemeni Astrolabe in the Metropolitan Museum of Art in New York City', *Zeitschrift für die Geschichte der arabisch-islamischen Wissenschaften*, 2 (1985), 99–122, with *addenda* in ibid., 4 (1987/8), 268–9. Repr. in id., *Islamic Astronomical Instruments* (London: Variorum, 1987), II. Updated in id., *SATMI* 1, XIVa.

———, *A Survey of the Scientific Manuscripts in the Egyptian National Library* (American Research Center in Egypt Catalogs, 5; Winona Lake/Indiana: Eisenbrauns, 1986).

———, 'Astronomie im mittelalterlichen Jemen', in Daum (ed.), *Jemen*, 276–302.

———, 'Universal Solutions to Problems of Spherical Astronomy from Mamluk Egypt and Syria', in Farhad Kazemi and Robert D. McChesney (eds.), *A Way Prepared: Essays on Islamic Culture in Honor of Richard Bayly Winder* (New York: New York University Press, 1988), 153–84. Updated in id., *SATMI* 1, VIb.

———, 'A Survey of Medieval Islamic Shadow Schemes for Simple Time-Reckoning', *Oriens*, 32 (1990), 191–249. Updated in id., *SATMI* 1, III.

———, *Astronomy in the Service of Islam* (London: Variorum, 1993).

———, 'Astronomie im Dienste des Islam', in Anton von Gotstedter (ed.), *Ad radices: Festband zum fünfzigjährigen Bestehen des Instituts für Geschichte der Naturwissenschaften der Johann Wolfgang Goethe-Universität Frankfurt am Main* (Stuttgart: Steiner, 1994), 99–124.

———, *World-Maps for Finding the Direction and Distance to Mecca: Innovation and Tradition in Islamic Science* (Islamic Philosophy, Theology and Science. Texts and Studies, 36; Leiden: Brill, 1999).

———, 'Mathematical Astronomy in Islamic Civilisation', in Helaine Selin (ed.), *Astronomy across Cultures: The History of Non-Western Astronomy* (Dordrecht: Kluwer Academic Publishers, 2000), 585–613.

———, 'Essay Review: Notes on Yemeni Astronomy in the Rasulid Period', *Yemen Update*, 44 (2002), 44–8. Also available on <http://www.aiys.org/webdate/afdking.html>. Updated in id., *SATMI* 2, XIVa-B.

———, *In Synchrony with the Heavens: Studies in Astronomical Timekeeping and Instrumentation in Medieval Islamic Civilization. 1: The Call of the Muezzin* (Studies I–IX) (Islamic Philosophy, Theology and Science. Texts and Studies, 55; Leiden: Brill, 2004). (Study III is an updated version of id., *Shadow Schemes*, study VIb of id., *Universal Solutions*).

———, *In Synchrony with the Heavens: Studies in Astronomical Timekeeping and Instrumentation in Medieval Islamic Civilization. 2: Instruments of Mass Calculation* (Studies X–XVIII) (Islamic Philosophy, Theology and Science. Texts and Studies, 55; Leiden: Brill, 2005). (Study XIVa is an updated version of id., *Yemeni Astrolabe*, study XIVa-B of id., *Notes on Yemeni Astronomy*).

———, *The Frankfurt Catalogue of Medieval Astronomical Instruments* (in preparation). Summarized briefly in id., *SATMI* 2, XVIII.

———, Samsó, Julio, and Goldstein, Bernard R., 'Astronomical Handbooks and Tables from the Islamic World (750–1900): An Interim Report', *Suhayl*, 2 (2001), 9–105. Also available on <http://usd.proves.ub.edu/suhayl/volums/volum2/paper%201.pdf>.

Lee, Samuel, 'Notice of the Astronomical Tables of Mohammed Abibekr Al Farsi, Two Copies of which are Preserved in the Public Library of the University of Cambridge', *Transactions of the Cambridge Philosophical Society*, 1 (1822), 249–65. Repr. in *IMA*, 77, 315–31.

Macdonald, D.B., 'Budūḥ', *EI*^{2}, suppl. (2004), 153a–154a.

Pellat, Ch., 'Anwā'', *EI*^{2}, I (1960), 523a–524a.

Pingree, David, *The Astronomical Works of Gregory Chioniades. 1: The Zīj al-Alā'ī. Part 1: Text, Translation, Commentary* (Corpus des astronomes byzantins, 2; Amsterdam: Gieben, 1985).

——— (ed.), *Picatrix. The Latin Version of the Ghāyat al-Ḥakīm: Text, Appendices, Indices* (Studies of the Warburg Institute, 39; London: The Warburg Institute, 1986).

Porter, Venetia, 'Die Kunst der Rasuliden', in Daum (ed.), *Jemen*, 225–36.

———, 'Islamic Seals: Magical or Practical?', in Alan Jones (ed.), *University Lectures in Islamic Studies* 2 (London: Altajir World of Islam Trust, 1998), 135–49, and figs. 8.1–8.13. Repr. in Savage-Smith (ed.), *Magic and Divination*, 179–200.

Price, D. de Solla, Gibbs, Sh.L., and Henderson, J.A., *A Computerized Checklist of Astrolabes* (New Haven/Conn.: Yale University, Departement of History of Science and Medicine, 1973).

Ritter, Hellmut (ed.), *Pseudo-Maǧrīṭī: Das Ziel des Weisen. 1. Arabischer Text* (Studien der Bibliothek Warburg, 12; Leipzig: Teubner, 1933).

———, and Plessner, Martin (trans.), *"Picatrix". Das Ziel des Weisen von Pseudo-Maǧrīṭī* (Studies of the Warburg Institute, 27; London: The Warburg Institute, 1962).

Ruska, J., and Carra de Vaux, B. (Bosworth, C. E.), 'Tilsam', *EI*², X (2000), 500a–502a.

al-Ṣanʿānī, Šaʿbān Ibn Salīm/Schopen, Armin, and Kahl, Oliver (eds. and trans., with a commentary), *Die Natāʾiǧ al-fikar des Šaʿbān b. Salīm aṣ-Ṣanʿānī: Eine jemenitische Gesundheitsfibel aus dem frühen 18. Jahrhundert* (Wiesbaden: Harrassowitz 1993).

Savage-Smith, Emilie (ed.), *Magic and Divination in Early Islam* (The Formation of the Classical Islamic World, 42; Aldershot: Ashgate Variorum, 2004).

Schmidl, Petra G., 'Two Early Arabic Sources on the Magnetic Compass (Revised Translation of a Master Thesis, Johann Wolfgang Goethe-University Frankfurt 1994)', *Journal of Arabic and Islamic Studies,* 1 (1997), 81–132. Also available on <http://www.uib.no/jais/v001ht/01-081-132schmidl1.htm>.

———, 'al-Ashraf ʿUmar', *BEA*, 1, 66a–67b.

———, 'al-Fārisī', *BEA*, 1, 357b–359a.

———, *Volkstümliche Astronomie im islamischen Mittelalter: Zur Bestimmung der Gebetszeiten und der Qibla bei al-Aṣbaḥī, Ibn Raḥīq und al-Fārisī* (2 vols.; Islamic Philosophy, Theology and Science. Texts and Studies, 68; Leiden: Brill, 2007).

———, *'Lunar Elections in Ibn Raḥīq's Folk Astronomical Treatise'*, to appear in the Proceedings of the colloquium on "From Masha'allah to Kepler: The Theory and Practice of Astrology in the Middle Ages and the Renaissance" held at Warburg Institute of the University of London, School of Advanced Study, in November 2008.

Schmidt, Arno (ed. and trans.), *Ps.-Galeni liber de humoribus critice editus, adnotationibus instructus*. Dissertation zur Erlangung des Doktorgrades der Philosophischen Fakultät der Georg-August-Universität zu Göttingen (Göttingen, 1964).

Schopen, Armin, *Traditionelle Heilmittel im Jemen* (Wiesbaden: Steiner, 1983).

Sésiano, Jacques, 'Wafḳ', *EI*², XI (2002), 28a–31a.

———, 'Herstellungsverfahren magischer Quadrate aus islamischer Zeit (I)', *Sudhoffs Archiv,* 64 (1980), 187–96.

———, *Les carrés magiques dans les pays islamiques* (Lausanne : Presses polytechniques et Université, 2004).

Sezgin, Fuat, *Geschichte des arabischen Schrifttums* (9 vols.; Leiden: Brill, 1967–84), with *Mathematische Geographie und Kartographie im Islam und ihr Fortleben im Abendland* (3 vols.; Frankfurt am Main: Institut für Geschichte der Arabisch-Islamischen Wissenschaften, 2000).

———, *Science and Technology in Islam: Catalogue of the Exhibition of the Institute for the History of Arabic-Islamic Science (at the Johann Wolfgang Goethe University, Frankfurt, Germany), Frankfurt Book Fair 2004* (Frankfurt am Main: Institut für Geschichte der Arabisch-Islamischen Wissenschaften, 2004).

———, and Neubauer, Eckhard, *Wissenschaft und Technik im Islam: Katalog der Instrumentensammlung des Institutes für Geschichte der Arabisch-Islamischen Wissenschaften* (5 vols.; Frankfurt am Main: Institut für Geschichte der Arabisch-Islamischen Wissenschaften, 2003), 2: *Astronomie.*

Smith, G. R[ex], 'Rasūlids', *EI*², VIII (1995), 455a–457b.

———, 'Taʿizz', *EI*², X (2000), 118a–b.

Strunz, Franz, *Astrologie, Alchemie, Mystik: Ein Beitrag zur Geschichte der Naturwissenschaften* (Munich: Barth, 1928).

Suter, Heinrich, 'Die Mathematiker und Astronomen der Araber und ihre Werke', *Abhandlungen zur Geschichte der Mathematischen Wissenschaften mit Einschluß ihrer Anwendungen,* 10 (Leipzig: Teubner, 1900). Repr. in Fuat Sezgin (ed.), *Beiträge zur Geschichte der Mathematik und Astronomie im Islam. Nachdruck seiner Schriften aus den Jahren*

1892–1922 (2 vols.; Frankfurt: Institut für Geschichte der Arabisch-Islamischen Wissenschaften, 1986), 1, 1–285, and repr. in *IMA*, 82, 1–288.

———, 'Nachträge und Berichtigungen zu "Die Mathematiker und Astronomen der Araber und ihre Werke"', *Abhandlungen zur Geschichte der Mathematischen Wissenschaften mit Einschluß ihrer Anwendungen*, 14 (Leipzig: Teubner, 1902), 157–85. Repr. in Fuat Sezgin (ed.), *Beiträge zur Geschichte der Mathematik und Astronomie im Islam. Nachdruck seiner Schriften aus den Jahren 1892–1922* (2 vols.; Frankfurt am Main: Institut für Geschichte der Arabisch-Islamischen Wissenschaften, 1986), 1, 286–314, and in *IMA*, 82, 289–317.

Ullmann, Manfred, *Die Medizin im Islam* (Handbuch der Orientalistik, 1. Abt., VI:1; Leiden: Brill, 1970).

———, *Die Natur- und Geheimwissenschaften im Islam* (Handbuch der Orientalistik, 1. Abt., VI:2; Leiden: Brill, 1972).

———, *Islamic Medicine* (Edinburgh: University Press, 1978).

Varisco, Daniel Martin, 'Rasūlidische Landwirtschaft und traditionelle Almanache', in Daum (ed.), *Jemen*, 303–5.

———, 'Arzneikunde und Heilpflanzen im mittelalterlichen Jemen', in Daum (ed.), *Jemen*, 306–7.

———, *Medieval Agriculture and Islamic Science: The Almanac of a Yemeni Sultan* (Seattle: University of Washington Press, 1994).

———, 'The Magical Significance of the Lunar Stations in the 13th Century Yemeni *Kitāb al-Tabṣira fī 'ilm al-nujūm* of al-Malik al-Ashraf', *Quaderni di Studi Arabi*, 13 (1995), 19–40.

———, 'Islamic Folk Astronomy', in Helaine Selin (ed.), *Astronomy across Cultures. The History of Non-Western Astronomy* (Dordrecht: Kluwer Academic Publishers, 2000), 615–50.

Wiedemann, Eilhard, 'Auszüge aus arabischen Enzyklopädien und anderes', *Sitzungsberichte der Physikalisch-Medizinischen Sozietät zu Erlangen*, 37 (Erlangen: Palm & Enke 1905), 392–455. Repr. in Wolfdietrich Fischer (ed.), *Aufsätze zur arabischen Wissenschaftsgeschichte* (2 vols.; Collectanea, 6; Hildesheim: Olms, 1970), 1, 109–72.

———, 'Über die Zeichen für die Planeten usw. auf Astrolabien', *Byzantinische Zeitschrift*, 19 (1910), 145–6. Repr. in Fuat Sezgin (ed.), rev. by Dorothea Girke, *Gesammelte Schriften zur arabisch-islamischen Wissenschaftsgeschichte* (Veröffentlichungen des Instituts für Geschichte der Arabisch-Islamischen Wissenschaften, Reihe B: Nachdrucke 1, 1-3; Frankfurt: Institut für Geschichte der Arabisch-Islamischen Wissenschaften, 1984), 1, 449–50, and in *IMA*, 34, 48–9.

———, 'Zu den magischen Quadraten', *Der Islam*, 8 (1918), 94–7. Repr. in Fuat Sezgin (ed.), rev. by Dorothea Girke, *Gesammelte Schriften zur arabisch-islamischen Wissenschaftsgeschichte* (Veröffentlichungen des Instituts für Geschichte der Arabisch-Islamischen Wissenschaften, Reihe B: Nachdrucke 1, 1–3; Frankfurt: Institut für Geschichte der Arabisch-Islamischen Wissenschaften, 1984), 2, 870–3.

Winkler, H.A., *Siegel und Charaktere in der muhammedanischen Zauberei* (Studien zur Geschichte und Kultur des islamischen Orients. Zwanglose Beihefte zu der Zeitschrift "Der Islam", 7; Berlin, Leipzig: de Gruyter, 1930).

QĀT AND TRADITIONAL HEALING IN YEMEN[1]

Daniel Martin Varisco

1. Origin and Spread of *Catha edulis* in Yemen

> It is quite impossible to talk about Yemen without mentioning qāt.[2]
> Qat is as indispensable to the southern Arabian's existence as the Koran.[3]

Much has been written, pro and con, about the chewing of *qāt* leaves in Yemen. There is, to be neologistic about it, a virtual '*qāt*-alog' of source material in Arabic and Western languages.[4] Unfortunately there is also a fair amount of misinformation in the literature, including the entry for *qāt* in both editions of the *Encyclopaedia of Islam*.[5] This is not surprising, given the nature of the plant as a possible 'drug' or at the very least a 'bad habit' in the eyes of many Western observers. In addition, the use of *qāt* in Yemen is often conflated with its use in Ethiopia, thus providing virtually no comparison to consumption in other African contexts. It is also important to note that most Western scholars have had limited access to Arabic source material on *qāt*, which is a relatively recent import into Yemen, and is not discussed in the major *materia medica* tradition in Arabic. The purpose of this essay is to focus on one of the major gaps in the literature, assessing the traditional medical and pharmacological assessment of *Catha edulis* (Vahl) Forsk. ex Endl. (Celastraceae) in the humoural system with the findings of modern scientific investigation of the plant. At present there is

---

1 I thank Muhammad Gerhoum for assistance in finding Arabic references on *qāt* in Yemen and Dina Dahbany-Miraglia for references and information on the use of *qāt* in Israel.

2 Seager, 'The Yemen', 221.

3 Helfritz, *The Yemen*, 82.

4 The important references in Western languages by Kennedy, *The Flower of Paradise*; Schopen, *Qāt;* and Weir, *Qat in Yemen*, are in need of updating and should be used with caution, especially in regards to the historical origins of the plant. I have previously published on the origin and spread of *Catha edulis* in Yemen (Varisco, 'Turning Over a New Leaf'), the legitimacy of chewing *qāt* leaves (id., 'The Elixer of Life') and the social significance of *qāt* chewing in Yemen (id., 'On the Meaning of Chewing'). For a valuable early reference based on medical work in Yemen, see Mancioli and Parrinello, 'Il gat'. There are numerous works by Yemenis, including the anthologies of al-Ḥibshī, *Thalāth rasā'il*, and al-Mu'allimī, *al-Qāt*.

5 Hess, 'ḳāt'. Rodinson, 'Esquisse', published an update of the original *EI* article, but his knowledge was based primarily on experience with the plant in Ethiopia.

a wide gap between the two sets of data—an academically created *barzakh* (barrier) that needs to be bridged in the here and now.

As background, there are two primary ways in which *qāt* has been used as a stimulant. In Yemen the most common method, although perhaps not the original use, is by storing the tender new leaves and shoot ends in one side of the mouth. This process is literally labelled 'storage' (*takhzīn*), although earlier legal texts consistently cite the verb *akala* with the generic sense of 'eating' or 'consuming.' A second mode is by using the powder from the dry leaves to make a drink, a kind of 'tea' in this sense, often mixed with other ingredients such as honey or sugar.[6] Fresh leaves can also be pounded in a mortar into powder or juice that is consumed by old men who can no longer chew the leaves properly.[7] Based on al-Jazīrī's mid-sixteenth-century treatise on coffee, it seems that the Sufis who introduced *qāt* at first made a drink from it, but came to prefer coffee to obtain the same effect.[8] The passage suggests that *kafta*,[9] a term referring to the *qāt* leaves, was not readily available in Aden and was not as simple to use as were coffee beans.

Given the fragmentary textual evidence available, it may never be possible to set the record straight on the historical trajectory of *qāt*'s introduction to Yemen. However, several important pieces of the puzzle now seem to have a credible fit. First, there is no doubt that the botanical origin of *Catha edulis* is in Ethiopia. From the Ethiopian highlands it spread through human use to other parts of Africa, as well as to Yemen.[10] Second, the earliest evidence for *qāt* in Arabic is from a historical text by Ibn Faḍl

---

6 Schopen, *Qāt*, 85–6, discusses the drinks and pastes made of *qāt* and other ingredients in Ethiopia, Somalia, and Tanzania. In South Africa a *qāt* drink is called 'Bushman's tea.' In Israel there is a drink made of *qāt* for use as an aphrodisiac (Ben-Ami, 'The Yemeni Book'). In May 2009 the Israeli Knesset outlawed use of a capsule form of synthetic cathinone called 'hagigat,' which was sold in 2004 for 6.5 British pounds per capsule as an aphrodisiac, but allowed the fresh leaves to be chewed (Siegel-Itzkovich, 'Knesset Dubs "Hagigat"', Urquhart, 'Drugs and Dance'). It is worth noting that in contemporary Scotland an infusion is made by blending the leaves with water and lemon for use as a 'high' at 'Rave' dance parties (Brown et al., 'Use of Drugs').

7 Brooke, 'Khat', 53.

8 al-Jazīrī/al-Ḥibshī (ed.), *'Umda*, 48.

9 The eighteenth-century Yemeni lexicographer al-Zabīdī (*k-f-t*) does not mention the term *kafta* in reference to *qāt* leaves, but does note that the term *kaft* can refer to food or anything that sustains life; nor does this late dictionary refer to *qāt*, although the author wrote a *qaṣīda* on *qāt* that has not yet surfaced; see Reichmuth, *The World*, 137.

10 The flawed claim for a Yemeni origin, with the plant being taken to Ethiopia before the Islamic era and then reintroduced, was made by Revri, Catha Edulis. I address this misidentification in Varisco 'Turning Over a New Leaf', 243.

Allāh al-ʿUmarī (d. 1349) for Ethiopia.[11] The earliest mention of the plant in a Yemeni text is in a poem from Jamāl al-Dīn Muḥammad b. Saʿīd al-Ṭabarī, known as Ibn Kabban (d. 1438).[12] The Zaydi imam Yaḥyā Sharaf al-Dīn (d. 1557/8) claimed that *qāt* had been known in Yemen since the end of the eighth century AH, i.e. around 1350–1400 CE or near the end of the Rasulid era.[13]

A third puzzle piece is the vector of transmission. As is the case for coffee, also a stimulant plant introduced from Ethiopia at about the same time, the most likely source for bringing the plant to Yemen is the Sufis. The Yemeni poet ʿAbdallāh al-Baraddūnī is representative of most Yemeni scholars in attributing the origin to Sufi mystics who used the plant for its stimulant qualities and labelling it "the sustenance of the righteous" ("*qūt al-ṣāliḥīn*").[14] A number of specific candidates have been suggested, including Shaykh ʿAlī b. ʿUmar al-Shādhilī (d. 1418), who is said to have preferred drinking coffee to a concoction made from *qāt* leaves. This religious trajectory is also the most logical explanation by a process of elimination. Unlike coffee, there was no commercial value to *qāt* in the historical record apart from local demand. Both the Ottoman Turks and the Dutch traders could have taken the dried leaves of *Catha edulis*, as in the case of tea in China and India, but only coffee beans left Yemeni ports. The primary motivation for Sufis in the fourteenth or fifteenth centuries would be the stimulant property inherent in the leaves. This would also explain the rather long incubation period for widespread use of the plant in Yemen, especially in the Zaydi north where mystical practices were not well tolerated. As al-Baraddūnī notes, it was probably used most by the upper

11 This is his *Masālik al-abṣār fī mamālik al-amṣār*. The information is copied in a later historical text of al-Maqrīzī. Several scholars (e.g. Schopen, *Qāt*, 44, 87) claim that the earliest reference is by al-Bīrūnī (d. *c.*1050), who describes a certain plant called *qāt* in Turkestan. However, from the description provided by al-Bīrūnī this is not in reference to *Catha edulis*, nor is there evidence of its cultivation in Central Asia. This spurious claim is oft repeated and appears in the ill-informed Wikipedia entry on "khat" (<http://en.wikipedia.org/wiki/Khat>). Misinformation on the origins of *qāt* chewing is common in articles by scientists and medical experts; e.g. Saha and Dollery ('Severe Ischaemic Cardiomyopathy', 318) claim "The practice of chewing khat leaves has been a part of the culture in areas of East Africa and the Arabian Peninsula since the 7th century."

12 As noted by al-Ḥibshī, 'Mushkilat ẓuhūr al-qāt', 82; see Schopen, *Qāt*, 176, n. 4.

13 Sharaf al-Dīn, 'al-Risāla', 11.

14 al-Baraddūnī, 'al-Qāt', 44. For example, in the poetry of Muḥammad al-ʿUjaylī, quoted in Yemen Center for Research and Studies (ed.), *al-Qāt*, 196. See Wagner, 'The Debate', 125.

classes rather than the common people, given its price and the frequent famine conditions.[15]

A fourth and compelling point is the origin of the term. Most of the speculation on the origin of the term *qāt* in Arabic is based on a fundamental misunderstanding of the relation of the Arabic term to the Amharic term *tchat*. The obvious similarity in sound suggested to many that the two terms were cognates, but which came first?[16] The total lack of reference in Arabic lexical sources belies a formal Arabic origin, despite attempts to relate the term to *qūt* (i.e. food).[17] Linguistic purists, such as Maxime Rodinson, were convinced that the Arabic *qāf* could not be derived from the relevant Amharic letter.[18] I literally stumbled on the most probable linguistic trajectory while reading an eighteenth-century edition and Latin translation of a text by the Egyptian historian al-Maqrīzī, who was quoting Ibn Faḍl Allāh al-ʿUmarī.[19] Here the reference is to *jāt* with no mention of *qāt*. Indeed, the earlier author specifically claims that the first letter in his transcription is pronounced between the Arabic *jīm* and the Arabic *shīn*. I suggest that the written term was pronounced with a hard [g], as in Cairene and some other dialects, and entered Yemen orally. The earliest Yemeni texts we have were written by Zaydis in the north, where it is the *qāf* that is pronounced with a hard [g]. Having heard about the plant but not seeing the term written down, as in the text of Ibn Faḍl Allāh, it was only natural that it be transcribed as *qāt* in Yemen's north and continued in pronunciation as *gāt*.

By the sixteenth century Yemeni scholars were embroiled in a debate over the licitness of the use of *qāt*—both the chewing of fresh leaves and the drying of its leaves for a drink. As a newly introduced substance there was no direct guidance from the Qurʾān, traditions or previous legal and medical texts.[20] This was not just the case for *qāt*, as the treatise by Yaḥyā

---

15 al-Baraddūnī, 'al-Qāt', 44.

16 This is clearly what happened with Ethiopian teff (*Eragrostis tef*), a grain that became *ṭahaf* in Arabic.

17 Even Lane, *An Arabic-English Lexicon*, 2572, places the term *qāt* under the trilateral *q-w-t*, although his only source is the Swedish botanist Forskål.

18 Rodinson, 'Esquisse', 75. The problem was unresolved in the entries for the *Encyclopaedia of Islam* and the etymological survey by Powels, 'Herkunft'.

19 This is al-Maqrīzī/Rinck (ed. and trans.), *Macrizi Historia regum Islamiticorum*. Rodinson, 'Esquisse', 77, n. 19, had examined this text, but inexplicably did not realize the significance of the rendering as *jāt* rather than *qāt*. Neither did Schopen, *Qāt*, 46. Burton, *First Footsteps*, 196, recorded the term *jāt* during his visit to Ethiopia in 1854.

20 While there was obviously no direct evidence in the Qurʾān, some Yemenis see an indirect reference. A farmer in al-Ahjur in 1979 referred to the plant as *shajarat al-zaqqūm*

b. al-Ḥusayn (d. 1689) on the three plants of coffee (*qahwa*), tobacco (*ṭabāq*), and *qāt* well illustrates. The primary issue from a religious standpoint was whether or not the effects of consuming *qāt* could be considered as producing the inebriating effect of an intoxicant (*muskir*) or the numbing impact of a narcotic (*takhdīr*). Claims were being made by devout Muslims that use of the plant was actually a godsend, allowing them to overcome fatigue and hunger in order to better perform their religious duties. As Yaḥyā b. Muḥammad al-Iryānī notes in his *qaṣīda*: "[I]t drives away sleep when I want to stay awake for devotions and has an excellent distinction when performing beyond what is required" ("*wa-yaṭrudu nawman in aradtu tahajjudan, fa-niʿma l-muʿīnu idh tuqāmu l-nawāfilu*").[21] An example of the devotional approach to the use of *qāt* is provided in the poem of the Yemeni Sufi Muḥammad b. Aḥmad al-ʿUjaylī (d. 1602), who argued that the effect of its use brought a Muslim closer to Allah.[22] The fact that many of the users were Sufis no doubt made the plant suspect to some interpreters, especially those conservative legal minds concerned with innovation (*bidʿ*) in worship rituals. Yet even today, Yemenis cite the *qāt* session as an occasion for discussion of religious matters, especially during the fasting month of Ramadan. It is reported that Yemeni women cite learning about religious matters as a reason for attending a session.[23]

My concern in this essay is not to update the discussion about the positive and negative health impact of using *Catha edulis* with a scientifically based argument. Nor is the legal issue of treating *qāt* as an intoxicant or narcotic in accordance with Islamic opinions one that needs to be renegotiated by anyone outside Yemeni society. I am struck by the almost total lack of cross fertilization between the historical texts, limited as the medical information in these is, with scientific research undertaken both in the laboratory and among users.[24] While the pioneering social research

---

in reference to a bitter plant growing in the midst of hell and the fruit of sinners (sūrat al-Ṣaffāt, Q 37:62–4).

21 Quoted by al-Ḥibshī, 'al-Qāt', 151. The term *nawāfil* is often used in Islamic texts for supererogatory prayers.

22 This poem is translated by Schopen, *Qāt*, 196–200, into German, with a facsimile of the Arabic provided on 241. The Arabic is also provided in the publication by the Yemen Center for Research and Studies, *al-Qāt*, 196–7. Schopen has translated into German a number of the Arabic poetic excerpts documented by al-Ḥibshī, 'al-Qāt', 143–54. Wagner, 'The Debate', provides an English translation of some *qāt* poetry.

23 Khalīl, *al-Marāt*, 167.

24 There has been little research done on the pharmacological and therapeutic use of *qāt* in Yemen, in part because most discussions are still in manuscript form or the oral folklore of healers. Radt, 'Contribution à l'histoire', 52, noted the same lack of study on the

by anthropologist John Kennedy provides a solid foundation for examining the use of *qāt* in Yemen, there was little analysis of the medical debate over *qāt* in the Arabic sources. In the following sections I focus on the historical debate over the negative and positive aspects attributed to the use of the plant in the indigenous humoural system and suggest ways in which this information can be better understood in the light of relevant contemporary scientific study.

2. The "Qāt Fatwā" by Ibn Ḥajar al-Haytamī

wa-lā ta'kulanna l-qāta raṭban wa-yābisan
fa-dhāka muḍirrun dā'uhu fīhī a'ḍalan
fa-qad qāla a'lām mina l-'ulamā'i
inna hādhā ḥarāmun lil-taḍarruri ma'kalā[25]

Never consume *qāt*, fresh or dry
For that is harmful, the malady with it difficult.
An authority among the scholars has said
That this is forbidden due to the harm from its consumption.[26]

The late introduction of *Catha edulis* into the Arabic *materia medica* genre presented a problem for anyone attempting to determine the role of the plan in the prevailing humoural system and the possibility that it could be a forbidden substance. The crux of the debate begins, at least in extant sources, with the extensive commentary by the well-known Meccan jurist Ibn Ḥajar al-Haytamī (1504–67). This scholar provides an early and extensive analysis of the alleged harmful effects of *qāt* in an inquisitive and relatively balanced discussion. His *Taḥdhīr al-thiqāt min akl al-kafta wa-l-qāt* [Studiously Preparing Confidence in the Consumption of Dry and Fresh *Qāt*] is included in his massive *al-Fatāwā l-kubrā* in the "Bāb al-ashriba wa-l-mukhaddirāt" [Section on Drinks and Narcotics].[27] Unlike the case of opium or wine, for which there were by this time established legal restrictions, this newly introduced plant had devout men who praised it as well

traditional therapeutic use in Ethiopia. See Ulrike Lindequist's chapter in this volume for references to recent investigations of the pharmacological effects of *qāt*.

25 Ḥamza al-Nāshirī, quoted in Ibn Ḥajar al-Haytamī, *al-Fatāwā*, 226.

26 Translation by the author.

27 I consulted both Ibn Ḥajar al-Haytamī, *al-Fatāwā*, 223–8, and the reproduced passage in al-Ḥibshī, *Thalāth rasā'il*, 19–49, and al-Mu'allimī, *al-Qāt*, 93–113. His text was completed in 1553. Rosenthal, *The Herb*, 12, notes that the material on *ḥashīsh* here is taken from an earlier treatise by the *shāfi'ī* scholar Ibn al-'Imād al-Aqfahsī (d. 1405/6).

as those who found it harmful. The fact that Ibn Ḥajar al-Haytamī wrote an extended personal commentary illustrates the seriousness of the confusion over conflicting views on the effects of its use.

The reason cited for the commentary is the arrival in Mecca of scholars from Ṣanʿāʾ and Zabīd with several writings and differing opinions on the consumption of a previously unknown plant called *qāt*. Since Ibn Ḥajar had no personal knowledge of the plant, he was forced to determine which of the facts communicated about it were trustworthy. As he notes near the start of his analysis, Ibn Ḥajar was told: "It results in noxious qualities (*maḍarr*), including yellowing of the face (*taṣfīr al-wajh*), decreasing the desire for food, weakening libido (*taftīr al-bāh*), and causing urine dripping (*wady*) after urination."[28] When asked how he knew this, Ibn Ḥajar's source indicated it was based on the experience of those who used it, to which the renowned jurist responded that such evidence was not sufficient. The problem was that there was disputing testimony based on experience, nor were the specific contextual conditions of time and place spelled out.

The issue noted here is medicinal, although none of these specific problems would seem to warrant its total prohibition. Extolling the virtue of a scientific assessment of the issue, since the plant was unknown in the earlier medical tradition, Ibn Ḥajar conducted an investigation and questioned a number of individuals in Mecca in addition to the written reports brought to him from Yemen. He was keen to resolve the issue and separate any deception from the true impact of the plant. The last thing he wanted to do was fall into the trap of offering a dubious legal opinion (*shubha*). This was no easy task, since at the time of his writing there was an abundance of legal writing about other intoxicants and narcotics, especially marijuana (*ḥashīsh*).[29]

A *shāfiʿī* imam explained to Ibn Ḥajar that he had visited Zabīd and Taʿizz some thirty years earlier and personally found *qāt* to pose no harm (*ḍarr*), neither for its moistness or dryness in the humoural system. Similarly, several *shāfiʿī* teachers in Mecca confided that there was no narcotic effect (*takhdīr*) or direct harmful impact on the understanding (*ghībat al-dhihn*). Since it weakened their libido (*shahwa*) due to its dryness, they had consumed it. On the other hand, some of the *ḥanafī* teachers had sampled *qāt* brought by several Yemeni Sufis visiting the Great Mosque in Mecca. The Yemenis offered it, saying it was blessed (*mubārak*). But

[28] Ibn Ḥajar al-Haytamī, *al-Fatāwā*, 224.

[29] Rosenthal, *The Herb*, 6, cites the text *Zahr al-ʿarīsh fī taḥrīm al-ḥashīsh* of Muḥammad b. Sulaymān al-Shāṭibī (d. 1274) as the oldest known monograph on the subject.

when one of the *ḥanafī* scholars tried it, he found it to be narcotic (*takhdīr*) and recollected that it caused faulty speech (*kalām dhayn*).[30] Noting that his own bodily composition was moderate (*muʿtadil*), he admitted it may not have the same impact on someone with a different composition. But he felt a narcotic effect and dizziness (*dawarān al-raʾs*), so he would not consume it ever again. Some of the notables in Mecca noted that it had a negative effect on sensory perception, so that one person for a length of time could not tell the sky from the ground or length from width, a key defining element of an intoxicant.[31] This is the same rationale provided by the Zaydi imam Sharaf al-Dīn in an anecdote about a scholar who, while chewing *qāt*, went on a journey towards a town called Manqadha but did not come to his senses until he had gone far beyond it to the town of Riṣāba.[32]

Part of the problem facing Ibn Ḥajar was that some scholars who had forbidden the plant based on what they were told then changed their minds after trying it themselves. For example, Imam al-Ṣafī al-Muzajjad (d. 1524) concluded: "As for the fresh and dry leaves of *qāt*, I do not think that it alters the mind or dissuades from compliance [with religious duties]. Indeed, it produces energy and spirituality and pleasant thoughts, without resulting in any harm. Furthermore, sometimes it is an aid for increased work."[33] Similar praise was provided to Ibn Ḥajar from the scholar Aḥmad b. Muḥammad al-Bakrī al-Tandāwī (d. 1541) and Ibn Kabban (d. 1438). Clearly, it was not sufficient to rely solely on testimony, given the differences of opinions among respected authorities.

The argument for banning *qāt* is outlined in detail in the written opinion of a certain Ḥamza al-Nāshirī (d. 1519), quoted by Ibn Ḥajar.[34] The basis of his argument hinges on the meaning of *muskir* and *mufattir*, both

---

[30] According to Yaḥyā b. al-Ḥusayn, 'al-Mustakhrajāt', 96, *ḥanafī* scholars considered the use of coffee lawful. Unlike the case of *qāt*, an attempt was made by the Sufi Shaykh al-Shādhilī to link the origin of coffee to the time of the Prophet. However, al-Shādhilī is said to have observed that the name of Allah had been written on some *qāt* leaves, because it was one of the trees brought down from Paradise with Adam (al-Ḥibshī, *Maqāmāt*, 347).

[31] The specific reference that *sukr* refers to not knowing the earth from the sky, in the sense of down from up, or a man from a woman is attributed to the *faqīh* Abū Ḥanīfa (d. 767) (al-Jazīrī/al-Ḥibshī (ed.), *ʿUmda*, 88; al-Shawkānī, 'al-Baḥth', 37).

[32] Sharaf al-Dīn, 'al-Risāla', 12. Kennedy, *The Flower of Paradise*, 120, records a similar anecdote about a Yemeni who left a chewing session to get coals for the water pipe and kept walking in a daze until he entered another house rather than his own.

[33] This passage, translated from Ibn Ḥajar, is also copied in al-Jazīrī/al-Ḥibshī (ed.), *ʿUmda*, 77–8.

[34] Ibn Ḥajar al-Haytamī, *al-Fatāwā*, 226.

of which are prohibited by the Prophet Muḥammad.[35] A substance is considered *mufattir* when it heats the body so that it breaks down ("*mā yakūn minhu ḥarāra fī l-jasad wa-inkisār*"). This is said to be observable (*mushāhad*) with the use of *qāt* as it is in the use of other intoxicants.[36] *Qāt* is also claimed to have the properties of an intoxicant (*muskir*), including tremors (*riʿsha*), addiction (*idmān*), partial paralysis (*fālij*), drying of the brain and lasting alteration of the mind. For al-Nāshirī it appears that *qāt* is worse than other intoxicants, since it has no redeeming humoural qualities; specifically it has no heat in it. The health consequences mentioned include drying the brain, being opposed to what is natural, lessening the appetite for food and sex, drying and cooling the intestines and stomach, and the like. Indeed, the negative qualities of *qāt* are said to be worse than opium. Similarly all the bad qualities associated with marijuana are said to be found in greater abundance in *qāt*, according to al-Nāshirī.[37]

Ibn Ḥajar's treatise demonstrates the extent of the author's quandary, given the conflicting evidence provided to him. At the very least it could be argued that those who received a negative effect should refrain from using it and those who did not should not forbid it. Ibn Ḥajar acknowledges that one of the characteristics of consuming the plant is an increase in energy, but the issue is whether this ultimately causes harm.[38] After a lengthy discussion of how to reconcile the conflicting views, he notes that the case of *qāt* is not like that of marijuana that has been known to be an intoxicant for centuries and has been widely discussed in the science of medicine. Even in this case there may be a difference in the effect of the

---

35 For a discussion of the legal aspects of defining both terms, see Rosenthal, *The Herb*, 105–17. Kueny, *The Rhetoric*, 33–52, discusses the definition of wine as an intoxicant. al-Jazīrī/al-Ḥibshī (ed.), *ʿUmda*, 88–100, provides an informative discussion on the debate over intoxicants.

36 The Zaydi imam Sharaf al-Dīn, 'al-Risāla', 15, includes the same passage quoted by Ibn Ḥajar and attributed to *al-Nihāya fī gharīb al-ḥadīth*. In his discussion of the term, al-Shawkānī, *al-Baḥth*, 41, describes the term as referring to drinks which create weakness (*futūr*) and numbness (*khadar*) in the extremities, noting that this is the beginning of intoxication.

37 This claim, which is clearly prejudicial, is also made by the French traveller Louis du Couret/S., C. D. (trans.), *Life in the Desert*, 22, who confounds his description by calling "kaad" betel as well. Both claims should be examined in comparison to the extensive earlier literature on the harmful effects of using marijuana, such as the comment by al-Zarkashī (d. 1392) that there were 120 harmful effects in a religious sense (quoted in Rosenthal, *The Herb*, 177).

38 Ibn Ḥajar al-Haytamī, *al-Fatāwā*, 227. As al-Jazīrī/al-Ḥibshī (ed.), *ʿUmda*, 39, notes, one of the main arguments for the use of coffee is its ability to create energy and aid memory.

fresh marijuana leaves from those that have been prepared. Similarly, the fact that scholars disagree over its effects is like the case of nutmeg (*jawz al-ṭīb*) that some condemn and others do not. Thus, there is no sure way to resolve the issue apart from personal experience. Although Ibn Ḥajar does not definitively condemn the use of *qāt*, as he does other known intoxicants, his treatise is largely devoted to the alleged harmful effects.[39]

3. *Qāt* in the Humoural System

> All of this is deduced from God's words: *eat and drink and do not be excessive* (Q 7:31). He thus guided His servants to consume such food and drink as will support the body, replacing what has been dissolved and to such quantity and quality as is beneficial to the body.[40]

The evaluation of *qāt* on a medicinal basis by Muslim scholars depends on its placement in the cumulative humoural system at the time of its appearance. The humoural system offered a complete guide to all aspects of health and was seen by Muslim scholars as a sign of Allah's creative mercy to humans. The limited commentary on health and diet in the Qur'ān was coupled with statements attributed to the Prophet Muḥammad to form a genre known as the Prophet's medicine (*al-ṭibb al-nabawī*).[41] The theory underlying the humoural system is a simple notion of balance in nature, although achieving consistency in the details was fraught with difficulty. Every substance was defined according to a grid of hot or cold and wet or dry, in varying degrees. The four natural humours (*akhlāṭ*) were blood (*dam*), which was hot and wet, yellow bile (*mirra ṣafrā'*), which was hot and dry, phlegm (*balgham*), which was cold and wet, and black bile (*mirra sawdā'*), which was cold and dry. These four basic humours could be associated with organs in the body, moods, seasons, and a host of other qualities.

The key to the health regime was balance or a proper mixture (*i'tidāl al-mizāj*), thus countering each humoural property with its opposite. Specific types of foods are recommended for balancing each humour in

[39] The Yemeni scholar al-Shawkānī (in al-Muʿallimī, *al-Qāt*, 117) suggests that Ibn Ḥajar's account is full of information from those who did not know what *qāt* was.

[40] Ibn Qayyim al-Jawziyya/Johnstone (trans.), *Medicine*, 158.

[41] For a concise description of this system, see Pormann and Savage-Smith, *Medieval Islamic Medicine*, 44–5. Penelope Johnstone provides an informative introduction to the subject in her translation of *Medicine of the Prophet* by Ibn Qayyim al-Jawziyya. This tradition was not a simple borrowing of Greek medicine, but included local folk methods throughout the region.

order to ensure good health and mitigate or cure illness. Thus yellow bile is checked with sour (*ḥāmiḍ*) tasting foods and black bile with fatty meat dishes (*tharāʾid dasima*). Since *qāt* is defined as cold and dry, thus linked to black bile in this system, the best foods for balancing the effect of *qāt* consumption are hot. In fact, most Yemenis say that it is proper before chewing *qāt* to eat hot foods, such as lamb, fenugreek (*ḥulba*), hot pepper, white radish, wheat bread, and sorghum porridge (*ʿaṣīd*).[42] For rural Yemenis in the north these are the traditional staples, although the introduction of *qāt* chewing can also affect dietary choice.[43] In principle, foods to be avoided for causing an excess of black bile include salty and sour tasting foods, broad beans, and lentils. Drawing on the humoural qualities of food, for the purist there were in fact a number of foods that should or should not be used prior to chewing *qāt*, as illustrated in Table 1. Another way of preparing the body for the cooling action of *qāt* is vigorous exercise or a visit to the public hot bath, although this is seldom practised today.[44] In his autobiography, Qāḍī Muḥammad al-Akwaʿ recollects that his father's passion for *qāt* was combined with an equal passion for walking a mile or two; this was said to counter the heat raised in the body from drinking scented cold water during the chew.[45] In addition, the cooling nature of *qāt* on the body can be counteracted by keeping the room where it is chewed warm, usually by closing windows to stop the flow of air.[46] The drying action of *qāt* is assuaged by the custom of drinking cool water while one chews.[47]

The existing literature does not explain the rationale for classifying *qāt* as cold and dry in the humoural system. Stemming back to Galen, the classification for living things was based on the relative share of heat versus cold and dryness versus wetness. For Galen, the most important aspect was the relative balance in each case.[48] Arab physicians accepted the four

---

42 For a description of the typical highland Yemeni foods eaten before chewing, see Gingrich, 'The Guest Meal', 137–8, and Schopen, *Qāt*, 121–6.

43 Gingrich, 'The Guest Meal', 143.

44 Kennedy, *The Flower of Paradise*, 81–2.

45 al-Akwaʿ, *Ṣafḥa*, 61.

46 Mackintosh-Smith, *Yemen*, 17, records a Yemeni joke about the ability of Yemeni chewers to withstand intense heat, even in hell.

47 Kennedy, *The Flower of Paradise*, 89, notes, "In Taiz and the Hujjariyya area of the southern part of the country, tea, coca cola, and other soft drinks are increasingly being substituted for water in the qat sessions, but Sanani purists believe that such beverages spoil the taste of the qat." Drinking sugar-loaded beverages can lead to hypoglycemia and other disorders, especially in combination with the chemical impact of *qāt*.

48 In his treatise on mixtures, Galen (in Singer, *Galen*, 209) argues that while the season of spring is both hot and wet, it is not as hot as summer nor as wet as winter: "Spring is

Table 1. Humoural properties of major foods and substances, according to al-Azraq (15th century)[49]

Hot and dry	Hot and wet	Cold and wet	Cold and dry
basil	almond (sweet)	Christ's thorn	barley
cheese (dry)	banana	(*nabq*)	beef
coriander	cheese (wet)	cucumber	broad bean (*fūl*)
cumin	chickpea	egg white	camel
dill	chicken	fish	date (unripe)
egg yolk	date (ripe)	goat	dolichos bean (*kishd*)
eggplant	fenugreek	melon	henna
garlic	fig	peach	lentils (*ʿadas*)
gazelle	grapes	purslane	locust
ginger	milk	radish (white)	millet (*dukhn*)
honey	onion	sour milk	orange (sour)
lamb	pomegranate (sweet)		quince
nigella seeds	raisins		sesame
(*al-ḥabba al-sawdāʾ*)	sugar cane		sorghum
leek (*kurrāth*)	wheat		tamarind
nutmeg	yogurt		thyme
pepper (hot)			vinegar
pepper (long)			
rabbit			
saffron			
salt			
senna			

possible combinations, but in fact at times disagreed on the designation for a specific plant and also noted that the state of the plant (e.g., used fresh, as a powder or in liquid) could change the classification. The primary reason for classifying *qāt* as dry would appear to be its physical state as a leaf with no surface moisture and limited wetness within. At the same time, the designation would apply if the effect of consuming *qāt* produced a drying effect in the body, as one would expect from a plant associated symbiotically with black bile. As noted by the Yemeni poet ʿAlī b. ʿAbdallāh al-Iryānī (d. 1905), "Drying harms the body, as the body becomes emaciated" ("*yabis yaḍurr al-jism wa-l-jism nāḥil*").[50] An excess of the cold and dry black bile produces insomnia and induces thirst, two of the major effects with *qāt*. Given that *qāt* reduces the libido, this would imply it has a cooling effect, since 'hot' substances (e.g., fennel, long pepper, and onion) are more likely to be aphrodisiacal.

well-balanced in all respects." Galen concludes that attributing heat and wetness to spring is not because these are dominant, but in relation to the other seasons.

[49] al-Azraq, *Tashīl al-manāfiʿ*, *passim*.

[50] Quoted in al-Ḥibshī, 'al-Qāt', 149.

The Yemeni scholar al-Ḥārithī notes that *qāt* is cold and dry to the second degree.[51] In a less formal sense, Yemenis distinguish four main types of *qāt* in terms of their effect on the body; these are slight (*khafīf*), moderate (*muʿtadil*), strong (*qawī*), and very strong (*qawī jiddan*).[52] The amount and frequency of chewing is also relevant. Although critical of *qāt* use, the poet ʿAlī b. ʿAbdallāh al-Iryānī cautions the reader to chew in moderation, at best only half of a bundle (*rubṭa*). In response, his nephew Yaḥyā b. Muḥammad al-Iryānī says that there is no harm in limited use but only from overuse.[53] According to Yaḥyā b. Muḥammad al-Iryānī, *qāt* is beneficial for anyone who is fearful of diseases caused by an excess of moisture (*ruṭūba*).[54] As the case of coffee illustrates, the designation of humoural property depends in part on one's view of the substance. Thus, al-Jazīrī notes that many physicians consider coffee to be hot and dry, but those who censor (*ahl al-dhamm*) its use consider coffee cold and dry, qualities that are related to the condition of death.[55] The politics of humoural identity is further illustrated in the assessment of lentils (*ʿadas*) by Ibn Qayyim al-Jawziyya (d. 1350), who insists the Prophet Muḥammad could never have praised this food that—as cold and dry—is harmful in several ways to the constitution.[56]

4. Positive Health Aspects

Pass ruby branches of qāt *with verdant topaz leaves!*
Its greenness resembles the Garden of Paradise,
Its scent puts that of the flowers of the Garden to shame,
Its intoxication makes one forget the drunkenness of wine and the goblet,
Consuming it clears my mind and seeing clears my eye—It sweetens my life and my times.[57]

---

51 This is the only reference (al-Ḥārithī, as quoted in Serjeant, '*Qāt*', 174) I have found thus far as to the degree of coldness and dryness attributed to *qāt*. Levey, *Pharmacology*, 125, observes: "After the middle of the eleventh century, the four degrees of each humour were of little or dying significance in writings on medical therapy."

52 Schopen, *Qāt*, 97–102, gives a description of the varieties associated with the level of effect.

53 al-Ḥibshī, 'al-Qāt', 151.

54 Ibid.

55 al-Jazīrī/al-Ḥibshī (ed.), *'Umda*, 41.

56 Ibn Qayyim al-Jawziyya/Johnstone (trans.), *Medicine*, 245.

57 ʿAbdallāh b. Sharaf al-Dīn/Wagner (trans.), 'The Debate', 124 (emphasis in the original).

The literature on *qāt* is replete with admirers of the plant. On the whole Yemeni scholars have positive things to say about the chewing of *qāt* or its use in some way as a medicant. Yet there has long been ambiguity about its use, as the Yemeni proverb suggests: "*qāt* is wonderful but there's nothing worse than it" ("*al-qāt ṭayyib mā akrah minhu*").[58] The first admirers, evident in Ibn Ḥajar's commentary, were *shāfiʿī* scholars and Sufis. The major problem with the use of *qāt* was one that had both legal and medicinal aspects in determining if the use of *qāt* should be considered an intoxicant (*muskir*) or narcotic (*takhdīr*) for Muslims. This is clearly laid out at the beginning of the Zaydi imam Yaḥyā Sharaf al-Dīn's treatise condemning the use of *qāt*.[59] Writing just prior to Ibn Ḥajar's *fatwā*, Sharaf al-Dīn has no doubt about the identification of the substance as an intoxicant. Citing the Qurʾān and linguistic usage, he argues that the problem is that the intoxicant obscures the awareness in the minds of those who use it. While the Qurʾān specifically forbade drinking *khamr*, a tradition of Muḥammad elaborated this to include every intoxicant (*muskir*) and anything that weakens or results in overheating (i.e. *mufattir*) of the body.[60] As for *qāt*, he concludes that it leads to altering, inebriating, and confusing the mind as is found among those who drink alcoholic beverages or use narcotics such as wheat or barley beer (*amzār*), opium (*afyūn*), and marijuana (*ḥashīsh*).

When a delegation of scholars went to the court of the Tahirid ruler al-Malik al-Ẓāfir ʿĀmir b. ʿAbd al-Wahhāb (d. 1517), he consulted the Sufi *shaykh* Muḥammad b. ʿAlī (known as Ibn ʿAbd al-Hādī al-Sūdī, d. 1526), who found upon consuming *qāt* that there was no conclusive evidence for its harm and no appropriate legal analogy.[61] The *shaykh* ruled, contrary to Imam Sharaf al-Dīn, that the use of the plant was *ḥalāl* and only forbidden to individuals who would be harmed by it, as in the case of honey.[62] Such harm would appear from actual use of the plant, rather than

---

[58] Sources for this proverb include Rossi, *L'Arabo*, 165.

[59] The title is 'al-Risāla al-māniʿa min istiʿmāl al-maḥramāt al-jāmiʿa fī ʿillat al-taḥrīm bayn al-ḥashīsh wa-l-qāt wa-ghayrihā min sāʾir al-muskirāt' [Preventative Treatise on the Use of General Forbidden Substances: On the Cause of the Prohibition between Marijuana and *Qāt* and Other of the Various Intoxicants]. The text is edited in al-Ḥibshī, *Thalāth rasāʾil*, 7–18.

[60] Quoted by Sharaf al-Dīn, 'al-Risāla', 13, and Yaḥyā b. al-Ḥusayn, 'al-Mustakhrajāt', 54. The banning of intoxicants is found in all the major *ḥadīth* collections, e.g. al-Bukhārī, 9, book 89, #284.

[61] Yaḥyā b. al-Ḥusayn, 'al-Mustakhrajāt', 57.

[62] Honey can cause tempers to rise for those who have yellow bile, according to Yaḥyā b. al-Ḥusayn, 'al-Mustakhrajāt', 62. The author also mentions musk and ambergris as two

any legal analogy to a known intoxicant. Indeed, the *shaykh* was incensed by the license of those who were trying to ban *qāt*, as evidenced in the lines of a *qaṣīda* he wrote:

> *ʿajību li-shakhṣin laysa yaʿrifu ismahu*
> *yaḥramuhu jahlan bi-ghayri dalālāti*
> *bi-ayyi kitābin am bi-ayyi sunnatin*
> *yaqūlu ḥarāmun qūtu ahli l-karāmāti.*[63]

> How incredible that one who knows not its name
> ignorantly prohibits it without evidence.
> By what writing or by what sacred tradition
> does one say the food of respected saints is forbidden.[64]

In his defence of the use of *qāt*, Yaḥyā b. al-Ḥusayn cites a quranic injunction about caution in prohibiting that which Allah has made lawful (al-Naḥl, Q 16:116–17): "Do not say falsely, 'This is lawful and that is forbidden,' inventing a lie about God: those who invent lies about God will not prosper—they may have a little enjoyment, but painful punishment awaits them."[65] His point is that the plant itself is ambiguous, so the focus should only be on specific varieties that cause harm, since some do not.[66] Yet the harm here is said to be that overuse results in a drying (*nashāf*) of the body rather than intoxication.

The case of *qāt* use is interesting, because a major part of the rationale for its use is the positive value it has on the Muslim both for performing his ritual duties and for creating a proper sense of well-being. This was clearly the attraction for Sufis, as had been the case previously with marijuana. In Ethiopia the plant itself was considered holy to the extent that the harvesters would wash their bodies before picking the leaves.[67] Several of the texts refer to the effect that *qāt* has on the heart, mostly in a figurative sense. Yaḥyā b. al-Ḥusayn, for example, quotes an earlier text that describes the plant as blessed (*shajara mubāraka*) because it makes one

---

substances as intoxicating for some individuals. See also al-Jazīrī/al-Ḥibshī (ed.), *ʿUmda*, 122, for a similar argument.

63 This is quoted by Yaḥyā b. al-Ḥusayn, 'al-Mustakhrajāt', 58.

64 Translation by the author.

65 Abdel Haleem, *The Qur'an*, 173–4.

66 Yaḥyā b. al-Ḥusayn, 'al-Mustakhrajāt', 61, cites several known examples of varieties that are harmful, including ones from Bilād al-Jabāmī [al-Jabābī?] in Wuṣāb ʿAlī near Jibla and Jabal Ṣabir near Taʿizz. Kennedy, *The Flower of Paradise*, 118, discovered that there are certain varieties and even specific trees that are said to produce harmful effects like anxiety, loss of semen, or impotence.

67 Getahun and Krikorian, 'Chat', 356.

more compassionate or merciful (literally, *taraqqu l-qulūb*).[68] Indeed, this quality is said to have encouraged Ethiopian Christians to convert to Islam.

The famed Yemeni scholar Muḥammad b. ʿAlī al-Shawkānī (d. 1834) defended its use: "As for *qāt*, I have consumed various kinds and have done so frequently, and as a result I have not found an effect of weakening (*taftīr*), narcotic (*takhdīr*) or mind alteration (*taghyīr*)."[69] He was quick to add, however, that if a variety of *qāt* not known to him did impact to the level of an intoxicant or weakening of the body, then that specific variety should be banned.[70] Like his predecessors, al-Shawkānī quotes the Prophetic tradition that every intoxicant was forbidden; a small amount of wine was forbidden, even if it did not cause intoxication. Not only is *qāt* not an intoxicant, but there should be no prohibition of its sale, as is the case for wine, improperly slaughtered meat, or pork. For al-Shawkānī the restriction on selling an item is only if it furthers something prohibited. Thus, it is permissible to sell a donkey or a mule even though it is unlawful to eat its meat, unless that is the express purpose of the sale.

The contemporary Qāḍī ʿAbd al-Raḥmān b. Yaḥyā al-Iryānī concurred with the opinion of al-Shawkānī that there was no offense (*taʾthīm*) in its consumption.[71] In response to those who would condemn the use of *qāt*, he reminds his readers of a saying by Imam ʿAlī that whoever gives a legal opinion without knowledge will be cursed by the angels of heaven and earth.[72] The thrust of his argument, drawing on such notables as Muḥammad ʿAbduh and Rashīd Riḍā (d. 1935), is that what Allah has created is permissible (*ibāḥa*) unless there is a known reason to forbid something. Indeed, some substances, like poisons, are harmful in some ways and helpful in others. A committee of twelve Yemeni religious scholars reviewed the previous commentaries and concluded with al-Shawkānī that *qāt* should not be banned as an intoxicant or narcotic in the Islamic legal sense.[73]

Some aspects of the plant have both a negative and positive impact, depending on the context. The most obvious effect is the stimulant quality, due to the phenylpropylamines cathinone and cathine (= norpseudo-

---

[68] Yaḥya b. al-Ḥusayn, 'al-Mustakhrajāt', 61.

[69] al-Shawkānī, *al-Baḥth*, 49. Also quoted in al-Muʿallimī, *al-Qāt*, 117.

[70] Ibid., 40, 50.

[71] Quoted ibid., 119.

[72] This comment is also quoted by Qāḍī ʿAbd al-Raḥman al-Iryānī in his introduction to the privately published *fatwā* by al-Shawkānī, *al-Baḥth*, 9.

[73] This was published in the newspaper *al-Rāʾī* on 8 June 1982, and is reproduced at the end of the published text of al-Shawkānī, *al-Baḥth*, 55–62.

ephedrine) in the fresh leaves that allow the user to stay alert and awake. This has long had a practical application in Yemen, where life required substantial physical exertion. Farmers built and maintained terrace walls on steep slopes, cultivated crops by hand or through use of animal draft power, and performed all crop production and processing by hard physical labour. Certain occupations, such as stone cutters and other construction jobs, were exhausting. Since most travel in the mountainous areas was by foot, *qāt* could serve as a welcome burst of energy. Even today truck drivers chew *qāt* to counteract drowsiness on long hauls, although it may be that extended use can impair driving ability.[74]

One of the most vaunted, pleasurable aspects of chewing *qāt* is the sense of well-being or euphoria that can result. An Adeni *qāḍī* confided to the visiting poet Ameen Rihani (d. 1940) that *qāt* "is one of the bounties of Allah. We chew it, and through it we recover our strength. We obtain a little keif [*kayf*] too—not the keif that wine affords, but a keif of the spirit, which otherwise we do not feel, except, of course, through religion."[75] The Arabic term *kayf* has a wide semantic range, from the general sense of one's state or mood to pleasure, well-being, and even the sense of an opiate. The Yemeni al-Ḥārithī describes this state as one that "expands the soul, rejoices it, removes depression and melancholy (*al-waḥshah wa-'l-waswās*), hot palpitation (*khafaqān*), introspective thoughts (? *al-khawāṭir al-nafsāniyyah*), and removes anxieties (*kurab*) when taken in a known quantity."[76] In his assessment of the various stages of *kayf*, Kennedy comments, "The principle qualities of experience which informants identified for us as constituting the *kayf* were increases in alertness, ability to concentrate, the flow of ideas, contentment, confidence and friendliness."[77] In clinical terms, Kennedy describes the state as a mild hypomania transforming into meditative concentration. The French botanist Paul Botta, travelling through Yemen in 1836, found chewing to result in "un grand plaisir dans l'excitation douce."[78] Not long after that James Vaughan observed that *qāt* produces "great hilarity of spirits and an agreeable state of wakefulness" and a century later another British gentleman, B.W. Seager, labelled it a "feeling of contentment and well-being."[79]

---

74 Toennes and Kauert, 'Influence of Khat', 89.
75 Rihani, 'Under the Roofs', 878.
76 Quoted in Serjeant, '*Qāt*', 174.
77 Kennedy, *The Flower of Paradise*, 112.
78 Botta, *Relation*, 76–7.
79 Vaughan, 'Notes,' 269, and Seager, 'The Yemen', 221.

Yemeni descriptions of the overall sense of well-being include phrases such as "harmony of the inner person" (*insijām al-nafs*) and "relaxing of the nerves" (*irtiḥā' al-a'ṣāb*) and descriptive words such as contentment (*riḍan*), happy (*fāriḥ*), peacefulness (*hudū'*), and withdrawal (*imtināʿ*).[80] As Ḥamūd Manṣūr phrases it, *qāt* is refreshing to the soul (*rūḥ*), personality (*nafs*), and intelligence (*ʿaql*).[81] Yemenis will commonly say that chewing at the end of the day, after one has worked hard, takes away the fatigue (*tisḥab al-taʿb*). Coinciding with the increased alertness is the tendency for *qāt* to ward off sleepiness, a positive for those who want to stay awake and perform religious duties but a problem for those who suffer from insomnia. The French botanist Albert Deflers (d. 1921) describes the effect as an "insomnie agréable" rather than a burden.[82]

Although *qāt* was not known in the earlier *materia medica* texts, later scholars did discuss its therapeutic value in addition to known side effects. Unfortunately, very little research has been done on this aspect and most of the relevant textual material remains unpublished. One of the few pharmacological accounts is by Aḥmad b. ʿAbdallāh al-Waqīdī al-Ḥārithī.[83] The alleged health benefits of *qāt* in some form that he cites are summarized in Table 2.

The prescriptive commentary by al-Ḥārithī considers *qāt* both as a simple (i.e. non-compound) drug and in combination with other medicinal substances. His note about its use for various eye problems indicates that *qāt* could become a substitute for other known medicants in the literature.

Western travellers provide limited and anecdotal details on the medicinal value of *qāt*, both for its use in Yemen and Ethiopia. The botanist Peter Forskål (d. 1763), as narrated through the work of Carsten Niebuhr (d. 1815), notes that the plant is useful against infectious disease (*infectos peste*).[84] This observation is followed by James Vaughan, who claims that *qāt* carried in one's bosom is a "safeguard against infection" and that land where it was grown was secure from plague.[85] Niebuhr remarks that *qāt*

---

80 These terms are taken from Schopen's, *Qāt*, 94, and based on personal experience.
81 Manṣūr, *Aḍrār al-qāt*, 11.
82 Deflers, *Voyage*, 122.
83 Serjeant, '*Qāt*', 174, translates an excerpt from a manuscript in Rome. There is no indication from his comments of the date of the text. According to al-Ḥibshī, *Maqāmāt*, 351, who provides an excerpt, there is a manuscript of his medical work in the Great Mosque in Ṣanʿā'.
84 Quoted in Schopen, *Qāt*, 87–8, from Forskål's *Flora Aegyptiaco-Arabica*, 64.
85 Vaughan, 'Notes', 270.

Table 2: Alleged therapeutic value of *qāt* as a medicant, according to al-Ḥārithī[86]

Specific diseases	• cures epilepsy (*ṣarʿ*)
Health conditions	
Body surface	• against hot swellings and pustules (*buthūr*), especially in combination with vinegar and ceruse (*isfidāj*) • against smarting of scrofula (*nākhis al-khanāzīr*)[87] in combination with fava bean (*bāqillā*) flour and wheat/barley gruel (*sawīq*); reduces swelling if mixed with coriander • heals and dries wounds and ulcers (*qurūḥ*), especially if roasted and applied in rose oil • stops nosebleeds if powder of dry leaves is combined with vinegars
Eyes	• for sharp sight, itching, tumours [mycosis?] of the eyelid (*sulāq*), vascular opacity of the cornea (*sabal*), throbbing of the eye, and to dry watering of the eye, use a sprig of *qāt* burned with a sprig of quince (*safarjal*); this recipe substitutes for flowers of zinc (*maghsūl al-tūtiya*) • application of leaves prevents eyes from running
Fevers	• crushed leaves combined with vinegar and opium alleviate throbbing from temperature
Internal organs	• prevents rising of vapour from phlegm to the head • for throbbing due to being too cold, crush leaves with egg yolks and saffron • effective for nausea (*ghathayān*) • dries up wateriness of stomach (*bullat al-maʿida*) and hardens it • alleviates haemorrhage when a *mithqāl* of powder from its leaves is added to four ocques of tamarind water and applied to a hernia (*fatq*) along with cypress (*sarw*) leaf • brings heart complete relief[88]
Mouth	• ameliorates lesion (*nakba*) in mouth if powder of dry leaves is combined with vinegar • freshens bad breath if powder of dry leaves is combined with vinegar
Psychological	• cures nightmares • removes depression (*waḥsha*) and melancholy (*waswās*)[89]

fortifies the body against "infectious distempers" and also serves as an aid for digestion.[90] These claims are also made by Yemeni writers, such as Yaḥyā b. Muḥammad al-Iryānī, who said use of *qāt* lessens the danger in

86 As quoted in Serjeant, '*Qāt*', 174, and al-Ḥibshī, *Maqāmāt*, 351.
87 This is rendered *nākhir* (decay) (ibid.).
88 See ibid., 348, for a poem on the influence of *qāt* on the heart.
89 Also reported in a debate between coffee and *qāt* by al-Muʿallimī (ibid., 347).
90 Niebuhr/Heron (trans.), *Travels*, 2, 352.

an area with infectious disease (*wabāʾ*).[91] It is not unusual to hear Yemenis cite *qāt* as useful for relief of colds, fevers, and headaches,[92] or as a laxative.[93] Based on research in the far north of Yemen, Shelagh Weir suggests that Yemenis do not make strong correlations between *qāt* use and the many prevalent diseases, either as a causal or mitigative factor.[94] However, a wide-ranging study of *qāt* use among Yemeni women by Najāt Khalīl found that 46% of chewers were interested in learning about the role of *qāt* in traditional medicine.[95]

One of the chief combination effects of *qāt* chewing is retarding the appetite and inducing thirst. This is widely reported in the literature and easily observed from experience. The loss of appetite is due mainly to the norpseudoephedrine in the fresh leaves.[96] However, while there are, indeed, high levels of malnutrition in Yemen, it would be difficult to blame *qāt* as a major causal factor. The traditional *qāt*-chewing session is held in the late afternoon, after the main meal of the day, so the evening meal is minimal at any rate. There also does not seem to be any negative effect on the next day's breakfast.[97] But there is no question that chewing contributes to keeping down one's weight and to a diet necessary to combat the now more sedentary life of Yemenis in comparison to their more active past.[98] The *shāfiʿī* scholar Abū Bakr b. Ibrāhīm al-Muqrī al-Ḥarāzī (d. 1558) deplores that *qāt* takes away the pleasure (*ladhdha*) in eating.[99]

There is some nutritional value in chewing. The French traveller Deflers claims the benefit of *qāt* on a long march, giving a minimum amount of nourishment.[100] A study conducted in 1959 found that consumption of 100 grams of fresh leaves introduced significant amounts of ascorbic acid, beta-carotene, calcium, and iron into the diet.[101] It has been alleged that

---

91 al-Ḥibshī, 'al-Qāt', 151.

92 Kennedy, *The Flower of Paradise*, 11.

93 Rihani, 'Under the Roofs', 879.

94 Weir, *Qat in Yemen*, 44.

95 Khalīl, *al-Marāt*, 167.

96 McKee, 'Aspects', 763. The Arabic *materia medica* recognize a number of foods that retard the appetite, such as saffron, *baqla*, and sesame combined with honey (al-Azraq, *Tashīl al-manāfiʿ*, 58).

97 Kennedy, *The Flower of Paradise*, 130, observes: "However, in the opinion of informants, and according to my own experience, hunger inhibition is a temporary condition which is compensated for when the drug effects wear off."

98 Manṣūr, *Aḍrār al-qāt*, 11.

99 Quoted in Ibn Ḥajar al-Haytamī, *al-Fatāwā*, 225.

100 Deflers, *Relation*, 122.

101 Quoted in Getahun and Krikorian, 'Chat', 372.

qāt chewing may supply a beneficial amount of vitamin C to Yemenis.[102] Recent studies suggest that *qāt*'s active ingredients can be antibacterial and thus be of therapeutic value.[103] *Qāt* has been reported to lower blood sugar and may stimulate insulin for individuals with diabetes.[104]

5. Negative Health Aspects

> That Qat is a habit-forming drug and injurious to health goes without saying, but, as the Prime Minister once said to me, it keeps people out of trouble.[105]

In the writings of Western travellers, *qāt* has long received a bad reputation. British administrators who could barely function without a hot toddy in the officers' club were quick to bemoan the drug addiction of any Yemeni who chewed *qāt*. "It reminds one very much of the cocaine habit of the West," complains Charles Crane.[106] Precisely; the problem is that chewing *qāt* always reminds Westerners of other things they do not like, or may even secretly admire, like "lotus eaters."[107] For others it was simply an either/or, as in C. Craufurd's assumption that "[s]ince his religion forbids the juice of the grape, he chews *Khat Edulis*."[108] It is not uncommon to find Western writers referring to *qāt* as a narcotic, although its immediate effect is the opposite.[109] Arab authors trained in the West are often as condemnatory, as in Sami Hamarneh's ethnocentric conclusion that *qāt* "demoralized and degenerated the people and kept them in the darkness of the Middle Ages for more than six centuries."[110] Then there are the non-tobacco related pipe dreams, as in Abbas Faroughy's wish that chewing gum might supplant the use of *qāt*.[111]

---

102 Mustard, 'Ascorbic Acid Content', 34; see also Fleurentin, *Guérisseurs*, 147, and Kennedy, *The Flower of Paradise*, 185.

103 Al-Hebshi and Skaug, 'Khat', 305.

104 Ramadan et al., 'Effect', 9, and see the discussion in 'Nadwat al-qāt', 218–23.

105 Robertson, 'San'a', 52.

106 Crane, 'Visit', 62. The earlier traveller, Charles Millingen, 'Notes of a Journey', 124, more accurately noted that Yemenis chew *qāt* leaves "in the same way and with the same advantages as the natives of Peru use the coca plant."

107 Forbes, 'Visit', 278.

108 Craufurd, 'Yemen', 574.

109 Wendell Phillips, *Qataban and Sheba*, 89, adds that it "has proved one of the scourges of that region." Seager, 'The Yemen', 221, calls it a "noxious form of drug-addiction." For other negative comments, see the citations in Kennedy, *The Flower of Paradise*, 13–14. As Kennedy argues (ibid., 176), the experience of *qāt* use is "precisely the opposite" of drowsiness-producing opiates.

110 Hamarneh, 'Pharmacy', 236.

111 Faroughy, *Introducing Yemen*, 18.

Most Yemenis themselves generally do not view moderate chewing as a threat to health, although negative health aspects are attributed to those who chew excessively.[112] The primary argument against the traditional use of *qāt* is socio-economic, that too much agricultural land and irrigation water are devoted to this non-food crop and that the market costs drain family budgets. As Kennedy has well-observed, the minority of Yemenis who see harmful health effects from chewing are those who have been educated or travelled abroad and picked up Western notions of "drug use."[113] Indeed, his anthropological study in the 1970s was motivated by the "apparent paradox" that "such a mild stimulant could be so rewarding that millions of people would ignore the terrible medical consequences which are alleged."[114] His review of the literature available at the time concluded that many of the allegations of adverse health effects (Table 3) were exaggerated or not fully supported by the data, but that some do have sufficient evidence to be taken seriously. However, his analysis totally ignored the medical reading of *qāt* in the traditional humoural system that combined its supposed nature as a cold and dry substance as well as the reported experience of users.[115]

Qāt chewing has a number of internal gastrointestinal effects, recognized by earlier Yemeni scholars and confirmed through more recent scientific analysis. One of the most obvious is constipation (*qabḍ*).[116] al-Ḥārithī observed that *qāt* "binds the bowels and inhibits movement."[117] The infusion from dried leaves is said by this author to be more constipating than chewing the fresh leaves. As Kennedy observes, because *qāt* inhibits urination and defecation, one can sit for hours without moving—useful for

---

[112] This conclusion is based on personal experience by several anthropologists, including Kennedy, and also as a result of surveys (e.g., Date et al., 'Qat Chewing', 410). There are, however, a number of intellectuals (e.g., al-Aghbarī, *al-Qāḍī al-ʿallāma*, 130) who oppose *qāt* as one of the most abominable Yemeni customs (*min ashnaʿ al-ʿādāt*). The Yemeni sociologist Ḥamūd al-ʿAwdī, *al-Turāth al-shaʿbī*, 299, wishes that the Prophet Muḥammad would come to earth again to make it clear to Yemeni religious scholars how dangerous *qāt* is.

[113] Kennedy, *The Flower of Paradise*, 213.

[114] Ibid., 214.

[115] Most of this literature remains unpublished. One of the more important texts is *Nūr al-abṣār fī shifāʾ khawāṭir al-afkār* of Aḥmad b. ʿAbdallāh al-Wāqidī (18th century); see Wagner, 'The Debate', 127.

[116] Reported by the 1958 *Qāt* Commission of Inquiry in Aden, Serjeant, '*Qāt*', 172, Halbach, 'Medical Aspects', 25, and long recognized both in the Arabic literature and by Western travellers (e.g., Bury, *Arabia Infelix*, 152). Fleurentin, *Guérisseurs*, 146, remarks that the ban on *qāt* in Aden in 1957 led to a 90% reduction in the sale of laxatives.

[117] Quoted in Serjeant, '*Qāt*', 174.

Table 3. Alleged negative health effects of *qāt* use in Yemen[118]

anaemia	hypothermia	paralytic ileus
angina pectoris	insomnia	pellagra
anorexia	ischemic stroke	periodontal disease
cerebral haemorrhage	leukoencephalopathy	pulmonary oedema
constipation	liver damage	stomach cancer
disjointed speech	low birthweight infants	stomach ulcers
duodenal ulcer	migraine	stomatitis
esophagitis	mucosal lesions	tachycardia (elevated heart rate)[119]
gastritis	mydriasis	
gingivitis	myocardial infarction	testicular degeneration
haemorrhoids	oral carcinoma	tuberculosis
hypertension	palpitation	xerostomia

the traditional mode of chewing in Yemen.[120] al-Ḥārithī also notes that its use causes borborygmi or stomach growling and farting. The astringent quality of the tannins is a primary cause of gastritis, but the active alkaloids in the fresh leaves can impact secretory, muscular, and absorptive activities.[121] Eating fenugreek (*ḥulba*) sauce is said by Yemenis to counteract the indigestion caused by chewing.[122] The use of modern medicine presents a new problem for *qāt* use; studies, for example, have shown that chewing interferes with the absorption of amoxicillin and ampicillin.[123]

In Kennedy's study of male and female chewers, six specific gastrointestinal problems were found among the sample: chronic gastritis, haemorrhoids, colitis, ulcers, esophagitis, and avitaminosis.[124] As might be expected, given the extremely poor health conditions in Yemen, there was a high prevalence of gastrointestinal problems and the data from their survey suggested that *qāt* use did contribute to these. The harmful impact on those with haemorrhoids was recognized by the Yemeni scholar al-Ḥārithī and confirmed by recent clinical analysis.[125] A major negative factor attributed to use of *qāt* relates to the urinary system, at least for

118 There is a broad scientific literature on the pharmacological effects of *qāt*. For a recent review of the medicinal claims, see Al-Hebshi and Skaug, 'Khat'.

119 I note, with unintended irony, that the official website of the US Drug Enforcement Administration (<http://www.usdoj.gov/dea/concern/khat.html>) misspells this as tahycardia [*sic*].

120 Kennedy, *The Flower of Paradise*, 115.

121 Ibid., 218.

122 Bornstein, *al-Zohra*, 12.

123 E.g. Attefa et al., 'Khat Chewing'.

124 Kennedy, *The Flower of Paradise*, 219.

125 al-Ḥārithī is quoted in Serjeant, '*Qāt*', 174. See Al-Hadrani, 'Khat', for the recent analysis.

males.[126] al-Ḥarāzī, quoted by Ibn Ḥajar, claimed that something like the urine drip (*wady*) is released after consuming it and this does not stop until after awhile.[127] The problem of urinary incontinence is noted by al-Ḥārithī and also for cases in Somalia.[128]

One of the more obvious negative effects of *qāt* chewing, due to the storing of the leaves in the inside cheek, is the harm caused to teeth and gums. In a poetic duel between tobacco and *qāt*, the tobacco warns that chewing will destroy the teeth (*yikhrab al-aḍrās*).[129] The traveller Wyman Bury (d. 1920) observed that "[t]he teeth are much affected, becoming permanently discoloured and loose, for the gums become flaccid."[130] Oral cancer is also recorded, although this appears to be due mainly to combination of chewing *qāt* and use of tobacco. Damage to the tongue is probably due to extended contact with the *qāt l*eaves.[131] An early study of Yemenite Jews in Israel found evidence of a high percentage of periodontal disease.[132] Among other symptoms, it is said by some Yemenis that *qāt* can cause colic (*qawlanj*).[133] The same is indicated for coffee and colds (*zukām*).[134] al-Ḥārithī reports deprivation of sensation (*takhdīr*) accompanied by a slight rise in temperature.[135]

The analysis of *qāt* as a consumable substance often revolves around the issue of addiction. So is *qāt* chewing addictive? The 1958 *Qāt* Commission of Inquiry in Aden, conducted after a legislative ban in the British controlled colony, concluded emphatically that it was not. "*Qāt* does not create an addiction, like opium or hashish, in that those who are suddenly deprived of it, do not suffer physical consequences."[136] Earlier analyses of the possibility that *qāt* was a dangerous drug were inconclusive. An advisory committee to the League of Nations concluded in 1936 that there was no proof one way or the other of the alleged negative effects;

---

126 Kennedy, *The Flower of Paradise*, 235, reports negative effects on the urinary and hepatic systems of females as well.

127 Ibn Ḥajar al-Haytamī, *al-Fatāwā*, 226.

128 al-Ḥārithī is quoted in Serjeant, 'Qāt', 174, and al-Ḥibshī, *Maqāmāt*, 352. For Somalia, see Peters, 'Khat', 36.

129 al-Ḥibshī, *Maqāmāt*, 366.

130 Bury, *Arabia Infelix*, 152.

131 Sawair et al., 'High Relative Frequency', 193.

132 Rosenzweig and Smith, 'Periodontal Health'.

133 Yaḥyā b. Muḥammad al-Iryānī in al-Ḥibshī, 'al-Qāt', 151.

134 al-Ḥibshī, *al-Maqāmāt*, 351, 366.

135 Quoted in Serjeant, '*Qāt*', 174.

136 Quoted ibid., 172, with a personal note by Serjeant: "[...] yet the Yemenis are a sturdy race upon which the writer has seen no apparent general ill effect."

nor did the UN Commission on Narcotic Drugs in 1956 find evidence that there were harmful effects.[137] A major difficulty in answering this question is the definition of 'addiction.' There is no denying the pharmacological effects on most users and that the derivative form methcathinone (known as 'cat') is highly addictive, similar to the relation of cocaine to the fresh coca leaf. But, as Kennedy and others have observed, there is no physiological addiction from chewing for most users, nor is there anything like the addiction to nicotine in tobacco.[138]

Another claim in the literature, and one that is echoed in some of the early criticism of its use in the legal literature, is that it leads to psychological problems, including insanity.[139] Manṣūr describes the case of three youth in Shahāra who are said to have gone crazy due to their overindulgence in *qāt*.[140] There are alleged cases of excessive use of *qāt* leading to schizophrenic psychosis.[141] The problem with most of these claims is that it is difficult to separate out other causal factors on behaviour. A study of one Somali *qāt* user in The Netherlands is a case in point, since his clinical paranoia could as easily be due to his alcohol abuse.[142] In a survey of 800 adults (aged 15 to 76) in Yemen during 2001–2, Nabil Numan found no link between *qāt* chewing and psychological morbidity as measured in the Symptoms Checklist-90.[143] This included hostility, interpersonal sensitivity, somatisation, depression, anxiety, phobia, obsession, paranoia, and psychoticism. He concludes, along with Hans Halbach, that one reason for the lack of a causal link is the method of chewing that would rarely yield plasma levels needed for the development of psychosis. Similarly, a survey of 136 Yemenite Jews in Israel by A. Litman et al. found no link between chewing *qāt* and psycho-pathology or social deviance.[144] This is not to say that individual cases of severe psychological issues do not arise in specific individuals, a possibility recognized in the *fatwā* literature and suggested by anecdotal evidence. Hallucinations are reported, although

137 Halbach, 'Medical Aspects', 21.

138 Fleurentin, *Guérisseurs*, 147, concludes: "Tous les auteurs sont unanimes pour reconnaître qu'il n'y a pas de dépendance physique, alors qu'elle est reconnue pour les drogues dures comme l'héroïne."

139 An example is Jawhar and Ayyūb, *al-Yaman*, 121. Mackintosh-Smith, *Yemen*, 20, was told to avoid *qāt* inadvertently being planted over a grave, because it would bring sorrow.

140 Manṣūr, *Aḍrār al-qāt*, 21.

141 Gough and Cookson, 'Khat-induced Schizophreniform Psychosis', 455.

142 The case is described in Nielen et al., 'Khat and Mushrooms', 50.

143 Numan, 'Exploration', 64.

144 Litman et al., 'The Use of Khat', 394.

rare, especially the sense of insects crawling over one's body, if one overindulges.[145]

Ironically, these studies confirm those earlier Yemeni scholars who argued that the use of *qāt* did not produce the negative effects of known intoxicants and narcotics in the existing medical literature. Yaḥyā b. al-Ḥusayn, for example, states that the plant is permissible in general, unlike the case for opium, nutmeg, marijuana (*shahdānij*), and henbane (*banj*).[146] In popular usage, however, some Yemenis compare the effect of *qāt* as similar to or slightly less than that of marijuana.[147] Based on his experience in southern Yemen, the traveller Bury claimed that "those who use alcoholic stimulants at all fail to notice the subtleties of kât," adding that those who drink do not chew.[148] Whatever sample Bury was citing from personal experience, there is ample evidence that in the past four decades some Yemenis drink whiskey to counter the stimulant impact of the *qāt*. There has been a substantial illicit trade in hard liquor, especially whiskey, mainly for use by the educated elite and recently returned immigrant workers. The motive for drinking such prohibitive intoxicants is that they counteract the negative effects of chewing, especially insomnia. Yet, as Ḥamūd al-ʿAwdī complains, drinking begins after up to six to eight hours of the chewing session and continues until God only knows what time.[149]

One of the studies specifically targeting Yemeni women who chew *qāt* was conducted in 1984 as part of a broader study on maternal mortality and morbidity.[150] The data were collected on 1181 consecutive deliveries in maternity units in seven locations in the Yemen Arab Republic. The authors found statistical evidence for an association between *qāt* chewing and decreased birthweight of infants. At the time no specific mechanism was proposed, although it was noted that one of the active substances (norpseudoephedrine) had been shown to have an adverse effect on placental blood circulation. To the extent the use of *qāt* was anorectic and reduced food intake, especially in a population where malnutrition was not uncommon, lower birthweights could also be expected. However, it should also be noted that the combination of *qāt* with smoking a water

145 Kennedy, *The Flower of Paradise*, 121.

146 Yaḥyā b. al-Ḥusayn, 'al-Mustakhrajāt', 62.

147 For example, al-ʿAwdī, *al-Turāth al-shaʿbī*, 170.

148 Bury, *Arabia Infelix*, 153.

149 al-ʿAwdī, *al-Turāth al-shaʿbī*, 297, uses the term *khamr*, but in reference to alcoholic drinks in general. His literal phrase is *wa-ilā mā shāʾ Allāh*. He has an extended commentary (297–302) on the dangers in combining *qāt* and alcohol.

150 Abdul Ghani et al., 'The Influence'.

pipe would make it difficult to separate the effect of tobacco from that of the *qāt*.

A recent factor contributing to the negative health impact of *qāt* use is the application of chemical pesticides since the early 1980s. These tend to be applied more during the winter. Many Yemenis assume that the chemical residues can be cleaned by washing the leaves, but in fact chemical components are absorbed by the tissues of the leaves.[151] In their analysis of over 120 chewers in the Ṣanʿāʾ region, Junko Date et al. recorded that the conditions resulting from *qāt* grown with pesticides included body weakness, dizziness, headache, stomach ache, stomach bulge, vomiting, and nasal problems. In the Taʿizz area there is a disease called *ṭāwiya* due to chewing *qāt* leaves that have fungus.

Part of the rationale for condemning *qāt* relates to the problem it was said to create for doing the proper ablutions for prayer. As Ibn Ḥajar explains, *qāt* chewing caused urine to flow out on the clothes, thighs, and legs when a chewer was in the mosque, thus making it difficult to perform prayers.[152] Similarly, al-Ḥarāzī complains that pieces of *qāt* would be wedged between the teeth and were difficult to remove.[153] Arguments about the uncleanness of tobacco use, especially dirtying the beard and moustache, were employed by later Ottoman authors.[154] Another criticism levelled against the chewing session itself is that individuals delay their prayers because they are too engaged with the effect of the *qāt*.[155]

6. Conclusion

> I have frequently eaten kât, when offered to me in audience, at the courts of certain sultans in the Aden hinterland. It has a somewhat bitter, but not disagreeable taste, and the only after-effect I noticed was slight insomnia. Other Europeans say the same, and I never yet heard of one who liked it.[156]

More so than any other single plant discussed in the Islamic legal tradition, *Catha edulis* may be the most ambiguous substance. Several intoxicants, including wine and beer, have been defended at times and others have since been almost universally exonerated by Muslims, such as coffee, but

---

151 Date et al., 'Qat Chewing', 412.
152 Quoted in al-Ulughkhānī/Ross (ed.), *An Arabic History*, 357.
153 Quoted in Ibn Ḥajar al-Haytamī, *al-Fatāwā*, 226.
154 Grehan, 'Smoking', 1361.
155 al-Aghbarī, *al-Qāḍī al-ʿallāma*, 130.
156 Bury, *Arabia Infelix*, 153.

qāt remains *arbor incognita.* Like all substances which have either a stimulant or narcotic effect on people, the use of *qāt* in any form cannot be reduced to its chemical properties any more than human behaviour can be explained by DNA. The issue of whether or not Muslims are allowed to use *qāt*, as with any other substance, depends on observation of the behaviour resulting from its use. Since *qāt* was not used at the time of the Prophet Muḥammad, there is no mention of it in the sacred texts, nor did it merit commentary in any of the major *materia medica* due to its late introduction in Yemen. The debate over the legitimacy of *qāt* was complicated because there was no definitive scientific placement of the plant in the humoural framework, nor experimentation beyond anecdotal evidence of its potential healing properties. Thus, the debate over its use succumbed to the inevitable politics of how one viewed those who used the plant.

The judicial reasoning of Ibn Ḥajar al-Haytamī, who was faced with conflicting and at times heated points of view from Muslim scholars, demonstrates a desire to be objective and look to the findings of the science of his day, rather than apply a knee-jerk ban based on a weak analogy or rejection of the plant simply because of who used it. Lacking any prior experience with the plant, there was clearly a need to place its properties scientifically into the prevailing humoural system of medicine. In the medicine of the day this was reduced to working back from the observed or alleged effects on those who consumed the plant. Being a leaf with no food value, it is not surprising that it was considered to be dry and moist. But this placed it in a problematic category alongside the known banned substances of marijuana and opium, also accepted by some Sufis. As al-Haytamī concluded, there really was no conclusive evidence, so the cautious approach would be to avoid it even though it did not warrant an outright ban. This reasoning supported those Yemeni scholars, like al-Shawkānī, who over the years accepted *qāt* as legitimate except in the case of varieties that were known to intoxicate or for individuals with inappropriate humoural natures.

Sifting through the accounts of Western travellers over the past several centuries, a proper understanding of the use of *qāt* is clouded by the obvious disdain of most of these European visitors. Not surprisingly, much of the available literature contains a discernible bias and frequent errors of fact. Similarly, discussions in Arabic often approach *qāt* in a defensive mode, stimulated in part by the negative views of most non-Yemeni Muslims, or else associate its use with a backward mentality. Today there are numerous reports of clinical studies on the use of *qāt* and the chemical structure of the plant's active constituents is well established, but in the past a major problem in assessing the 'scientific' literature on the study of *qāt* was the wide range of claims. The broad survey in Yemen conducted by Kennedy in the 1970s challenged many of the standard claims about effects from *qāt* use, noting that much of this was based on hearsay and did not take into account the specific variety of *qāt*, the extent of its use, and other psychological and health aspects of those chewing it. Just as one should not define all wine drinkers by the actions of an alcoholic, it is problematic to say that there is a specific set of effects for any user. Another problem affecting the reliability of studies is that many take place outside the country of origin of the chewer, where there may be other stress factors at play.

My aim here has been to pull together the scarce information on the ascribed health impacts of *qāt* use in the traditional Yemeni system. I have also reviewed some of the main clinical findings about the health impacts of contemporary users of *qāt* in order to highlight the need for further study that brings both sets of data together. The most obvious conclusion I find from the literature surveyed is that there can be no single medical profile of a *qāt* user. There are simply too many contextual variables to consider. First, there are chemical differences in the leaves of different varieties, as recognized in the qualities attributed to some varieties over others. Research needs to be conducted on varietal differences in the context of cultivation.[157] For example, the Yemeni poet 'Alī b. 'Abdallāh al-Iryānī noted that the effect on the intellect was due to the qualities of the soil (*khawāṣṣ al-arḍ*) in which it was grown.[158] Second, future study of the use of *qāt* should carefully discriminate the various ways it has been consumed, both for the pleasure of chewing as a stimulant and as a medicant. What is the effect if chewing occurs simultaneously with use of tobacco, either in the water pipe or with cigarettes? What is the role of diet, a factor of major importance in the humoural tradition? Third, what other aspects of *qāt* use influence the health impact, such as chewing leaves contaminated with pesticides and sharing a water pipe or containers of water? Fourth, what is the differential impact on males and females? Kennedy analyzes results of a survey given to male and female chewers.[159]

---

157 Yemeni scholars and physicians are well aware of the local differences of *qāt* varieties, as well as the distinction from *qāt* grown in Ethiopia; see, for example, the comments of Dr. al-'Udāyā in 'Nadwat al-qāt', 222.

158 Quoted in al-Ḥibshī, 'al-Qāt', 153.

159 Kennedy, *The Flower of Paradise*, 116–20.

Yet his casual conclusion that "Female tasks are not *regarded* as particularly taxing of mind or body, or even as 'work' in the male sense of that term" raises the issue of how women view their work. Certainly the workload of rural women is not light. Indeed, women in the central highland valley of al-Ahjur complained that they were often too busy with their work to take time off for chewing on a regular basis. Finally, and this is not a variable independent of the others listed here, what is the role of the 'attitude' of the chewer, the psychological factors that create moods and desires in combination with the chemical impact?

Bibliography

Abdel Haleem, M. A. S. (transl.), *The Qur'an* (Oxford: Oxford University Press, 2004).

Abdul Ghani, N., Eriksson, M., Kristiansson, B., and Qirbi, A., 'The Influence of Khat-chewing on Birth-weight in Full-term Infants', *Social Science and Medicine*, 24/7 (1987), 625–7.

al-Aghbarī, 'Abd al-Raḥmān 'Abdallāh, *al-Qāḍī al-'allāma Muḥammad b. Ismā'īl al-'Amrānī* (Ṣan'ā': Maktabat al-irshād, 2002).

al-Akwa', Muḥammad b. 'Alī, *Ṣafḥa min ta'rīkh al-Yaman al-ijtimā'ī wa-qiṣṣat ḥayātī* (Damascus: Maṭba'at al-kātib al-'arabī, 1979).

Attefa, Omer A., Alib, Abdul-Azem A., and Alic, Hassan M., 'Effect of Khat Chewing on the Bioavailability of Ampicillin and Amoxycillin', *Journal of Antimicrobial Chemotherapy*, 39 (1997), 523–5.

al-'Awdī, Ḥamūd, *al-Turāth al-sha'bī wa-'alāqatuhu bi-l-tanmiya fī l-bilād al-nāmiya: Dirāsat taṭbīqiyya 'an al-mujtama' al-Yamanī* (Cairo: 'Ālam al-kutub, 1980).

al-Azraq, Ibrāhīm b. 'Abd al-Raḥmān b. Abī Bakr, *Tashīl al-manāfi' fī l-ṭibb wa-l-ḥikma* (Beirut: al-Maktaba al-sha'biyya, 1978).

al-Baraddūnī, 'Abdallāh, 'al-Qāt... min ẓuhūrihi ilā isti'mālih', in Yemen Center for Research and Studies (ed.), *al-Qāt*, 41–8.

Bornstein, Annika, *Al Zohrah: An Agricultural Village in the Tihama* (unpublished paper, Yemen: FAO Nutrition Program #13, March 1972).

Botta, Paul Emile, *Relation d'un voyage dans l'Yémen* (Paris : de Soyte, 1880).

Brooke, Clarke, 'Khat (*Catha edulis*): Its Production and Trade in the Middle East', *Geographical Journal*, 126/1 (1960), 52–9.

Brown, E.R., Jarvie, D.R., and Simpson, D., 'Use of Drugs at "Raves"', *Scottish Medical Journal*, 40 (1995), 168–71.

Burton, Richard, *First Footsteps in East Africa* (reprint New York: Praeger, 1966).

Bury, G. Wyman, *Arabia Infelix: Or, the Turks in Yamen* (London: MacMillan, 1915).

Crane, Charles R., 'Visit to the Red Sea Littoral and the Yaman', *Journal of the Royal Central Asian Society* 15/1 (1928), 48–67.

Craufurd, C., 'Yemen and Assir: El Dorado?', *Journal of the Royal Central Asian Society*, 20/4 (1933), 568–77.

Date, Junko, Tanida, Noritoshi, and Hobara, Tatsuya, 'Qat Chewing and Pesticides: A Study of Adverse Health Effects in People of the Mountainous Areas of Yemen', *International Journal of Environmental Health Research*, 14/6 (2004), 405–14.

Du Couret, Louis/S., C. D. (trans.), *Life in the Desert, or Recollections of Travel in Asia and Africa* (New York: Mason, 1860).

Faroughy, Abbas, *Introducing Yemen* (New York: Orientalia, 1947).

Fleurentin, Jacques, *Guérisseurs et plantes médicinales du Yémen : Au pays de l'encens, de l'aloès et du café* (Paris : Karthala, 2004).
Forbes, Rosita, 'A Visit to the Idrisi Territory in 'Asir and Yemen', *Geographical Journal*, 62/4 (1923), 271–8.
Forskål, Petrus/Niebuhr, Carsten (ed.), *Flora Aegyptiaco-Arabica. Sive descriptiones plantarum, quas per Aegyptum inferiorem et Arabiam felicem detexit* (Hauniae [Copenhagen]: Möller, 1775).
Getahun, Amare, and Krikorian, A.D., 'Chat: Coffee's Rival from Harar, Ethiopia. I. Botany, Cultivation and Use', *Economic Botany*, 27/4 (1973), 353–77.
Gingrich, Andre, 'The Guest Meal among the Munebbih: Some Considerations on Tradition and Change in *'aish wa milh* in Northwestern Yemen', *Peuples méditerranéens*, 46 (1989), 129–49.
Gough, S.P., and Cookson, Ian B., 'Khat-induced Schizophreniform Psychosis in UK', *The Lancet*, 323 (1984), 455.
Grehan, James, 'Smoking and "Early Modern" Sociability: The Great Tobacco Debate in the Ottoman Middle East (Seventeenth to Eighteenth Centuries)', *American Historical Review*, 111/5 (2006), 1352–77.
Al-Hadrani, Ahmed M., 'Khat Induced Hemorrhoidal Disease in Yemen', *Saudi Medical Journal*, 21/5 (2000), 475–7.
Halbach, Hans, 'Medical Aspects of the Chewing of Khat Leaves', *Bulletin of the World Health Organisation*, 47 (1972), 21–9.
Hamarneh, Sami, 'Pharmacy in Medieval Islam and the History of Drug Addiction', *Medical History*, 16 (1972), 226–37.
Al-Hebshi, Nezar N., and Skaug, Nils, 'Khat (Catha edulis): An Updated Review', *Addiction Biology*, 10 (2005), 299–307.
Helfritz, Hans, *The Yemen: A Secret Journey* (London: Allen & Unwin, 1958).
Hess, J.J., 'ḳāt', *The Encyclopaedia of Islam* (New Edition), (VI; Brill: Leiden, 1978), 741a–b.
al-Ḥibshī, 'Abdallāh, 'al-Qāt fī l-adab al-Yamanī', in id., *Dirāsāt fī l-turāth al-Yamanī* (Beirut: Dār al-'awda, 1977), 141–57.
———, 'Mushkilat ẓuhūr al-qāt... wa-fuqahā' al-qarn al-'āshir', in Yemen Center for Research and Studies (ed.), *al-Qāt*, 73–9.
——— (ed.), *Maqāmāt min al-adab al-Yamanī* (Ṣan'ā': Dār al-Yaman al-kubrā, 1984).
——— (ed.), *Thalāth rasā'il fī l-qāt* (Beirut: Dār al-tanwīr, 1986).
Ibn Faḍl Allāh al-'Umarī, *Masālik al-abṣār fī mamālik al-amṣār* (Casablanca: Tawzī' Sūshibrīs, 1988).
Ibn Ḥajar al-Haytamī, *al-Fatāwā l-kubrā l-fiqhiyya* (4; Beirut: Dār al-kutub al-'ilmiyya, 1983).
Ibn Qayyim al-Jawziyya/Johnstone, Penelope (trans.), *Medicine of the Prophet* (Cambridge: The Islamic Texts Society, 1998).
Jawhar, Ḥasan Muḥammad, and Muḥammad al-Sayyid Ayyūb, *al-Yaman* (Cairo: Dār al-kātib al-'arabī lil-ṭibā'a wa-l-nashr, 1967).
al-Jazīrī, 'Abd al-Qādir b. Muḥammad/al-Ḥibshī, 'Abdallāh (ed.), *'Umdat al-ṣafwa fī ḥall al-qahwa*, (Abu Dhabi: Cultural Foundation, 1996).
Kennedy, John G., *The Flower of Paradise: The Institutionalized Use of the Drug Qat in North Yemen* (Dordrecht: Reidel, 1987).
Khalīl, Najāt, *al-Mar'a al-Yamaniyya wa-majālis al-qāt* (*al-tafriṭa*) (Ṣan'ā': Dār al-majd lil-ṭibā'a wa-l-nashr, 1998).
Kueny, Kathryn, *The Rhetoric of Sobriety: Wine in Early Islam* (Albany: SUNY Press, 2001).
Lane, Edward, *An Arabic-English Lexicon* (London: Williams and Norgate, 1877).
Levey, Martin, *Early Arabic Pharmacology* (Leiden: Brill, 1973).
Litman, A., et al., 'The Use of Khat: An Epidemiological Study in Two Yemenite Villages in Israel', *Culture, Medicine and Psychiatry*, 10 (1986), 389–96.
Mackintosh-Smith, Tim, *Yemen: Travels in Dictionary Land* (London: Murray, 1997).

Mancioli, Massimo, and Parrinello, Antonino, 'Il gat (*Catha edulis*)', *La Clinica Terapeutica*, 43/2 (1967), 103–72.
Manṣūr, Ḥamūd, *Aḍrār al-qāt fī l-jumhūriyya al-ʿarabiyya al-Yamaniyya* (Beirut: Dār al-fikr al-muʿāṣir, 1988).
al-Maqrīzī, Aḥmad b. ʿAlī/Rinck, Fridericus Theodorus (ed. and trans.), *Macrizi Historia regum Islamiticorum in Abyssinia* (*Kitāb al-Ilmām bi-akhbār man bi-arḍ al-Ḥabash min mulūk al-Islām*] (Lugduni Batavorum [Leiden]: Luchtmans, 1790).
McKee, C.M., 'Medical and Social Aspects of Qat in Yemen: A Review', *Journal of the Royal Society of Medicine*, 80/12 (1987), 762–5.
Millingen, Charles, 'Notes of a Journey in Yemen', *Journal of the Royal Geographical Society*, 44 (1874), 118–26.
al-Muʿallimī, Aḥmad ʿAbd al-Raḥman, *al-Qāt fī l-adab al-Yamanī wa-l-fiqh al-islāmī* (Beirut: Manshūrāt Dār maktabat al-ḥayāt, 1988).
Mustard, M., 'Ascorbic Acid Content of Some Miscellaneous Tropical and Subtropical Plants and Plant Products', *Food Research*, 17 (1952), 31–5.
'Nadwat al-qāt', *Dirāsāt Yamaniyya*, 8/9 (1982), 211–28.
Niebuhr, M. [Carsten]/Heron, Robert (trans.), *Travels Through Arabia, and Other Countries in the East* (2 vols.; Edinburgh: R. Morison and Son, 1792).
Nielen, Roman J., et al., 'Khat and Mushrooms Associated with Psychosis', *World Journal of Biological Psychiatry*, 5/1 (2004), 49–53.
Numan, Nabil, 'Exploration of Adverse Psychological Symptoms in Yemeni Khat Users by the Symptoms Checklist-90 (SCL-90)', *Addiction*, 99 (2004), 61–5.
Peters, Derek, 'Khat: Its History, Botany, Chemistry and Toxicology', *Pharmaceutical Journal*, 169 (1952), 16–18, 36–7.
Phillips, Wendell, *Qataban and Sheba* (London: Gollancz, 1955).
Pormann, Peter E., and Savage-Smith, Emilie, *Medieval Islamic Medicine* (Washington, DC: Georgetown University Press, 2007).
Powels, Sylvia, 'Zur Herkunft des Wortes Qāt (Catha Edulis Forsk.)', *Zeitschrift für arabische Linguistik*, 24 (1992), 7–20.
Radt, Christine, 'Contribution a l'histoire ethnobotanique d'une plante stimulante : Le Kat', *L'Ethnographie*, 65 (1971), 38–65.
Ramadan, Mohyi El-Din A., Abul-Kheir, Fathi A., and Labib, Shadia, 'Effect of Cath Edulis (Khat) on Glucose Tolerance in Diabetcs [*sic*]', *Dirāsāt Yamaniyya*, 2 (English section, 1979), 15–22.
Reichmuth, Stefan, *The World of Murtada al-Zabidi (1731-91): Life, Networks and Writings* (Exeter: Gibb Memorial Trust, 2009).
Revri, Raman, Catha Edulis *Forsk. Geographical Dispersal, Botanical, Ecological and Agronomical Aspects with Special Reference to Yemen Arab Republic* (Göttinger Beiträge zur Land- und Forstwirtschaft in den Tropen und Subtropen, 1; Göttingen: Institut für Pflanzenbau und Tierhygiene, 1983).
Rihani, Ameen, 'Under the Roofs of Sanaa', *Asia*, 29 (1920), 878–83, 918–20.
Robertson, William, 'San'a and the Qat-Eaters', *The Scottish Geographical Magazine*, 58/2 (1942), 49–52.
Rodinson, Maxime, 'Esquisse d'une monographie du qât', *Journal Asiatique*, 265 (1977), 71–96.
Rosenthal, Franz, *The Herb: Hashish versus Medieval Muslim Society* (Leiden: Brill, 1971).
Rosenzweig, Kurt A., and Smith, Patricia, 'Periodontal Health in Various Ethnic Groups in Israel', *Journal of Periodontal Research*, 1 (1965), 250–9.
Rossi, Ettore, *L'Arabo parlato a Ṣanʿāʾ* (Rome: Instituto per l'Oriente, 1939).
Saha, Sagar, and Dollery, Claire, 'Severe Ischaemic Cardiomyopathy Associated with Khat Chewing', *Journal of the Royal Society of Medicine*, 99/6 (2006), 316–18.

Sawair, Faleh A., et al., 'High Relative Frequency of Oral Squamous Cell Carcinoma in Yemen: Qat and Tobacco Chewing as Its Aetiological Background', *International Journal of Environmental Health Research*, 17/3 (2007), 185–95.

Schopen, Armin, *Das Qāt. Geschichte und Gebrauch des Genussmittels Catha Edulis Forsk. in der Arabischen Republik Jemen* (Wiesbaden: Steiner, 1978).

Seager, B.W., 'The Yemen', *Journal of the Royal Central Asian Society*, 42 (1955), 214–30.

Serjeant, R.B., '*Qāt*', in R.B. Serjeant and Ronald Lewcock (eds.), *Ṣan'ā': An Arabian Islamic City* (London: World of Islam Festival Trust, 1983), 171–5.

Sharaf al-Dīn, Yaḥyā, 'al-Risāla al-māni'a min isti'māl al-maḥramāt al-jāmi'a fī 'illat al-taḥrīm bayn al-ḥashīsh wa-l-qāt wa-ghayrihā min sā'ir al-muskirāt', in al-Ḥibshī (ed.), *Thalāth rasā'il fī l-qāt*, 7–18.

al-Shawkānī, Muḥammad b. 'Alī, *al-Baḥth al-musfir 'an taḥrīm kull muskir wa-muftir* ([s.l.]: Aḥmad b. 'Alī Ḥasan, 1984).

Singer, P.N., *Galen. Selected Works* (Oxford: Oxford University Press, 1997).

Toennes, Stefan W., and Kauert, Gerold F., 'Driving under the Influence of Khat: Alkaloid Concentrations and Observations in Forensic Cases', *Forensic Science International*, 140 (2003), 85–90.

al-Ulughkhānī, 'Abdallāh Muḥammad/Ross, Denison (ed.), *An Arabic History of Gujarat, Ẓafar al-Wálih bi Muẓaffar wa Ālih* (Indian Texts Series, 2; London: Murray, 1910).

Varisco, Daniel Martin, 'Turning Over a New Leaf: The Impact of *Qât* (*Catha edulis*) in Yemeni Horticulture', in Michel Conan and W. John Kress (eds.), *Botanical Progress, Horticultural Innovations and Cultural Changes* (Washington, DC: Dumbarton Oaks Research Library and Collection, 2007), 239–56.

———, 'The Elixer of Life or the Devil's Cud: The Debate over *Qāt* (*Catha edulis*) in Yemeni Culture', in Ross Coomber and Nigel South (eds.), *Drug Use and Cultural Context: Tradition, Change and Intoxicants beyond 'The West'* (London: Free Association Books, 2004), 101–18.

———, 'On the Meaning of Chewing: The Significance of *Qât* (*Catha edulis*) in the Yemen Arab Republic', *International Journal of Middle East Studies*, 18 (1986), 1–13.

Vaughan, James, 'Notes upon the Drugs Observed at Aden, Arabia', *Pharmaceutical Journal and Transactions*, 12 (1853), 268–71.

Wagner, Mark, 'The Debate Between Coffee and Qāt in Yemeni Literature', *Middle Eastern Literatures*, 8/2 (2005), 121–49.

Weir, Shelagh, *Qat in Yemen: Consumption and Social Change* (London: British Museum, 1985).

Yaḥyā b. al-Ḥusayn, 'al-Mustakhrajāt al-bayyanāt 'alā taḥlīl al-ashyā' al-musta'malāt min al-qahwa wa-l-ṭabāq wa-l-qāt', in al-Ḥibshī (ed.), *Thalāth rasā'il fī l-qāt*, 51–103.

Yemen Center for Research and Studies, *al-Qāt fī ḥayāt al-Yaman wa-l-Yamāniyyīn* (Ṣan'ā', 1981–2).

Internet Sources

Ben-Ami, Yuval, 'The Yemeni Book of Living and Dying', *Everywhere*, 18 November 2007 <http://yuvalbenami.blogspot.com/2007/11/yemeni-book-of-living-and-dying.html>, accessed September 2009.

Deflers, Albert, *Voyage au Yemen : Journal d'une excursion botanique faite en 1887 dans les montagnes de l'Arabie heureuse* (Paris : P. Klincksieck, 1889) <http://www.archive.org/details/voyageauyemenjouoodefl>, accessed September 2009.

Siegel-Itzkovich, Judy, 'Knesset Dubs "Hagigat" and Amphetamines Illegal', *The Jerusalem Post*, 19 May 2009 <http://www.jpost.com/LandedPages/SearchResults.aspx?q=knesset dubs>, accessed September 2009.

Urquhart, Conal, 'Drugs and Dance as Israelis Blot out Intifada', *The Guardian*, 4 September 2004 <http://www.guardian.co.uk/world/2004/sep/04/israel>, accessed September 2009.

<http://en.wikipedia.org/wiki/Khat>, accessed September 2009.

<http://www.usdoj.gov/dea/concern/khat.html>, accessed July 2009.

THE ALOE AND THE FRANKINCENSE TREE IN SOUTHERN ARABIA: DIFFERENT APPROACHES TO THEIR USE[1]

Miranda Morris

Both aloe and frankincense have a status that extends far beyond the areas in which they grow. Frankincense has been renowned over millennia for its fragrant gum and its perceived protective and supernatural properties; whilst the sap of aloe, more pragmatically, has long been appreciated for its medicinal value. Much has been written about the uses of both plants, historically and in modern times.[2] But how do those who live where they grow regard the plants?[3]

Both plants grow in Soqotra, other parts of Yemen, and in Dhofar (in the Sultanate of Oman)—areas whose people are linked culturally, often linguistically[4] and who share many distinctive traditions. This paper examines the differing uses made of these two plants by the people who live in the drier, more remote areas in which the most valuable representatives of both plants flourish, rather than the ways the plants are utilized in the more heavily populated and cosmopolitan towns of the region. Here the uses of the commercial products—dried frankincense gum and dried aloe sap—are similar to those of much of the wider Middle Eastern region, and these have been well described elsewhere. The paper also looks at contrasting local attitudes towards the plants, and examines the role of aloe and frankincense today.

---

[1] Transliteration of Modern South Arabian languages follows the system of the Seminar for Arabian Studies, London: <http://www.arabianseminar.org.uk/ArabianSeminarLatestGuidelines2010.pdf>.

[2] For instance, simply googling 'aloe' comes up with an amazing 12,900,000 hits, and 'frankincense' with some 4,800,000 hits (January 2010).

[3] Those parts of the text that examine the different uses of the plants are written in the past tense for the sake of consistency, but also to reflect modern reality: many of these uses are now historical.

[4] See below n. 6.

1. Frankincense

1.1. *The Frankincense Tree*

The frankincense tree is a member of the Burseraceae family, one which contains many shrubs and trees producing balsams, resins and gums. The gum produced by the frankincense tree is more accurately an oleo-gum resin comprising essential oils, water-soluble gums, and alcohol-soluble resins which are contained in reservoirs in the bark. These are extracted by tapping: using a spatulate chisel to make deep, longitudinal incisions in the bark. The initial cuts grow a 'scab' that is peeled off at regular intervals to make the tree 'bleed' more gum. This exudate then has to be dried for two to three months before being ready for sale.

Only one species of frankincense grows in the South Arabian mainland: *Boswellia sacra*, the 'sacred Boswellia,' whereas on Soqotra no fewer than eight species have been distinguished by botanists to date.[5] On the mainland the frankincense tree is called *shajarat al-lubān* in Arabic, or in the MSA languages[6] spoken in southern Yemen, Soqotra, and Dhofar, *meġerót* or *meġerāt*. Not surprisingly, on Soqotra there is more than one name for the many species of frankincense tree: *emġīro* or *emʿīro* (where /ġ/ is realized as /ʿ/ in some of the island dialects), clearly related to the *meġerót, meġerāt* of the mainland, but also *ṣamaʿáno* and *tilīyə*, while the cliff-growing trees are called *źífḥa*, meaning 'squeezed, crouched.' The islanders believe that only one of the species, *Boswellia socotrana*, was specifically tapped for its gum in the past. The gum resin, which all species produce, is referred to by the same term on the mainland as on the island, namely *lubān* in Arabic and *śáḥaz, śēḥez* in the MSA languages. This term is not restricted to the gum resin of frankincense trees, but is also used for that of various *Commiphora* species[7] (of the same Burseraceae family as the frankincense tree), as well as for the latex produced by various tree euphorbias and wild fig species that coagulates and hardens on exposure to air.

---

[5] *Boswellia ameero; B. bullata; B. dioscorides*; *B. elongata; B. nana; B. popoviana; B. socotrana;* and another species which is still under taxonomic discussion. In Arabia, *Boswellia sacra* grows from Ḥāsik in eastern Dhofar to Ḥabbān in the eastern part of the Ḥaḍramawt in Yemen. It is also found along the north eastern coast of Somalia. See Miller and Morris, *Plants of Dhofar*, 78, and eid., *Ethnoflora*, 457–64.

[6] Modern South Arabian languages, namely Śḥerɛ̄t, Mehriyɔ̄t, Hobyɔ̄t, Baṭḥari, Ḥarsūsi, and Sʌḳȯṭeri, spoken in southern Yemen and southern Oman.

[7] Indeed, Balfour reports that the resin of the endemic *Commiphora parvifolia* was sometimes used as an incense. See Balfour, *Botany of Socotra*, s.v. *Commiphora*.

We shall see that for many mainland usages of frankincense the Soqotran islanders often use one or other of the *Commiphora*[8] trees instead.

Apart from the trade in the dried gum, how were the frankincense trees exploited in the areas where they grow?[9]

1.2. *Foliage, Flowers, Wood, and Bark*

Throughout the region the foliage provided a key dry season fodder for livestock. On Soqotra leafy stems of *Boswellia ameero* were offered to cows and goats at milking to encourage them to let down their milk. In periods of severe drought, chunks were cut from the larger boughs of *Boswellia* spp. and *Commiphora* spp., the papery outer layer removed, and the rest chopped up small to feed sheep; hungry goats were left to gnaw at it for themselves. The bark of *Boswellia ameero* was rarely used for this, as it has the unpleasant side effect of causing the animals' noses to run. The bark of the small-leaved *Commiphora* spp. (*C. parvifolia, C. socotrana*) was also made into a nutritious feed for kids, lambs, and calves on Soqotra by crushing chunks of bark in water, leaving them to soak and then squeezing out the liquid into a leather feeding-bottle. Dead frankincense wood was burned on the smudges lit in byres and milking yards as an insecticide and to soothe livestock; the older and more rotten the wood the better, as this produced plenty of acrid smoke. Bees come to the flowers, and are said to use the gum in the construction of their nests, sometimes building these in holes and cracks in the trees themselves. The dead wood was considered to be one of the best for smoking out wild bees to rob them of their honey as it produces a lot of smoke. People liked to nibble the buds, fruit, and tender new growth for their pleasantly astringent taste, and chewed them to sweeten the breath. Women suffering from nausea in early pregnancy chewed pieces of the underbark or prepared a tea from it.

The red underbark provided an important red-brown colorant used to dye the imported unbleached calico from which clothing for men and women was made; also to dye the cotton twist for knotting fishing nets, or, on Soqotra, woven to make the coloured stripes in the local sheep wool cloth. A stronger extract provided a stain for the multi-strand belts plaited from goat- and lamb-skin and to decorate the local clay pottery. The underbark of frankincense (and *Commiphora*) trees was crushed to a paste

---

[8] Of the five species of Commiphora on the island, four are endemic: *Commiphora ornifolia, C. parvifolia, C. planifrons*, and *C. socotrana*.

[9] Uses of plants in Dhofar are based on research carried out there from 1976 to 1990, and of plants in Soqotra on research begun in 1987 and still ongoing.

for tanning leather; it was also rubbed into a stiffened or ill-smelling leather container to soften and deodorize it. For children, a twig of the tree with the core removed provided an excellent popgun.

However, on the mainland the main importance of the bark, for people as well as for livestock, was medicinal. Pieces of the underbark were simmered in water and the hot liquid applied to infected wounds. Alternatively they were ground to a paste, called *nefǵót*, which was applied as a dressing, as well as being rubbed all over the body as a remedy for generalized oedema. Another key medicinal preparation was made by charring pieces of the papery outer bark with some of the inner bark and then reducing them to a fine, black powder. This antiseptic dressing, called *themdít*, was an important component of the family medicine chest. On Soqotra, *Commiphora* bark[10] was used instead, the powdered preparation being called *naqf* and the liquid one, applied boiling hot, *ˊirziz*. The latter was important for treating the wound of circumcision.

1.3. *Fresh, Soft Gum*

Small pieces were inserted into a painful carious tooth to stop up the hole and relieve the pain, and fresh gum was chewed to strengthen the teeth and jaw muscles and to treat halitosis. It was also chewed to alleviate thirst and to treat various stomach complaints. The saliva stimulated by the chewing was believed to have a tonic effect and pieces of gum were given to stimulate the appetite of the sickly, especially children. Fresh *Commiphora* gum was often used in the same way.

On the mainland strips of the bark, coated with a layer of soft gum, were used to bind fractures. Fresh gum was boiled in milk to make a paste which was applied locally to treat mastitis in both women and livestock. People used the soft gum as a depilatory, and also as a hair lacquer, especially at the temples to give the hair a smooth and sleek appearance. The gum was moulded into cone-shaped 'candles' that were lit at dusk—more to keep vermin and the forces of evil at bay than for illumination. Fresh gum was used throughout the region as a general adhesive, in particular to repair cracked or holed clay vessels that were then held over the fire until the gum had set hard. Even the soot of the burning gum was collected for use by scraping it off a (clay) lid placed over a pot of smouldering gum. This soot was applied around the eyes as a *kuḥl*, on its own or mixed with

---

[10] *C. ornifolia* is used especially for the powdered preparation, and *C. parvifolia* and *C. socotrana* for the liquid one.

antimony, to improve vision and soothe sore eyes. It was added to water to make an ink, and was used in tattooing: patterns were pricked in the area of gum above and below the incisors with two needles bound together, and then the soot was rubbed in to produce a permanent stain. Some women also filed the incisors in parallel lines with slivers of flint and stained the abrasions with the soot. Very rarely this was done on Soqotra, mainly by 'Arab'[11] women of the northern coastal settlements, but here the stain was made by rubbing butter-oil into indigo-dyed cloth to produce a blue-black dye. An interesting use of frankincense trees on the island was as a soil fertiliser: small piles of the dead wood were mixed with animal dung and set alight, the ash then being mixed into the soil. Wood from *Jatropha*, *Euphorbia arbuscula*,[12] or *Commiphora* was also used for this purpose. This fertiliser was applied especially in the cultivation of the valuable tobacco or finger millet (*Eleusine coracana*).

1.4. *Root of a Young Plant*

Both on the mainland and on the island a young frankincense plant could be pulled up and its root (on the mainland called *téli* [Dhofari Arabic], *tiźót* [Śḥerēt] or, on Soqotra *kəndīyo* or *śerīxo, śerīḥo* (where /x/ is realized as /ḥ/ in some island dialects) chewed to quench thirst, or just for the sake of the flavoursome liquid it contained. On Soqotra the roots of other young plants, such as *Sterculia africana* (*bóhīn*), *Commiphora parvifolia, C. socotrana* (*léḳəhem*), and *Lannea transulta* (*kə́nəhor*),[13] were chewed in the same way.

1.5. *Dried Gum*

When it came to the crucial purpose of healing the sick, throughout South Arabia people would do their utmost to obtain gum of the very best quality. On the mainland those who harvested the gum would set aside the best pieces of gum, called *ḥánźob*, 'beads,' or *fiźźét*, 'silver,' or, in Arabic, *fuṣūṣ*, 'gemstones,' for separate sale for this purpose. On Soqotra this meant trying to obtain gum from overseas (*śáḥaz mən rínhem*, 'frankincense gum

[11] The islanders of the Soqotra interior generally referred to the more cosmopolitan inhabitants of the settled communities on the north coast as 'Arabs.' Indeed, pastoralists of the more arid western half of the island also referred to islanders who owned date palms or who were otherwise involved in cultivation as 'Arabs,' even where such people were principally pastoralists like themselves.

[12] The jatropha, *J. unicostata*, and *Euphorbia arbuscula* are also endemics.

[13] *Sterculia africana* is an endemic variety and the other plants are all endemic.

from the sea'), for any imported gum was considered to be superior to that produced locally: its droplets were larger and the perfume of its smoke stronger, and altogether it was regarded as much more potent.[14]

On Soqotra the attitude towards burning frankincense gum differed from that of the mainland. Here any burning of the gum was predominantly a matter for specialists and experts, and it was particularly associated with sorcery and the detection of sorcery. The gum was used under the guidance of the traditional healer or shaman, the *mékóli*, who was called in when a sickness in human or animal had not responded to other forms of treatment. The *mékóli* had many different methods of diagnosing and interpreting illness, either using his own unique powers unaided, or by going into a trance and thereby allowing his personal familiar (*jinn*) to take over and control his body. Muttering incantations, he burned a droplet of the gum, after wetting it with his saliva, or he ordered smoking gum to be carried around and underneath the patient. Sometimes he would chew the gum and then spray the afflicted object with his spittle; sometimes he would light a piece of gum and tell the patient to crouch down and inhale the smoke, covering his body with a rug or shawl. Date palm gardens and finger millet plots, pens, folds and byres, homesteads, cave living quarters, even the vital butter-skin, were all 'cured' in the same way by the *mékóli* to dispel the evil influences which had caused the damage and to uncover the identity of the spiteful witch.

On the mainland someone who had been struck down by the evil eye had a burner of smoking gum placed at their head while members of their family circumambulated the patient, carrying another smoking burner and reciting various invocations. This was done especially during the hours of darkness, and usually had to be carried out more than once. A similar ceremony was performed on Soqotra, but only in the presence of a *mékóli* or another man (it was always a man) with similarly recognized esoteric powers. Frankincense gum was used, but it was common to add other potent materials, such as trimmings from the horn of a goat, goat hair or donkey dung, and burn these together, the patient squatting in the smoke.

Due to these associations with malevolence and sorcery, the islanders were unwilling to burn the gum themselves or to make use of it casually, fearing that anyone smelling its unmistakable perfume might suspect them of too close an association with evil forces, or might credit them with

---

[14] Interestingly Carsten Niebuhr (d. 1815) noted that "Arabians hold their own incense in no estimation, and make use only of that which comes from India" (Niebuhr/Heron (trans.), *Travels*, 2, 356).

sinister powers of their own. If anyone did burn frankincense for protection or as a treatment then he or she did so in the greatest secrecy. Rarely, a husband and wife would carry out a minor version of the evil eye ritual in the privacy of their own home if they feared that one of them had inadvertently harmed something or someone in their household in this way.

Therefore, many of the ways the dried gum was used on the mainland would not have been considered appropriate on the island, and other materials were chosen instead. For instance, while on the mainland the smoke of burning frankincense was sniffed up to treat a headache or a severe head cold, on the island a piece of hoof, especially of a donkey (*ḥán'e, xéynə d-ḥə́mār*), pieces of horn (*ḳān d-šfāniś*), a vulture feather (*nə́frer d-sōʿīdo*), or a dried leaflet of the tree euphorbia, *Euphorbia arbuscula* (*éṣlaʿ d-ímtəhe d-ṣāmə*), was burned instead.[15] Where mainlanders burned frankincense to repel evil by throwing a piece of gum on the fire at sundown and sunrise—the two most dangerous times of the day when evil spirits are believed to be especially active—the islanders would burn instead dried leaflets from the tree euphorbia, dried *Adenium obesum* wood (*ísfəd d-ṣāmə*), or *Cissus hamaderohensis* or *C. subaphylla* fruit (*gəḥə́lo d-ʿáṭərhe*). Most powerful of all was sheep dung removed from the dung heap, for it was said that if evil spirits smelled '*ṭay' d-'ímiher,*' 'the odour of burning sheep dung,' they kept their distance. These materials were burned outside the living quarters in such a way that the wind blew the protective smoke over the livestock and homestead.

Mainlanders liked to burn frankincense gum for its pleasant smell, or to fumigate their clothing and bedding, but the islanders would burn instead the wood of *Cephalocroton socotranus*[16] (*d-ráḥmam, ṭan*), *Commiphora* or *Clerodendron leucophloeum*[17] (*sənémhen*). Burning the frankincense bark (*ḳɛ̄lifo*) was not viewed with the same suspicion on the island as burning the gum: bark was burned to fumigate clothing and bedding, and fragrant chunks of *Boswellia* bark, often with some gum adhering, were brought home and placed where they would catch the breeze to perfume the home. Nevertheless, other plants were more widely used to produce a pleasant smell, such as dried *Cephalocroton* or *Clerodendron* wood, or gum from *Commiphora ornifolia* (*íkšə*) or one of the small-leaved *Commiphora* spp. (*léḳəhem*).

---

[15] However, on ʿAbd al-Kūrī island, part of the Soqotra Archipelago, frankincense is used: the customs here are heavily influenced by those of the mainland.

[16] An endemic plant.

[17] An endemic plant.

Although not on Soqotra, on the mainland frankincense was burned to celebrate weddings and at major religious festivals, and burners of smoking gum were carried in processions that took place to mark the safe return of a ship from overseas, or the long-awaited arrival of the trade boats, or when transferring a bride to her new home. In the circumcision ceremony,[18] mainlanders carried smoking gum around the young man during and after the operation. On Soqotra instead, before the operation actually took place, the circumciser, the *mzēdihir*—another figure credited with certain occult powers—would place gum on a slip of pottery, light it, and place it at the base of the stone seat (*miskido*) where the young men would sit for the operation. Once the smoke had risen above the stone seat, the *mzēdihir* would give a signal and all those present would shout "*hob ʿayn*! *hob ʿayn*!" to rid the area of any inimical spirits, and only then would the first of the young men approach the seat to undergo the operation.

On the mainland it was customary to burn the gum to solemnize the swearing of an oath over the shrine of a sanctified person, or to ratify a pact made between two groups as they shared food and drink. This was not the custom on Soqotra, though the gum was sometimes burned when making supplications to the Creator. But again this was done only as instructed by a person considered to have a special relationship with the supernatural, such as the *mékóli*, or one of the *sāda*, a group respected for their relationship to the family of the Prophet Muḥammad.

Islanders would not grind the gum to a powder and mix it with other ingredients to make a body talcum, as was done on the mainland; nor would they pass around a burner of smoking gum at the end of a meal for guests to fumigate themselves before they departed. On the mainland frankincense gum was burned throughout childbirth to protect both mother and baby, and the post-partum woman would squat every day over a pot of the smoking gum for the forty day period of purification that follows a birth. On Soqotra women used *Lycium sokotranum*[19] wood instead during childbirth—indeed, the tree is commonly called *súhur d-bīrhítin*, '*Lycium* of childbed'—though if a woman suffered from a retained placenta she might squat over a chunk of smouldering frankincense bark as a remedy.

[18] Traditionally this operation was carried out on young men in a public ceremony accompanied by feasting, singing, and dancing. It marked their transition to manhood and allowed the young man to begin to think of marriage.

[19] An endemic plant.

In the settled coastal villages and towns of Soqotra, many of whose inhabitants originated from the mainland, some practices from the mainland have long been in use. Here it was common to burn the gum beside a woman during childbirth until the placenta had been safely delivered, and then to fumigate the clothing and bedding of childbed with frankincense. A lump of gum was often lit in the home after dusk to protect the house and those in it, especially during the rains. Many burned gum in their homes on a Wednesday evening, and pieces of gum were lit in the mosques on Wednesday and Thursday nights before being extinguished first thing on Friday morning. Frankincense was burned for the dead (from the moment of death until the bier reached the grave), or to celebrate a wedding, or to improve the memory[20] (usually in preparation for the recitation from memory of sections of the Qurʾān). However, such customs were not replicated in the Soqotra hinterland.

This rather restricted use of the gum on Soqotra has meant that the craft of making incense burners, so highly developed on the mainland, was negligible on Soqotra. Except for the towns of the north coast—Ḥắdiboh, Ḳāźeb, and Ḳalansiya—where potters did make clay incense burners and, in Ḥắdiboh especially, decorated them with crimson *Dracaena cinnabari*[21] resin, incense burners were rarely used, the gum being burned on any shard of clayware.

One of the few occasions on the island when the burning of the gum by a non-specialist was seen as acceptable was when moving into new living quarters, usually when transhuming to an empty cave or moving into a homestead which had been left empty for a period. At this time frankincense gum was burned to cense both living and livestock quarters in order to rid them of harmful vermin, *ré'ś*: scorpions, giant centipedes, wolf spiders, snakes, and certain other reptiles. It was believed that these cannot tolerate the smell of frankincense and are forced from their cracks

---

20 This was done by putting droplets of gum and a piece of iron in a pot of water and drinking the water the next day. In the settled communities of Soqotra, if a clay pot became foul-smelling, especially that used for storing butter-oil or water, it was filled with boiling water, left to stand for a while, then emptied and fumigated with the smoke of the burning gum. It was then turned the right way up and left open to the sunlight for the rest of the day. On mainland Yemen the large clay pots used to store water were fumigated with the smoke of the gum: this gave the water a distinctive flavour and perfume. Here too bowls and cups were often held inverted over frankincense smoke before being offered to visitors to drink from.

21 The most famous endemic tree of the island, often referred to as the 'dragon's blood tree.'

and crevices into the open to escape the smoke. Presumably it was hoped that any lurking evil spirits would likewise be driven out (*"ṭay' d-ṣamaʿáno: é'efo šíbi wə-iʿúmur śáḥaz d-ṣamaʿáno iṭārid dídəhe,"* "the smell of frankincense: people think that the smell of frankincense chases away evil spirits"). Yet even for this purpose it was seen as just as useful to burn the wood of other plants such as *Cephalocroton* or *Clerodendron*.

It was also considered acceptable for the ordinary person to burn gum as a remedy for aberrant behaviour, such as persistent sleep-walking, 'fits of madness', or even chronic insomnia. In the hope of forcing the malevolent spirit possessing the body to leave, the patient was held down firmly as the spirit struggled this way and that in its efforts to avoid inhaling the smoke. Nevertheless, even this treatment was best carried out under the supervision of the traditional healer. If he succeeded in uncovering what had caused the strange behaviour—that is, the identity of the witch—he would take some of the patient's hair and burn it with some frankincense to protect the patient from re-possession.

However, the truly respected traditional healers were few and far between, the charlatans were many, and each had to be paid for their ministrations by the slaughter of one or more of the precious livestock, or by a gift of butter-oil, or in later years, even with hard cash. So it is more than likely that in the remoter cave-settlements of the island many experiments were made to treat the sick without the guidance of a traditional healer.

1.6. *The Harvest*

The harvesting of the gum on the mainland was closely organized and followed a prescribed procedure. It involved coastal merchants who provided the food for the labourers in the harvest camps, headmen who organized the harvest in each site: giving each labourer an area of trees to harvest, drawing up a rota for fetching water and herding the camp milk-goats, deciding whose turn it was to fetch firewood or cook the evening meal and who should remain in camp to guard the ever-growing piles of harvested gum. It involved camel drivers who delivered the food supplies to the camp and took the harvested gum back down to the coast, and women who worked in the storehouses to clean and sort the gum: many different grades of gum were recognized, and the price varied accordingly. For many it was the main economic event of the year, when enough could be earned to pay off debts or to buy the necessities for the coming year. It was also a time when people of many disparate and distant communities met to work together, a time when marriages were arranged and news exchanged.[22]

In contrast, on Soqotra, collection of the gum was sporadic and opportunistic. A passerby might—or might not—stop to pick off droplets of gum oozing from the tree in the great heat of the summer months; at this season any break in the bark (caused by a herder lopping foliage for his livestock, for instance, or by browsing goats or by wild cats sharpening their claws) oozes gum. This gum has a particularly strong smell and is regarded as being of a superior quality. Anyone can collect gum like this: the trees are not specifically owned (other than in the general way of belonging to those who have grazing rights over the rangeland in which they grow), nor was the gum regarded as being of any particular value. After all, it was widely believed that the *mέkόli* was able himself to 'magically' produce any gum he needed, transforming a pebble, a date, or an ember into droplets of frankincense at will. Nevertheless, any active harvesting of the gum—by cutting into the bark—was always the prerogative of those who owned the land on which the trees grew and no-one could harvest a tree outside their own area without seeking permission to do so. When the gum still had some value, poorer people came up from the coast to harvest the trees and sell the gum to traders or to the people of the settled coastal communities. The greatest quantities of gum came from the north-west coastal area, especially from the seaward plains and foothills between Di-Ḥamź and Ḳalansiya, where *Boswellia socotrana* trees (*tilīyo, tilīyo ṣamaʿáno*) grow in the *Croton socotranus* shrubland. Some older islanders from this area remember a period when there was a rise in the demand for the gum from Aden; at this time the frankincense harvest was taken more seriously, and the scars on the tress are still visible today on many trees. The different species of *Boswellia* produced gums of different value, the most valuable being the gum from *tilīyə* trees, followed by that of *ṣamaʿáno* and finally of *emʿīro, emǵīro*. At this time of high demand even the gum of *Commiphora kua*[23] (*ḥárḥeyr*) was collected for sale, though the price for this was lower than for that of the *Boswellia* species.

So, to summarize, in the areas where the frankincense trees grow, we find, as might be expected, many uses for different parts of the tree as well as for the dried gum. We see too that, although all the people of southern

[22] See Camelin, 'Ash-Shiḥr', 21–3, for some details of the harvesting of frankincense in the mountains behind al-Shiḥr.

[23] Not an endemic plant. On 'Abd al-Kūrī it is the most important medicinal plant of the island (Miller and Morris, *Ethnoflora*, 465).

Arabia considered frankincense to have prophylactic, propitiatory and protective qualities, on the mainland the burning of the gum for such purposes was open to anyone and everyone, whereas on Soqotra it was the province of the specialist practitioner. Indeed, on Soqotra it was held that the gum could even be harmful in the wrong hands. On the island all *Boswellia* spp. were thought to shelter harmful creatures, both natural and supernatural; a stand of frankincense trees was the favoured haunt of evil spirits, and approaching a frankincense tree to remove anything from it was something that must be done carefully.

We also find that Soqotrans considered other plants to possess equally protective qualities. Thus *Euphorbia arbuscula* and *Lycium sokotranum* were used in place of frankincense for protection (indeed, a *Euphorbia arbuscula* was often planted close to the entrance to the living quarters): sprigs were hung over entranceways, tied to the all-important butter-churning skin, laid across pots of food, or suspended over a baby's hammock. On returning to a home left empty for a period, twigs were hung at the doorway of the goat- or sheep-fold. Nor were all frankincense-substitutes of plant origin: items such as the hair of a wild goat (*śfé d-ṭáḥrir*), pieces of horn, vulture feathers, well-matured sheep dung were equally valued.[24]

It is curious that, despite the number of frankincense species on the island, the proximity of the Soqotra Archipelago to the mainland and the great similarities in culture and language between the populations of the areas under discussion, the attitude on Soqotra towards the use of the gum differed so markedly from that on the mainland.

2. Aloe

Extracts of aloe have been used medicinally across the world for centuries, and much of the material has come from southern Arabia, the Soqotran sap (from *Aloe perryi*) being especially famous. Although the aloe also grows in wetter areas, it is the exudate of the plants of arid areas that is the most highly valued for its medicinal properties.[25] This sap is described by

[24] For other non-plant medicaments and treatments, see Morris, 'The Soqotra Archipelago.'

[25] In Dhofar, the large and fleshy aloes that grow in the monsoon rains and, on Soqotra, the tall, succulent aloes of the high, damp Ḥagəher mountains are not harvested at all commercially as their sap is considered to be inferior, and takes a very long time to dry out. However, in earlier times when aloe sap had a higher value these too may have been har-

harvesters as 'red,' 'orange' or 'gold,' while the sap of plants growing in the wetter areas is described as 'black.'

There are two products of the aloe leaf: gel and sap. The clear or light yellow gel is stored in the thin-walled parenchyma cells in the centre of the leaves. The golden to brown sap comes from the assimilating tissue just beneath the epidermis. When the leaf is cut from the plant the sap drains from this tissue and this is the main aloe product harvested.[26]

2.1. *The Aloe Plant*

A number of species of aloe grow on the mainland and on Soqotra.[27] All are called *ṣabr* in Arabic and *ṭayf* ('bitter') in the MSA languages. The leaf is called *ṣiź'ot* in the MSA languages of Dhofar and *əṣəlīʿo* on Soqotra; in Dhofar the fresh sap is called *josót* and on Soqotra *gis* or *gíso*, clearly related terms.

2.2. *The Harvest*

Although of commercial significance in the areas where the best aloes grow, the aloe harvest—at least according to local tradition—seems not to have been as organized as was the frankincense harvest. Aloes were harvested principally by women, who set up a temporary home in one of the many available caves of the aloe areas, and worked their way from plant to plant day after day with family members visiting to supply them with food and water. Harvesting was generally carried out in the month preceding the rains, to give the harvested plants maximum chance of recovery. On Soqotra, where aloes are still of commercial value, they are never cut in a period of drought, and if it has been a dry year the plants are rested for a year and not harvested until the following year. If it comes on to rain during harvesting, all work has to stop, as the plants become turgid, the quality of their sap deteriorates and it will not readily dry and harden. The harvesting method is the same across the region: the leaflets are snapped off at the base and placed in a ring around a hollow lined with a piece of leather or plastic. The sap drains out and collects at the bottom (the leaf is not squeezed because this would dilute the sap with gel). It is then

vested as well. Not all aloes, by any means, are regarded as being equally valuable medicinally. For instance, in Dhofar it is *Aloe dhufarensis* that is applied medicinally, whereas *A. inermis* is used mainly as a dye.

26 Christie et al., *An Aloe Case Study*, 46.

27 See Miller and Morris, *Plants of Dhofar*, 182–3, and eid., *Ethnoflora*, 297–303.

transferred to goatskins, and a complex system of drying follows: coating the goatskins with fine earth, sand, or ash and turning the skins at regular intervals until the juice has solidified.

2.3. *Medicinal Uses of Aloe*

Aloe was one of the most important and versatile medicinal plants of the region. However, in comparison to its extensive application in medicine elsewhere, its use on Soqotra was rather more limited: externally it was applied to treat eye and skin conditions, and internally it was taken to treat all sorts of stomach problems.

Although Soqotra has a unique and rich vegetation and the islanders have an intimate knowledge of the properties of their plants, it seems that the potential of plants as medicine was of less value than their potential as fodder for the livestock on which the islanders depended, and as a source of food, fuel, or timber. Although herbal medicine was certainly practised on the island, the *materia medica* was based on plants from the same rather small group, and other forms of treatment were more popular. In brief, the most prevalent remedies for illness were:

- cauterization (*ṣlḥir*), using mainly cauterizing irons (*móṣḥir*) but also hot ash, embers, or caustic plant latex;[28]
- sacrificing an animal (*múḥur*) in the name of the patient in supplication to the Creator, with the repeated chorus "*fé'es tok ḳanínhin ʎllʌh*," "I beg You, Lord God," the meat being shared amongst those in need;
- calling on the expertise of the specialist healer and 'witch-sniffer,' the *mékóli*, to discover who or what lay behind the illness;
- taking wild honey,[29] seen as the distillation of all that was beneficial in plants;
- taking a drink made by squeezing a handful of one-to-two year old dates (*tāmer mšórḳiḥ*) in water.

We shall examine how those who lived with the aloe plants made use of them, including material not available in the markets such as the fresh sap, leaves, and the root bark. The more common medicinal applications of the commercial product will not be discussed here, as these are well known and discussed in many publications.[30]

---

28 On cauterization, see also Ester Muchawsky-Schnapper's chapter in this volume.

29 On honey, see also Mikhail Rodionov's chapter in this volume.

30 The fullest study of aloe gel is perhaps that in Grindlay and Reynolds, 'The Aloe vera Phenomenon'.

2.4. *Flowers*

Bees love the flowers, and people too suck them for their sweet nectar. Indeed, in the hottest months it is possible in the early morning to run a hand along the inflorescence and gather nectar. The honey from this plant is described as 'hot' by the islanders, and it is highly appreciated for its medicinal properties, especially when made from aloes brought into flower by the rare summer rains.

2.5. *Fresh Sap*

This is more gentle in its purging effects than the dried product, and consequently was preferred by those with access to the plants. For children with stomach pains or constipation, a little fresh sap was inserted into a date or mixed with some sugar. Some mothers would give a small amount to their children every day prophylactically. Constipated livestock and animals with colic or worms were treated with the fresh material, and it was also taken as a vermifuge by people, first thing in the morning on an empty stomach. Women took the sap to induce or regulate menstrual discharge, and in higher doses to procure an abortion. Fresh sap was dripped into a sore or infected ear, and directly into the eyes to improve the sight, especially by the elderly as their sight began to deteriorate. To treat inflammation and a watering eye, drops directly into the eye were supplemented by painting more of the sap around the eye. For fresh injuries, a leaf was cut and the exudate applied directly to the injury. Dirty wounds and sores were washed with salt and water and then painted with sap to speed the healing process and to discourage flies. Cotton plugs soaked in the sap were inserted into the nose and more was painted around the nose to treat a severe nosebleed, and people with allergies and hay fever inhaled the sap through the nose.

In particular the fresh sap was used directly on the skin as a cooling and soothing agent: to the forehead as a remedy for a headache or head cold; to itchy or inflamed skin; to burns; to treat dry eczema and scabies; to reduce swellings, including the swellings of mumps and mastitis. It was painted all over the chest, sometimes with added salt and turmeric, to treat a persistent and painful cough: as it dries the sap pulls the skin taut and sets hard like a sticking plaster, which is said to relieve chest pain. A thick layer was painted over a painful back, knee, or other joint and left to set hard in the same way. Fresh sap was smeared over the affected part of the face in cases of a stroke twisting the mouth, a Bell's palsy, or any other affliction causing facial disfigurement. It was used on the thumb to discourage thumb-sucking, and on the nipple or teat to wean babies and young livestock. A parturient mother was anointed with a mixture of powdered indigo, turmeric, and myrrh, and her forehead bound with a length of material soaked in the sap, and her newborn baby was covered with a layer of aloe sap mixed with powdered indigo.[31] In some parts of the mainland fresh sap was applied cosmetically to the skin to make the skin glow and to stain the neck, bosom, lower arms, and legs a rich yellow[32] and to protect against cold and disease.

It was an important medicament too for treating livestock. For example, a suppurating abscess was washed with a strong salt and water solution and then a layer of sap applied, and a boil was painted with the sap to bring the pus to the surface. A large, fresh laceration was treated by packing it with a mixture of fresh sap and ground lichen or powdered, chalky stone, after first washing it with salt and water. The sap keeps flies away as well as speeding the healing process. When the bites of ticks, lice, or the biting flies of the rainy season became infected they were treated with an application of aloe sap. This property of deterring pests, insects, and other, was used to advantage on Soqotra: in the rainy season, shepherds have always to be alert to the possibility of blowfly or screw-worm attack. If they saw the characteristic signs around the tail or on a wound, they applied a dressing of fresh sap (or *Euphorbia arbuscula* latex), sometimes mixed with fine wood ash, to prevent the eggs from hatching, kill any larvae present, and to discourage further fly attack. Leather and clay grain containers were smeared with the sap mixed with ash to keep insects and rodents away, as were the emerging horns of young stock. Fresh aloe leaves were crushed and smeared around the neck and anus of young stock—kids and lambs—to protect them from raven and wild-cat attack.[33]

On Soqotra, someone who had suffered botfly[34] attack to the mouth, eyes, or nostrils took fresh or dried aloe sap immediately after the attack

---

[31] See Schönig, *Schminken*, 247–8, who also mentions the use of black aloes 'ink' to paint the newborn and the mother against the evil eye.

[32] This was done especially in areas where turmeric (*Curcuma longa*) was not readily available to be used for the same purpose.

[33] The aloe also had other non-medicinal uses: on Soqotra the fresh sap was applied as a glue, in particular to glue together handwritten sections of the Holy Qurʾān to make a booklet. Throughout the region it was customary to plant aloes on graves to 'shade' and 'cool' the dead.

[34] The botfly, *Oestrus ovis*, in Soqotri *di-ʿáṣer*, is attracted to goats and sheep in still, hot, and shady places. The flies are most prevalent in the early winter when the sun is fully up and then again in the late afternoon. The first-stage larvae, which are produced alive, are

to induce retching or vomiting, in the hopes of thereby expelling the injurious larvae. If no sap was available to be taken at once, it was still recommended to take it later, as the diarrhoea that ensues was believed to flush the larvae from the system.

2.6. *Entire Leaves*

On Soqotra an invaluable antiseptic dressing, like the one prepared from *Commiphora* bark (and on the mainland from frankincense bark),[35] was made from dried aloe leaves and was likewise called *naqf*. The leaves were charred and ground to a powder that was used especially to dress burns—both accidental and those resulting from cauterization.[36] A maggot-infested wound was washed with a strong salt and water solution and then treated with *naqf*, except in young children for whom this was considered too painful. In children the wound was washed out with fresh sap and then covered with another thick layer of sap; this was repeated daily until the wound healed. Generally it was said that a surface or fresh wound was best treated with sap and an older, deeper or infected one with the *naqf* powder. Infected multiple sores were especially common in children with scabies, head lice, or fleas and these were treated by charring a fresh aloe leaflet and then crushing it and applying the powder to the sores. The leaves, when green and swollen after rain, yield a liquid that can be drunk to relieve dehydration, the fleshy side of an opened leaf being placed on the upper stomach to 'cool' it. In the driest areas, goats when very thirsty search out the fleshier leaves to eat, though this can bring on abortion in early pregnancy.

---

usually deposited by the female flies near the nostrils of the sheep or goat. These then live parasitically on exudates in the nasal region and frontal or maxillary sinuses of the host. The fully mature larvae find their way out of the host, generally being sneezed out, to pupate in the soil. The botfly also 'spit' their larvae at humans, in the eye or mucous membranes of the mouth or nose, giving rise to a painful and inflamed eye or a long-standing cough. However, in humans the larvae are not able to develop beyond the first stage (see Wranik, *Fauna*, 397). Soqotran herders take various preventive measures against the fly, such as wearing a face mask (*maʿtímhim*) to cover the nose and mouth, or pulling a corner of the head shawl or beard across the lower face. Sometimes instead charcoal is daubed on the cheeks, chin, and mid-forehead to confuse the fly, and children are warned to avoid such areas at the dangerous times of day, or to cover the mouth and not talk.

35 See above p. 106.

36 See above p. 116.

2.7. *Stem Bark*

Strips of the bark were used on Soqotra to bind a fractured limb, much as frankincense bark was applied on the mainland.[37] The strips were beaten flat and spread out to form a cloth that was used to strap up the limb after setting the fracture. This binding was loosened and re-tied daily until the fracture had knit.[38] A sort of plaster-cast was made by mixing *Ficus* or *Euphorbia* latex with sheep wool or goat hair and laying a layer of this beneath the aloe bark bandage. Some healers instead made a paste by mixing fresh aloe sap with fine red earth that they moulded around the fracture: this set hard and supported the limb, and the sap was said to help it to heal more quickly and to prevent infection. Thick strips of stem bark were also used to support a bad sprain.

2.8. *Dried Aloe Sap*

Dried sap was regarded as more potent than the fresh. Lumps were kept in a small leather pouch, and when needed, a small piece was broken off and rubbed back-and-forth in water until it dissolved. This was the commonest aloe preparation wherever aloe plants were absent or rare.

For some conditions, the dried sap was preferred to the fresh. Thus on the mainland many preferred to treat a painful or purulent ear by applying a paste of the dried material around the ear and pressing a compress of hot cloth soaked in the paste to the ear to soothe the pain and draw the pus. On Soqotra the more potent dried material was used to treat livestock and humans with a distended belly or a swollen liver or spleen. An animal showing signs of a painful abdomen, particularly when tender over the region of the liver or spleen, was treated by smearing the belly and around the anus with reconstituted dried aloe. The same paste was inserted into the nostrils and anus of an animal that was unsteady on its feet and suffering from shivering attacks.

---

37 See above p. 106.

38 Elsewhere in Yemen aloe leaf-gel is applied directly to the site of a fracture to help the bone knit.

3. Fraudulent Augmentation of the Yield of Aloe and Frankincense

Given the commercial importance of the frankincense and aloe harvests to the local communities, it is perhaps not surprising that various means were tried to falsely inflate the yield. In the case of frankincense, harvesters would crush crystalline rocks or geodes and mix the crystals into the heaps of drying, newly-harvested gum. Although it was regarded as acceptable (indeed necessary, to prevent the piles of soft gum from congealing into a single sticky mass) to layer successive days' harvestings of gum with a powder made by crushing a type of soft stone, the unscrupulous would add much more than was necessary to increase the weight of their gum.

Aloe harvesters adulterated the sap to increase its weight by pounding the soft underbark of certain trees (such as *Boswellia* spp., *Commiphora kua*, wild fig (*ṭiḳ*) or *Hibiscus* shrubs (*dərʌ́ffān*) and adding the paste to the goatskins of sap. Others ground up whole aloe leaves to add bulk. These additions, however, interfered with the drying process and the adulterated sap never hardened completely as pure sap does, that in its dried form is rock hard. Less detectable methods were also used, for instance adding fine gravel or sand to the goatskin. Such ingredients became more or less indistinguishable from the sap itself once it had dried. If the sap were to be sold in liquid form, water could be added to the sap to make the skins heavier.

However, all these tricks were only likely to succeed at times of great demand and with an inexperienced buyer, usually someone from outside the growing region, for the local buyers were far too astute.[39] An obvious danger was that such adulterated material could be of harm to the person using it medicinally. That this was a risk recognized by the islanders is shown by their insistence on searching out a pure product from a reputable source for their own use.[40]

39 F.M. Hunter tells of the punishment meted out by the sultan to someone who had tried to trick him in this way, by "pouring the contents of impure aloes over the head of the culprit" ('Notes on Socotra', 367).

40 The same attitude is encountered today with islanders continuing to prefer, for medicinal use, wild honey robbed from bees to that currently being produced by the newly trained bee-keepers, despite the fact that the wild honey is much harder to come by.

4. Aloe and Frankincense in Southern Arabia Today

It might be supposed that in southern Arabia modern medicine, with its surgical intervention and great variety of specifically targeted drugs, would have replaced the trial-and-error 'folk medicine' of earlier times. In practice, however, in much of the region under discussion, modern medicine is expensive, poorly understood, and often misused. It may also not be available at all. So it is not perhaps surprising that an initial enthusiasm for 'modern medicine' has been superseded by a certain scepticism, and that people continue to use inexpensive and well-tried local remedies.[41] Aloe sap, for instance, is still taken as a purge to treat all sorts of illnesses. Indeed, since bodily well-being is held to depend on an internal equilibrium based on a properly functioning digestive system, it is perceived as desirable to eliminate any impurities through regular purging. Consequently many take a little powdered or fresh aloe regularly to cleanse the digestive system. Soqotrans also have a variety of other plants that they can use as a purge in place of aloe, from the mild tamarind fruit (*ḥibílə*) and various sennas (*ferlro*) to the more powerful root of *Euphorbia hadramautica* (*kidídhin*) or the leaves of *Gnidia socotrana*[42] (*ḳiṭəhər* or *lə'éffen*).[43]

Over the last fifty years or so, the island has become increasingly open to outside influence. The expertise of the traditional *mėkóli* healers has been discredited and these practitioners have largely faded from view, along with their old adversaries, the witches. Nor is cauterization as popular with the younger generation. Soqotran émigrés in the Gulf region now come to visit their former island home, and many islanders travel to the mainland as seasonal labourers or in search of further education or medical treatment. In addition many more mainland Yemenis spend time on the islands, and many have made their home there. All of this means that Soqotra's long isolation has now come to an end, and traditional remedies from the Arabian mainland have begun to infiltrate the Soqotran traditional health system, as well as new ideas about how to treat and

[41] That some conditions were recognized as very intractable and resistant to treatment is suggested by the various remedies proposed for someone suffering from *dyaḥś*, a skin condition that attacks the hands of milkers, especially where the skin comes into direct contact with the teats. The following remedies were collected by the author: cauterization (*ṣóḥor*); *Euphorbia arbuscula* latex (*dur d-ímtəhe*); *Euphorbia spiralis* sap (*dur d-ḳə́ššo*); *Euphorbia hadramautica* (*kədídhin*) root crushed directly onto the skin; vulture faeces (*ʿub/ġob d-sɔ̄ʿīdo*); chameleon fat (*śʌbḥ d-məśḥēbihi*); melted dolphin fat (*ṣīfə d-ʿə̄ləho*); imported chemical dye (*ring min rínhem*).

[42] An endemic plant.

[43] On purgative plants, see also Ingrid Hehmeyer's chapter in this volume.

interpret illness. For example, a 'malaria-like' illness was long recognized on the island as recurrent episodes of high fever accompanied by a severe headache. Under overseas influence this is now referred to as '*malāriya*' or, more commonly, '*marāra*,' i.e. 'bitterness' due to the bitter chloroquine used in its prevention and treatment. However, chloroquine is often replaced by bitter aloe—taking it dissolved in water or eating small pieces of fresh aloe leaf. This causes diarrhoea which is said to 'expel the illness.' Nowadays, aloe sap is widely taken, as a remedy and prophylactically, for anaemia—a widespread problem on the island—and to treat diabetes, an increasingly common diagnosis throughout the region. Recently another new treatment making use of aloe has arrived: if the damaged flesh around a fracture has become discoloured and infected, a whole aloe leaf is held at the fire until the fluid it contains begins to bubble and hiss. It is then carefully split in half along its length and strapped around the damaged area, the dressing being replaced daily until the condition improves.

In the new and very popular alternative medicine clinic on Soqotra opened in 2007, Ṭānuf Sālim Di-Kishin prescribes local plants and the different honeys derived from them. Here aloe sap is recommended for treating malaria and diabetes, in addition to its traditional use as a remedy for constipation and other stomach troubles. Mixed with honey it is given as an ointment to treat painful joints, itchy skin, and various other skin conditions. It is particularly recommended to treat patches of skin discoloration including the 'mask of pregnancy' (chloasma), where areas of skin on the face darken, or the depigmentation of vitiligo. Patients are also advised to rub fresh aloe sap on open sores and wounds to prevent infection and encourage healing, and to massage it into the lower limbs to treat feebleness and loss of strength. So there is still a demand for aloe in southern Arabia, and especially for the Soqotran product, and the plant continues to be harvested today.

As for frankincense gum, on Soqotra, with the collapse of the *mékóli* healing system and the weakening of the belief that frankincense smoke can repel evil, it is of even less importance than it was before, though some is gathered for tourists and visitors to buy. The islanders are bemused by the number of (mainly Arab) visitors who come to the island to scour it for the fabled *lubān dhikr*, 'male frankincense,'[44] for any news of which they are prepared to offer surprisingly large sums.[45] Not only is this gum

44 See also Schönig, *Schminken*, 166.

45 One enthusiast even pursued me with phone calls to Scotland, later turning up in person, keen to see the various types of frankincense I have collected over the years out of

believed to possess exceptional curative properties, but also, and possibly more importantly, to be a powerful aphrodisiac. Word has spread about Soqotra being home to an astounding number of unique plant species (over a third of its plants are endemic, a major factor in the recognition of the island by UNESCO in 2008 as a World Heritage Site).[46] This, coupled with the island's ancient reputation as a place of magic and sorcery, has encouraged many to visit the island in the hopes of discovering some new cure-all plant which will make their fortune.

On the mainland, frankincense gum continued to be harvested in a small way in Dhofar, principally by Somali labour,[47] until immigrant harvesting of frankincense trees was banned. These days little is gathered: it is hot, tiring, and not particularly profitable work for today's Omanis, and ironically most of the gum sold in the local markets is imported from Somalia. However, in 2000, part of Dhofar too was officially declared a UNESCO World Heritage Site: "The Land of Frankincense."[48] Now 'natural parks' of frankincense trees are being planted, one at Wādī Dawka and another at Wādī Danūn, as part of the 'Frankincense Trail,' and a new museum, costing many millions of dollars, has been opened in Ṣalāla, specially dedicated to this famous plant. Omani frankincense gum is exported worldwide and is burned in the international hotels of the region. A new and very expensive frankincense perfume—'Amouage' ('Waves')—has been developed, whose unique bottles sell at the very upper end of the market. The Amouage website states: "Amouage is a niche luxury fragrance house that draws inspiration from its birthplace of the Sultanate of Oman, infusing reference points from a rich and colorful heritage that fires the imagination of all who come into contact with its wonderful products."[49]

Smoking frankincense gum is still offered hospitably to guests at the conclusion of a meal in Dhofar, and its smoke still perfumes houses and mosques. Otherwise, here as on Soqotra, the trees are largely left to the

---

curiosity. He promised me huge sums if I were to tell him which tree produced *lubān dhikr*. Although I insisted that I knew nothing about this, and offered him samples from my collection to take and test, this only seemed to make him suspicious that I was somehow hiding something.

[46] See <http://www.worldheritagesite.org/sites/socotra.html>.

[47] Somalis have long made the journey to Yemen and Dhofar to work as seasonal labourers harvesting frankincense.

[48] See <http://whc.unesco.org/en/list/1010>.

[49] See <http://www.amouage.com>.

bees, to the browsing camels and goats,[50] and to the increasing number of tourists.

Bibliography

Balfour, Bayley I., *Botany of Socotra* (Transactions of the Royal Society of Edinburgh, 31; Edinburgh: Robert Grant and Son, London: Williams and Norgate, 1888).

Camelin, Sylvaine, 'À ash-Shiḥr, au Pays de l'encens', *Saba*, 2 : *Aromates & senteurs du Yémen* (1994), 21–3.

Christie, S.J., Dutton, R.W., Oakman, N.A., and Hannon, D.P., 'Sustainable Use of Natural Resources on Soqotra: An Aloe Case Study', *Proceedings: The Second International Symposium on the Developing Strategy of Socotra Archipelago and Other Yemeni Islands*, 2 (2003), 45–62.

Grindlay, D., and Reynolds, T., 'The *Aloe vera* Phenomenon: A Review of the Properties and Modern Uses of the Leaf Parcenchyma Gel', *Journal of Ethnopharmacology*, 16 (1986), 117–51.

Hunter, F.M., 'Notes on Socotra', *Journal of the Royal Anthropological Institute*, 7 (1878), 364–72.

Miller, Anthony G., and Morris, Miranda, *Plants of Dhofar, The Southern Region of Oman: Traditional, Economic and Medicinal Uses* (Sultanate of Oman: The Office of the Adviser for Conservation of the Environment, Diwan of the Royal Court, 1988).

———, and Morris, Miranda, *Ethnoflora of the Soqotra Archipelago* (Edinburgh: Royal Botanic Garden, 2004).

Morris, Miranda, 'The Harvesting of Frankincense in Dhofar, Oman', in Alessandra Avanzini (ed.), *Profumi d'Arabia, atti del convegno* (Saggi Di Storia Antica, 11; Rome: "L'Erma" di Bretschneider, 1997), 231–47.

———, 'The Soqotra Archipelago: Concepts of Good Health and Everyday Remedies for Illness', *Proceedings of the Seminar for Arabian Studies*, 33 (2003), 319–41.

Schönig, Hanne, *Schminken, Düfte und Räucherwerk der Jemenitinnen: Lexikon der Substanzen, Utensilien und Techniken* (Beiruter Texte und Studien, 91; Würzburg: Ergon, 2002).

Wranik, W. (ed.), *Fauna of the Socotra Archipelago: Field Guide* (Rostock: Universitätsdruckerei, 2004).

Internet Sources

Hunter, F.M., 'Notes on Socotra', *Journal of the Royal Anthropological Institute*, 7 (1878), 364–72 <http://www.jstor.org/stable/2841012?seq=1>.

Niebuhr, M. [Carsten]/Heron, Robert (trans.), *Travels Through Arabia and Other Countries in the East*, 2 (Edinburgh: R. Morison and Son, 1792) <http://books.google.de/books?id=4Zk4AAAAMAAJ&printsec=frontcover&dq=carsten+niebuhr+travels&source=bl&ots=28ukBq65TB&sig=mwvegK-7BlCglgy2hKIzJbdF-qo&hl=de&ei=4oaXS47ECouqsQa5wLzYCQ&sa=X&oi=book_result&ct=result&resnum=1&ved=0CAYQ6AEwAA#v=onepage&q=&f=false>, accessed 16 March 2010.

<http://www.worldheritagesite.org/sites/socotra.html>, accessed 21 January 2010.

<http://www.amouage.com>, accessed 24 January 2010.

<http://whc.unesco.org/en/list/1010>, accessed 21 January 2010.

[50] The hungry camel is especially destructive in its browsing, and on the mainland, where the pressure of camel numbers is high and natural grazing increasingly limited, there are fears that frankincense trees are being damaged by overgrazing.

Further Reading

Banti, Giorgio, and Contini, Ricardo, 'Names of Aromata in Semitic and Cushitic Languages', in Alessandra Avanzini (ed.), *Profumi d'Arabia, atti del convegno* (Saggi Di Storia Antica 11; Rome: "L'Erma" di Bretschneider, 1997), 169–92.

Cheung, C., and DeVantier, L., Science Editor Van Damme, K., *Socotra: A Natural History of the Islands and Their People* (Hong Kong: Odyssey Books and Guides, 2006).

Fleurentin, Jacques, and Pelt, Jean-Marie, 'Repertory of Drugs and Medicinal Plants of Yemen', *Journal of Ethnopharmacology*, 6 (1982), 85–108.

———, 'Cultural Background of the Medicinal Plants of Yemen', *Journal of Ethnopharmacology*, 7 (1983), 183–203.

———, 'Additional Information for a Repertory of Drugs and Medicinal Plants of Yemen', *Journal of Ethnopharmacology*, 8 (1983), 237–43.

Groom, Nigel, *Frankincense and Myrrh: A Study of the Arabian Incense Trade* (London: Longman, 1981).

Miller, Anthony G., and Morris, Miranda, *Conservation and Sustainable Use of the Biodiversity of the Soqotra Archipelago* (unpublished final report: Global Environment Facility YEM/96/G32, Edinburgh: Royal Botanic Garden, 2001).

Morris, M., 'Dhofar: What Made it Different', in B.R. Pridham (ed.), *Oman: Economic, Social and Strategic Developments* (London: Croom Helm, 1987), 51–78.

———, 'Plant Names in Dhofar and the Soqotra Archipelago', *PSAS*, 32 (2002), 47–61.

Muchawsky-Schnapper, Ester, 'The Use of Incense by Yemenite Jews', *Tema, Journal of Judeo-Yemenite Studies*, 6 (1998), III–XXX.

Müller, Walter W., 'Notes on the Use of Frankincense in South Arabia', *PSAS*, 6 (1976), 124–36.

———, 'Weihrauch', *Paulys Realencyclopädie der Classischen Altertumswissenschaft* (Suppl. 15; Munich: Druckenmüller, 1978), 700–77.

PSAS = *Proceedings of the Seminar for Arabian Studies.*

Rodionov, Mikhail, 'Field Data on Folk Medicine from the Ḥaḍramawt', *PSAS*, 26 (1996), 125–33.

Schopen, Armin, *Traditionelle Heilmittel in Jemen* (Wiesbaden: Steiner, 1983).

Serjeant, R.B., 'Folk-Remedies from Ḥaḍramawt', *Bulletin of the School of Oriental and African Studies*, 18 (1956), 5–8.

Simeone-Senelle, Marie-Claude, 'Aloe and Dragon's Blood, some Medicinal and Traditional Uses on the Island of Socotra', *New Arabian Studies*, 2 (1994), 186–98.

———, 'Suqutra : Parfums, sucs et résines', *Saba*, 2 : *Aromates & senteurs du Yémen* (1994), 9–17.

———, 'Magie et pratiques thérapeutiques dans l'îsle de Soqotra : Le médecin-guérisseur', *PSAS*, 25 (1995), 117–26.

———, 'Enquête au pays de l'encens, de l'aloès et du sang-dragon sur les langues sudarabiques modernes. 1. Au pays de l'encens—Le mehri', *Le gré des Langues*, 15 (1999), 58–71.

HEALING THROUGH MEDICINAL PLANTS: OLD YEMENITE THERAPEUTIC TRADITIONS AND THEIR APPLICATION IN JERUSALEM TODAY[1]

Ester Muchawsky-Schnapper

Pre-modern, traditional societies tend to heal illness, whether physical or mental, through natural products such as herbs, fruits, seeds, and resins, employing various forms and techniques. This is their only option. Such an approach was common in Yemen right up to the middle of the twentieth century, due to the near-absence of Western medicine. This paper gives an overview of the kinds of medicinal treatments practised by Jews in Yemen before their mass-immigration to Israel around 1950, and then describes which of the old customs can still be observed today. The data are based on interviews conducted in Israel since the early 1980s and in particular in preparation of this essay.

In modern Israel, where conventional medicine is *de rigueur*, some of the old-generation Yemenites who had brought seedlings and plants with them from Yemen when immigrating—as well as second-generation Yemenites—still practise traditional ways of healing, although some of the old methods are being progressively abandoned.

Today many people look for different ways of procuring health when conventional medicine fails. This is certainly the case for patients of Yemenite origin who prefer their familiar healing methods, but also for others who follow the contemporary trend of alternative or complementary medicine. What characterizes these methods is a holistic approach that looks at body and mind as a unit, not only at the place of affliction in isolation. This differs from modern medicine where hyper-specialization is the trend.

It is not my intention to elaborate on the ethnopharmacological and botanical aspects of the plants themselves since there has been significant research in Israel resulting in publications by Zohar Amar, Zecharia Dori, Efraim Lev, Zecharia Madar and Yocheved Raiany, and others.[2] In Raiany's

---

[1] The Hebrew transliteration follows Brill guidelines: <http://www.brill.nl/default.aspx?partid=162>.

[2] Dori, *Traditional Medicine*; Madar and Raiany, *Nutrition and Popular Remedy*; Lev and Amar, *Ethnic Medicinal Substances*; Lev, *Medicinal Substances*; see Efraim Lev's chapter in this volume.

pharmacological dissertation on Yemenite popular medicine, there are 219 examples of remedies quoted, 157 of them being various plants, the rest animal and mineral materials.[3] The medicinal efficacy of some of the plants has been analyzed by Prof. Zecharia Madar and Dr. Avinoam Tzabari.[4] While the focus of this paper is on medicinal plants in connection to Yemenite Jews, much work has been done on these subjects in a general Yemenite context.[5]

An important aspect should be singled out at this point and that is the existence of additional ways of healing practised by Yemenites, namely the ones having a 'magical' dimension that is often inseparable from the administration of herbal remedies.[6] Purely magical treatments such as writing amulets, preparing talismans or talismanic jewellery, or concocting magical potions that have the aim to influence others psychologically—like making one person love another or hurting a hated person—will not be dealt with here, although these methods constitute a fascinating subject in themselves.[7] Some of them enter the category of what Erich Brauer in his monograph on the ethnology of the Yemenite Jews called "black magic."[8] Magical treatment is not in the strict sense medicinal healing, although a healer using plants and herbs can concomitantly also employ these in 'magical' ways of treatment.

In the Israel Museum's Yemenite collection assembled by the German ethnographer Carl Rathjens in the 1930s and 1940s, there are examples of plants and other substances for medical use. Samples of incense, salt, fennel, senna, fenugreek seeds, and others were collected by Rathjens side by side with amulets and magic bowls[9] (which he significantly calls "Arzneischalen," i.e. medicinal bowls), all with the aim of curing illness.[10]

---

[3] Raiany, *Medicinal Drugs.*

[4] See below n. 43.

[5] E.g. Fleurentin, *Guérisseurs*; Martinez, Lohs, and Janzen, *Weihrauch und Myrrhe*, 125–51; Schönig, *Schminken*; Varisco, 'Arzneikunde'; Schopen, *Heilmittel.*

[6] For the methodological problems in this kind of research, see Matras, 'Ethnobotany and Folklore'.

[7] Brauer, *Ethnologie*, 387–8. For magic in Yemen in a general context, see Regourd, 'Transmission des sciences occultes'.

[8] Brauer, *Ethnologie*, 367–70, 387–8.

[9] See e.g. Canova, 'La *ṭāsat al-ism*'; Regourd, 'Deux coupes magiques'.

[10] Carl Rathjens was sent to Yemen on a mission by the Museum für Völkerkunde in Hamburg. There, he collected Muslim and Jewish material culture. Part of the collection was bought by Salman Schocken before WWII and later transferred to the Israel Museum; the remaining pieces are still in the Hamburg Museum.

1. Medical Treatments Practised in Yemen's Jewish Communities up to the Mid-twentieth Century

From Yemenite-Jewish records we can deduce that there were few Western physicians in Ṣan'ā' in the first half of the twentieth century. Frequently mentioned are an English and an Italian doctor, each having a clinic in Ṣan'ā'. Patients were treated there according to the European standards of the time. We know of a Jewish medical assistant by the name of Yiḥye Ḥaybi who worked in the Italian doctor's clinic in the 1930s and 1940s and became famous later for his photography.[11] He earned enough knowledge to give certain modern treatments like injections to members of his community in the Jewish ghetto of Ṣan'ā', the Gā'a al-Yahūd.

However, after interviews with many Yemenites who lived there at the time it became clear that one went to such Western doctors very rarely—usually when it was already too late. It was explained to me that they were afraid, and doubted the benevolent intentions of these doctors towards them. They preferred to seek help from healers within their own community, which happened to be in most cases the rabbi, called in Yemen *mori*.[12]

It has to be noted that before the middle of the twentieth century life expectancy was very low in Yemen,[13] and approximately 60% of children died as infants or in the first years of life, as I deduced from numerous interviews with Yemenite families.[14] Many women died in childbirth, yet what caused these early deaths has rarely been identified.

While Yomtob Sémach, a representative of the Alliance Israélite Universelle in Yemen, wrote in 1910[15] that there were many charlatans in this field—"les charlatans de toutes catégories sont nombreux dans tout le pays"—it cannot be said that that was always the case. There were also serious individuals who practised their profession according to old medical books and personal experience, as for instance the renowned seventeenth-century Jewish poet Mori Salim (Shalom) Shabazi from Ta'izz, and more recently Mori Yiḥye Qafiḥ and Mori Yiḥye al-Abyadh from Ṣan'ā',

---

[11] Muchawsky-Schnapper, 'Rare Photographs'.

[12] This oral information regarding the distrust of real physicians is confirmed by Sémach, *Mission*, 100, where he writes that a medical doctor was called by the Jews in Yemen 'tueur de malades,' i.e. killer of sick people, probably because when called to a patient, it was usually too late.

[13] According to the World Development Indicators of the World Bank, life expectancy in Yemen today is approximately 63 years. In 1960, it was slightly under 40 years.

[14] See also Brauer, *Ethnologie*, 180.

[15] Sémach, *Mission*, 98.

who both lived at the end of the nineteenth and the beginning of the twentieth century.

Mori al-Abyadh, who besides being a rabbi was also a famous silversmith working for the imam,[16] is still remembered and praised by my informants as having been very knowledgeable in medical matters. I was told that he gave, for instance, a specially prepared potent wine to women who had difficulties during childbirth.[17] Such strong wine may have increased blood circulation and as a consequence quickened the process of giving birth. In addition, it may have numbed the pain in the childbearing woman, but no doubt the mental conviction of the wine's efficacy—because of its provenance from the admired rabbi—played an important role. He, on the other hand, may have drawn his knowledge about the medicinal use of wine from the Babylonian Talmud: "At the head of all medicine am I, wine. Only where there is no wine are drugs required."[18]

An important factor to note is that, in Yemen, Jews were often accredited by Muslims with special knowledge in healing methods. They were believed to possess age-old secrets harking back to pre-Islamic, biblical times. This notion was reinforced by the respect felt towards Jews for being (like Christians) a People of the Book (*ahl al-kitāb*),[19] recognized as having *ergo ipso* special knowledge derived from these books. Muslims knew that Jews had books and Torah scrolls in Hebrew that they themselves could not read and in which they suspected hidden wisdoms.[20] The principle of going to healers and magicians of another religion or culture works both ways—each group visiting the other. It underlines the widespread phenomenon of attributing healing secrets and magic powers to another culture, imbuing the unknown 'other' with special supernatural qualities.[21] One can frequently observe that minorities and foreigners are credited with having such qualities. For instance, the Jews in Ṣanʿā' used to dress their children and brides with attributes usually only worn there by Muslims,[22] believing that in that way they would enjoy greater protection.

---

[16] About his craft, and for photographs of Mori al-Abyadh, see Muchawsky-Schnapper, 'An Exceptional Type of Yemeni Necklace', 188–91.

[17] Ead., 'Symbolic Decorations', 62–3.

[18] Baba Bathra 58b (Broshi, 'Wine in Ancient Palestine', 34).

[19] 'People of the Book' are people (such as Jews and Christians) who have received divine guidance in the form of scriptures (see Esposito, *The Oxford Dictionary of Islam*, 10).

[20] It was also known that all male Jews were literate. This was not the case with Muslims at the time.

[21] Eraqi-Klorman, 'Yemen: Religion, Magic, and Jews'.

[22] Muchawsky-Schnapper, 'Children's Attire', 354.

This seems also to have been the reason why Jews practised the profession of jewellery-making in Yemen and other Muslim countries. Since jewellery always had talismanic qualities, these were believed to be enhanced if made by foreigners because of the magic powers attributed to them.[23]

We know that Jews also used to look to Muslim healers for advice in matters of health through the work of Mori Salim Shabazi, the seventeenth-century poet, rabbi, and Kabbalist who quotes the superior knowledge of the 'sages of Arabia' and decided to become a healer in order to circumvent the habit of Jews going to Arab 'magicians.' He developed healing methods of a magical nature based on practical Kabbala like the Book of Raziel the Angel, a medieval Kabbalistic book with many recipes for healing. As a reaction to sand-magic, Salim Shabazi wrote *Sefer ha-ḥol* [The Sand-Book; Arab.: Kitāb al-Raml] in which he describes medicinal solutions reached through drawing with a stick in the sand.[24]

Additional insight into the use of medicinal practices employed by the Jews of Yemen in the first part of the twentieth century comes from Rabbi Salim (Shalom) ben Saʿadya Gamliel (d. 2001) who in his recollections dedicates two chapters to the nutrition and medicine of the Jews of Yemen.[25] In Ṣanʿāʾ, he had been responsible for the Jewish community vis-à-vis the imam, collecting the head-tax (*jizya*) for him and becoming his personal adviser, some even say his friend. According to Rabbi Gamliel, the health of the Jews in Yemen was at a high level because of a healthy diet with little consumption of fat and sugar, something that has changed drastically in Israel, leading to a significant rise in coronary diseases and diabetes. Furthermore, the rabbi writes that the fact people drank *qishr*, prepared from coffee husks and not from the beans, helped avoid kidney stones and arteriosclerosis. *Qishr* still belongs in the medicinal repertoire of the modern-day Yemenite healer.[26] Rabbi Gamliel also mentions the beneficial effects of strong physical work, the drinking of fresh water, and anointing the body regularly with oil (mostly sesame oil)—a custom

---

23 Ead., 'Les bijoux du Yémen'.

24 Brauer, *Ethnologie*, 348–62, 367–70, 379–84, 387–8. Generally speaking, geomancy is considered in Yemen, both today and in the past, as one of the most accurate sciences in regards to matters of daily life as well as to diagnosing sickness, see Regourd, 'Pratiques de géomancie au Yémen'.

25 Gamliel, 'A Gateway', XV–XVII (English section).

26 See below when discussing modern-day healers.

adopted from the Book of Ruth (3:3), where washing and anointing is advised.[27]

Rabbi Gamliel praises in his book the wisdom of Rabbi Yiḥye al-Abyadh who bought all the ingredients necessary for his medicines in the Sūq al-'aṭṭārīn (spice market). Besides 'inherited wisdom,' Rabbi al-Abyadh apparently also knew the medical books of Maimonides.[28] Rabbi Gamliel, who knew the imam personally, points out that Imam Yaḥyā by far preferred Mori al-Abyadh's medications to those administered by doctors who were specifically brought to Yemen from Europe to treat him.

Another source for medical procedures as practised by Yemenite Jews is Moshe Zadoc's personal account of his community's customs.[29] In the chapter entitled "Medicaments" there is only a short passage about Yemenite doctors using spices and herbs. He elaborates on two other ways of therapy involving cutting or burning the skin.[30]

Zadoc makes a distinction between women's and men's approaches to healing, thinking that men relied more on religion and prayers, while women were more superstitious, and preferred to use magical ways to eliminate disease they believed to have been caused by the evil eye. In one example of such a method, called *nakas*, the evil eye is expelled by burning salt in an open fire at the entrance of the home of the affected person, or by burning a piece of clothing belonging to the person suspected of having cast the evil spell. However, Zadoc's theory of attributing magical practices only to women seems unconvincing, especially in the light of Maimonides' prescriptions (often used by healers) that are in many instances of a 'magical' nature.

Much information on medicinal healing in Yemen is given in the recollections of the late Rabbi Yosef Qafiḥ (d. 2000), a renowned Maimonides-interpreter and grandson of the astronomer and healer, Rabbi Yiḥye Qafiḥ. Like his grandfather, who was the founder of the enlightened rationalist movement in Yemen at the end of the nineteenth century and who prea-

---

[27] According to my informants, anointing the body was practised by Yemenites until recently. One such example is the daily massaging of a baby with *samn* (clarified butter), believed to protect the child and avoid dryness of skin. Another example is massaging the stomach of a mother after childbirth to counteract the stretching of the skin caused by pregnancy (stretch-marks) and to avoid dryness of the skin resulting from binding the stomach for a few weeks after birth, which is practised to prevent sagging. These methods are still highly regarded by elderly Yemenite women. However, with the increasing pull towards modern medicine, these treatments are on the decline.

[28] Gamliel, 'A Gateway', XVI (English section).

[29] Zadoc, *History*, 158–60.

[30] See below n. 33.

ched against superstitions and Kabbala, he continued to expound rationalist ideas after immigrating to Palestine in 1943. In his memories on Jewish life in Ṣan'ā',[31] he writes—surprisingly in the same chapter in which he elaborates on medicaments—about amulets and superstitions, despite the fact that he himself was an advocate of rational thought, thus showing how closely related these topics were in Yemen. He writes that in his time there were only a few Jewish and Arab healers in Ṣan'ā' where he grew up, each one specializing in certain diseases. Their knowledge was based on old books and personal experience, and they prepared the medications from herbs grown by themselves. Their written sources of information were the medical books of Maimonides and the book *al-Wajīz* [The summary] by Rabbi Yiḥye al-Ṭabīb, called in Jewish sources Zekharya ha-Rofe ('the doctor'), who wrote philosophical and medical treatises in the fifteenth century. These and other sources were part of the private library of Rabbi Qafiḥ in Jerusalem.[32] He too writes that most of these "natural doctors" believed in two effective methods of healing not involving the use of herbs—namely cutting and cauterization.[33] In addition he states that other doctors employed natural herbal medications and prescribed their intake in connection with astronomical phenomena, a practice—so he says—already promoted by Ya'qūb b. Isḥāq al-Kindī, the early ninth-century Iraqi physician and astrologer.[34] Rabbi Qafiḥ also gives examples of how Yemenites used to protect their health through following a diet to

---

31 Qafiḥ, *Jewish Life*, 267–8.

32 Arab books of medicine are quoted by Rabbi Qafiḥ, ibid., 267, for example *Zād al-musāfir* [Provisions for the traveller] by Abū Ja'far Aḥmad b. Abī Khālid Ibn al-Jazzār (d. 1004/5).

33 These two Yemenite treatments should be included in this essay, though they are not connected to plants. They were used against fear, shock, worry, and trauma, so all informants told me, and were also mentioned in the book of Moshe Zadoc. The first involved making a 1 to 2 cm long incision on a person's back called *al-fushta*, or *fasht*. Some blood was drawn from the wound and it was then quickly closed with cold water. All fears were said to disappear immediately. It may be compared to the shock therapy used even today in psychiatric hospitals. In very serious cases where the fears were accompanied by depression, a stronger traumatic treatment was applied called *al-makwā*, where the skin was burned above the navel with a heated ironnail. The wound was then quickly closed with oil-covered leaves. Both methods, previously administered by Maimonides, were widely practised until ten to twenty years ago by Yemenite immigrants, but are now gradually being abandoned. They are still practised by Ethiopian, Bedouin, and Druze communities in Israel. A modern scientific explanation is that by inflicting a wound on the body in this dramatic way, antibodies are activated and start attacking the patient's ailments, be they physical or mental. Another interpretation explains these methods by comparing them to acupuncture, where needles are placed at certain important meridians of the body.

34 Qafiḥ, *Jewish Life*, 268, n. 30. See Petra Schmidl's chapter in this volume.

prevent illness. Most of his advice is related to the gall bladder, which may indicate that this organ frequently caused medical problems. For instance, he recommends that patients should eat almonds and bananas at late hours of the day in order to protect the gall bladder, and should reduce the intake of carrot cores and pomegranates. He also cautions against eating sweets, to avoid worms.

2. Present-day Yemenite Healing Methods in Israel

When analyzing Yemenite methods of healing used today in Israel, we encounter two kinds of healers. There are the older-generation so-called 'wise' women and men who grew up in Yemen and who use solely traditional Yemenite healing methods. They neither refer to themselves as 'healers,' nor put themselves into any of the modern-day categories. For them, it is not a profession but a God-given talent. Their knowledge is not advertised, but is made known by word-of-mouth. This group is dwindling as that generation dies out.

In the other category are what we might call 'modern Yemenite healers' who grew up in Israel and use eclectic methods, i.e. besides the Yemeni recipes they also borrow from non-Yemenite alternative (or complementary) medicine. In this category belongs the son of Rabbi Yosef Qafiḥ, David Qafiḥ, who grew up in Jerusalem where he works as an alternative healer.[35] Only part of his methodology is Yemenite, with the rest being a combination of various alternative healing methods typical for second-generation 'modern' Yemenite healers.[36]

We will focus only on the traditional Yemenite healing methods, as used by older-generation Yemenites who have learned them by the traditional manner of oral transmission from family members—treasured as family secrets through generations. David Qafiḥ, who is convinced that the capacity to heal runs in his family, defines these talents as 'genetic.'

All the healers whom I interviewed stressed as a first rule that body and mind have to be treated as one unit, a principle already held by the revered Maimonides (and before him by the Greek physician Hippocrates, d. *c.*370 BCE, who incidentally was not known to Yemenite Jews but was probably well-known to Maimonides). The healers are furthermore con-

[35] Qafiḥ, 'Yemenite Tradition'; id., *Natural.* I would like to express my thanks to David Qafiḥ for sharing his vast knowledge with me.

[36] See also Mizraḥi, *Mor u-Levona*, 331–8, 351, 363–80. Id. and Gundrass, 'Scientific Analysis'.

vinced that the natural forces in the patient have to be activated, and that the belief and trust of the patient in the capacity of the healer constitutes half of the treatment's success.

Many Yemenite herbs and plants traditionally used medicinally are still prescribed as medicinal treatment on their own or in concoctions today. It should suffice in the framework of this chapter to give an overview of the most prominent and popular medications still in use. A plant associated today in Israel with Yemenites is the *shadhāb* (Yemeni Arabic; Latin: *Ruta graveolens*), called in English 'common rue' or 'herb-of-grace'—a shrub with green delicate leaves and a strong, unique aroma believed to ward off the evil eye, and therefore considered to be a prophylactic medicine. For this reason it is used profusely in Yemenite homes where it is grown in pots in the garden, on the balcony, or on the window sill. After being cut, it is put into vases inside the house. A visitor entering a Yemenite home is enveloped by its unmistakable and all-pervasive aroma. *Shadhāb* is still included as a protective agent in a Yemenite bride's apparel.[37]

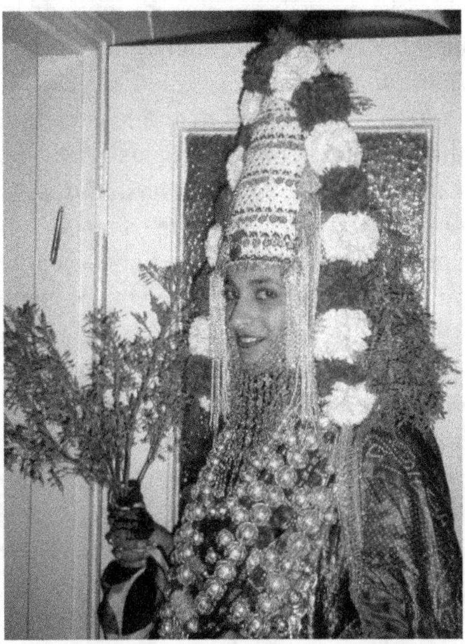

Figure 1. Yemenite Jewish bride in bridal apparel, holding a sprig of *shadhāb*, and with *shadhāb* tucked in the back of her head-apparel, Jerusalem 1980 (© Ester Muchawsky-Schnapper)

[37] For photos of rue on bride and bridegroom in Ṣan'ā', see Muchawsky-Schnapper, *The Yemenites*, 92–5.

Furthermore, it used to be an integral part of a room that was prepared festively for a woman after childbirth. It was placed in several vases on a shelf so that the room would be infused with its intense smell, to keep away evil spirits. However, the custom of preparing such a room is disappearing.[38]

Occasionally, a sprig of *shadhāb* is tucked into a baby's head covering or into its crib to give the child protection from the evil eye, but this custom, which is very common in Yemen, can be observed in Israel only in agricultural communities with a high concentration of Yemenites. Another aspect is rue's proven efficacy as an insect repellent, which makes it useful in a warm climate. As a Yemenite herbal remedy, David Qafiḥ cooks it for half an hour in oil, after which it apparently produces efficient anti-inflammatory eardrops.

Until recently a brew called *qahwat al-ṣufur* ('jaundice-drink'),[39] made of *Retama raetam* (Latin; Arabic: *ratam*, Hebrew: *rotem ha-midbar*, English: 'white weeping broom'), served as a remedy for hepatitis. A desert plant, *Retama raetam* is resistant to drought conditions and is poisonous when not applied properly. A Yemenite woman from Jerusalem, originally from Ṣanʿā', the late Shoshana Badiḥi bint-Cohen, worked all her life in a very discreet way as a healer.[40] She used to go regularly to hospitals to bring tea made from this plant for hepatitis patients (she had brought seedlings with her when she immigrated to Palestine in the early 1940s). She grew the plant in her garden, together with rue (*shadhāb*) and basil (*rayḥān*). All Yemenites knew about her and called her when necessary, but few knew how she prepared the drink. She called the straw-like plant in short *ṣfar* (i.e. *aṣfar* = yellow), which indicates a belief in sympathetic magic, namely fighting jaundice with a similarly yellow 'weapon.' She advised those with hepatitis to drink half a cup in the morning and half in the evening. Her family, she told me, was famous for knowing medicinal recipes. She insisted that this plant had been brought 2,000 years ago from the Land of Israel to Yemen. This is not a surprising claim, as in other cases, in order to prove the antiquity and legitimacy of a treatment or item, its ancient origin in the Holy Land is stressed by Yemenite Jews. In the case of *Retama raetam*, the plant grows in Israel, and is believed to be the

---

[38] For a reconstruction of a new mother's room including bunches of rue, see ibid., 58–9.

[39] Qafiḥ, *Natural*, 247.

[40] Shoshana Badiḥi bint-Cohen was one of my most reliable, patient, and generous informants who allowed me to learn from her precious knowledge over many years. I will always be grateful to her.

juniper of the Bible (I Kings 19:4–5, where it is called in the Hebrew singular *rotem*, and Job 30:4, in the plural *retamim*).[41]

David Qafiḥ, who treated hepatitis patients with the same boiled infusion, eventually stopped using this plant, fearful of a wrong dosage that could poison the patient. An anecdote illustrates the reason for his worry. He was called by the emergency ward of a Jerusalem hospital about a baby, seven days old, who was hardly breathing and blue. It turned out that the father had given the baby ten drops of this plant-concentrate instead of the correct single drop, in order to treat the baby's (common) neo-natal jaundice. The father wanted to make sure that the child would be healthy in time for its circumcision, that traditionally takes place on the eighth day after birth. He had received the drops from an old Yemenite woman who had specifically told him to give only one drop, the dosage that had healed many babies in the past. After David Qafiḥ alerted the doctors about the plant which must have caused the baby's critical condition, they pumped his stomach and saved his life.[42]

A common plant in Yemenite cuisine is *ḥilba* or fenugreek (*Trigonella foenum-graecum*), used as a key ingredient of a sauce added to soup and meat, or just as an additional dish in which one dips pita bread. *Ḥilba*, however, according to research carried out by Prof. Zecharia Madar and Dr. Avinoam Tzabari,[43] is also known as a remedy for diabetes, especially diabetes occurring during pregnancy. Large quantities have to be taken

---

[41] However, this does not mean that the plant was introduced in antiquity from Eretz Israel to Yemen, since it is indigenous to Yemen as well. It is a known phenomenon that immigrants take with them what is most important to them, be it simple household objects, food, or medicinal plants, even if there is a good chance of finding such things in the new place.

[42] For curing hepatitis, Yemenites have yet another custom known by all but not much talked about. Live doves are held firmly onto the sick person's stomach, placing the dove's anus on the umbilicus of the patient. The dove then exerts suction and starts rhythmically pulsating until it dies. I was told that between seven and fifteen doves are sometimes necessary to lower the bilirubin-level in the blood of the person with hepatitis. Male doves are used for men, and female doves for women. This method is of course not recognized by conventional medicine, but is firmly believed to be effective by most Yemenites I interviewed. When doctors allow this practice in the hospital (not in all hospitals), I was told that they do it out of respect for the patient's belief, and for the possibly positive response it may trigger. This healing custom of transferring a person's disease to a bird who has to die for it brings to mind the idea of scapegoat-sacrifice, a custom (not a religious duty) practised the day before Yom Kippur (Day of Atonement) when one's sins are symbolically transferred to a fowl (rooster for males and hen for females) that in Hebrew is called *kapparot*.

[43] Madar et al., 'Glucose-lowering Effect'. Arad, Abel, and Madar, 'Fenugreek'; Tzabari et al., 'The Effect of Fenugreek Seeds'.

in order to be effective, and therefore *ḥilba* is also produced in the form of a pill. The negative side effect patients complain about is the odour of the *ḥilba* emanating from urine and perspiration after consumption.[44] *Ḥilba* can also be used as a cream for eczema, and is smeared on the breast of mothers who want to stop breast-feeding.

One of the most widely advertised remedies in David Qafiḥ's list of beneficial plants is *qishr*, a beverage made from coffee husks and one that is still the regular drink of most older-generation Yemenites in Israel who do not drink coffee made from beans. In Yemen, he says, people did not suffer from kidney stones as *qishr* prevented the formation of calcium oxalate crystals, the most common type of kidney stone. He advises drinking at least three to four cups of *qishr* a day to prevent this condition as well as infections of the urinary tract.

Kurkum (*Curcuma longa*), known today in the West as a potent antioxidant against cancer,[45] is one of the ingredients of the spice-cocktail called *ḥawāyij* that Yemenites like to add to *qishr*; it also includes *qirfa* (cinnamon) and *zanjabīl* (ginger). Drinking *qishr* with a full teaspoon of *ḥawāyij* is believed to cure digestive problems, depression, and supposedly strengthens the body against disease.

Murr (myrrh, *Commiphora myrrha*) and *lubān* (frankincense, *Boswellia sacra*)[46] are resinous substances originating in Yemen and Somalia that are used frequently in Yemen. In Israel they can be bought in most open-air food markets and are still popular as incense (*bukhūr*) at Yemenite festive occasions like weddings. Before the onset of the Sabbath they are burned to purify the home: spiritually from evil spirits and physically from insects. A certain kind of *lubān*, called *muṣṭakā sulṭānī*, is chewed to cure stomach ache. When *lubān* is administered as a drink after it has been soaked overnight in water, it is believed to cure urinary tract infections. *Lubān* added to hot water has been compared by one informant to taking an aspirin for a headache.

Myrrh incense is believed, because of its bitter odour, to repel evil spirits and is therefore called *ḥijāb* (Arab.: amulet). It is sometimes still applied during the post-partum period. It is also said to possess medicinal properties. For example, a Jerusalem healer used to advise women to squat over

---

[44] I referred a colleague who got diabetes when pregnant with twins to a healer who prepared large amounts of *ḥilba* sauce for her that did, indeed, succeed in lowering her blood sugar level.

[45] Servan-Schreiber, *Anticancer*, 173–6.

[46] See Muchawsky-Schnapper, 'The Use of Incense', III–XXX; Brauer, *Ethnologie*, 182.

the hot fumes of *murr bukhūr* after childbirth so that the uterus would retract to its original form. In Yemen, it was a known treatment for women who experienced difficulties during childbirth to squat over an incense burner filled with myrrh. Since most women in Israel today give birth in hospitals, these methods are becoming rare. Daily massages and binding of the stomach were believed to avoid a protruding stomach after multiple births. Today these practices are only rarely observed among third-generation Yemenites.

Most intriguing of the Yemenite medicinal plants is the controversial *qāt* (Khat, *Catha edulis*),[47] a shrub whose leaves are chewed in Yemen every afternoon for several hours, comparable to coca-chewing in South America. *Qāt* is a stimulant drug and contains alkaloids of the ephedrine type. An interesting resurgence of the *qāt* chewing habit can be observed in areas in Israel with a high concentration of Yemenite Jews who grow *qāt*-bushes in fields near their homes and chew the leaves during social gatherings. Old-time Yemenite immigrants never stopped the habit of chewing *qāt*, but today we see second- and third-generation Yemenite men chewing the leaves ever more frequently. It has to be pointed out that *qāt* is usually chewed by Yemenites whose families come from areas outside Ṣanʿāʾ, because the rabbis in Ṣanʿāʾ always expressed their dislike of *qāt* and warned the community not to indulge in it, according to my informants from Ṣanʿāʾ.[48]

Part of the *qāt*-mystique is that its chewing not only triggers clarity of thought but also enhances sexual performance in men. Dr. Avinoam Tzabari, a gynaecologist of Yemenite descent, through interviews with both men and women has researched the efficacy of this plant as an aphrodisiac in men.[49] His results demonstrate that up to the age of about 50, there is not only an increased sexual desire, but also prolonged erection. On the other hand, *qāt*-chewers above the age of 50 feel only a greater wish for sexual activity, but no increase in potency. Dr. Tzabari points out that a stronger desire arises some half- to one hour after *qāt*-chewing, but never while chewing. During a *qāt*-session, which takes place in the company of other men, thoughts are said to be of a philosophical nature and infused with mystical spirituality. David Qafiḥ believes that *qāt*-chewing

47 See for a survey of *qāt*, including the psychological and medical aspects, Weir, *Qat in Yemen*; see Daniel Martin Varisco's chapter in this volume.

48 See Qafiḥ, *Jewish Life*, 222–5.

49 Tzabari et al., 'The Effect of Chewing Khat'. My thanks to Dr. Avinoam Tzabari for sharing with me his research on this subject.

can cause impotency, since after an initial euphoria a psychological down is often experienced.

A positive aspect of the renewed chewing of *qāt* is that cases have been reported where young drug addicts have been weaned from narcotic drugs on to chewing *qāt* that is not considered as dangerous, since it cannot cause death.

3. Conclusion

It is remarkable that many patients interested in being treated by Yemenite healing methods are not of Yemenite origin. As stated earlier, going to a healer of another culture underlines the notion that the 'other' possesses unique healing secrets. In a similar way, before the mass-immigration of the Yemenite Jews to Israel around 1950, a widespread belief in their healing capacities could be found among the Muslim population of Yemen. In the past as in the present, this includes explicitly practices that are inexplicable, such as those belonging to the realms of magic. Even today non-Yemenite Jews in Israel believe that the Yemenite Jews preserved their ancient traditions and old recipes through the vicissitudes of time during their 2000 year-long exile. The Yemenite Jew is perceived in Israel by many as the most direct descendant of the biblical Jew.

In any case, research in the field of traditional healing is just beginning to be recognized and appreciated. There is no doubt that we will benefit from the fruits of such research in the future.

Bibliography

Arad, J., Abel, R., and Madar, Z., 'Fenugreek as a Means of Reducing Glucose Levels in Diabetic Type II Subjects', *Advanced Diet Nutrition*, 2 (1988), 121–5.

Brauer, Erich, *Ethnologie der jemenitischen Juden* (Heidelberg: Winter, 1934).

Broshi, Magen, 'Wine in Ancient Palestine: Introductory Notes', *The Israel Museum Journal*, 3 (1984), 21–40.

Canova, Giovanni, 'La *ṭāsat al-ism*: Note su alcune coppe magiche yemenite', *Quaderni di Studi Arabi*, 13 (1995), 73–92.

Dori, Zecharia, *Traditional Medicine among the Jews of Yemen, Medicinal Plants, and Perfumes* [Hebrew] (Tel Aviv: Afiqim, 2003).

Eraqi-Klorman, Bat-Zion, 'Yemen: Religion, Magic, and Jews', *PSAS*, 39 (2009), 125–34.

Esposito, John L. (ed.), *The Oxford Dictionary of Islam* (Oxford: Oxford University Press, 2003).

Fleurentin, Jacques, *Guérisseurs et plantes médicinales du Yémen : Au pays de l'encens, de l'aloès et du café* (Paris : Karthala, 2004).

Gamliel, Shalom b. Sa'adya, 'A Gateway to the Lives of Yemenite Jews', in id., Mishael Maswari Caspi, and Shimon Avizemer (eds.), *Yemenite Paths: Studies on the Language, History, Literature and Folklore of the Jews of Yemen* [Hebrew with English summaries] (Jerusalem: The Shalom Research Center, 1984), XI–XXVII (English section).

Lev, Efraim, *Medicinal Substances in Jerusalem from Early Times to the Present Day* (Oxford: Archaeopress, 2003).

———, and Amar, Zohar, *Ethnic Medicinal Substances of the Land of Israel* [Hebrew] (Tel Aviv: Eretz; Jerusalem: Yerid, 2002).

Madar, Z., Abel, R., Samish, S., and Arad, J., 'Glucose-lowering Effect of Fenugreek in Non-insulin Dependent Diabetics', *European Journal of Clinical Nutrition*, 42 (1988), 51–4.

———, and Raiany, Yocheved, *Nutrition and Popular Remedy: Yemenite Tradition* [Hebrew], with contributions by Amar, Zohar and Yaniv, Zahara (Tel Aviv: Ministry of Defence, 2004).

Martinez, Dieter, Lohs, Karlheinz, and Janzen, Jörg, *Weihrauch und Myrrhe: Kulturgeschichte und wirtschaftliche Bedeutung. Botanik, Chemie, Medizin* (Berlin: Akademie-Verlag, 1989).

Matras, Hagit, 'Ethnobotany and Folklore—Methods of Collecting Data About Traditional Usages of Medicinal Plants' [Hebrew], *Jerusalem Studies in Jewish Folklore*, 4 (1983), 169–81.

Mizraḥi, Avshalom, *Mor u-Levona: The Living Habits, Health and Medicine in the Yemeni Jewish Community* [Hebrew] (Netanya: Focus, 2007).

———, and Gundrass, Shulamit, 'Scientific Analysis of Remedies Conventional among the Jews of Yemen' [Hebrew, Engl. summary: 236], *Tema, Journal of Judeo-Yemenite Studies*, 4, (1994), 200–6.

Muchawsky-Schnapper, Ester, 'Symbolic Decorations for a Woman after Childbirth in San'a', *The Israel Museum Journal*, 7 (Spring 1988), 61–74.

———, 'The Use of Incense by Yemenite Jews', *Tema, Journal of Judeo-Yemenite Studies*, 6 (1998), III–XXX.

———, *The Yemenites. Two Thousand Years of Jewish Culture* (Jerusalem: The Israel Museum, 2000).

———, 'Les bijoux du Yémen comme forme de symbiose socio-culturelle', *Perspectives. Revue de l'Université Hébraïque de Jérusalem*, 9 (2002), 184–95.

———, 'Children's Attire in Early 20th-century Ṣan'ā' as a Socio-cultural Paradigm', *PSAS*, 33 (2003), 343–55.

———, 'An Exceptional Type of Yemeni Necklace from the Beginning of the Twentieth Century as an Example of Introducing Artistic Novelty into a Traditional Craft', *PSAS*, 34 (2004), 181–92.

———, 'Rare Photographs from the 1930s and 1940s by Yiḥye Ḥaybi, a Yemenite Jew from Ṣan'ā': Historical Reality and Ethnographic Deductions', *PSAS*, 37 (2007), 135–55.

PSAS = *Proceedings of the Seminar for Arabian Studies.*

Qafiḥ, David, 'Yemenite Tradition in Complementary Medicine in Israel' [Hebrew], *Tehuda*, 24, (2007), 35–7.

———, *Natural. Medicinal Plants for Home Use* [Hebrew] (3 vols.; Jerusalem: David Qafih, 2007–8).

Qafiḥ, Yoseph, *Jewish Life in Ṣan'ā'* [Hebrew] (Jerusalem: Kiryat-Sefer, 1978).

Raiany, Yocheved, *Medicinal Drugs of the Yemenite Jews* [Hebrew] (PhD thesis, School of Pharmacy; Jerusalem: Hebrew University, 1963).

Regourd, Anne, 'Transmission des sciences occultes et société au nord du Yémen', in ead. (coord.), *Divination, magie, pouvoirs au Yémen. Quaderni di Studi Arabi*, 13 (1995), 213–26.

———, 'Pratiques de géomancie au Yémen', in Albert de Surgy (ed.), *Religion et pratiques de puissance* (Paris : L'Harmattan, 1997), 105–28.

———, 'Deux coupes magiques, biens de fondation pieuse (Nord du Yémen) : Transmission du savoir et efficacité', in C. Hamès (ed.), *Coran et talismans. Textes magiques en milieu musulman* (Paris : Karthala, 2007), 309–45.

Schönig, Hanne, *Schminken, Düfte und Räucherwerk der Jemenitinnen: Lexikon der Substanzen, Utensilien und Techniken* (Beiruter Texte und Studien, 91; Würzburg: Ergon, 2002).

Schopen, Armin, *Traditionelle Heilmittel in Jemen* (Wiesbaden: Steiner, 1983).

Sémach, Yomtob, *Une Mission de l'Alliance au Yémen* (Paris : Siège de la Société, [1910]).

Servan-Schreiber, David, *Anticancer : Prévenir et lutter grâce à nos défenses naturelles* (Paris : Laffont, 2007).

Tzabari, Avinoam, Peleg, David, Teper, Avraham, and Shalev, Eliezer, 'The Effect of Chewing Khat on Sexual Behaviour', lecture given at *The 3rd International Congress of Yemenite Studies*, Nordholan Folkehogskule (Bergen/Norway, 1–3 August 1993).

———, Peleg, David, Ben-Ami, Moshe, and Shalev, Eliezer, 'The Effect of Fenugreek Seeds (Trigonella) on Blood Glucose in Gestational Diabetes: Preliminary Study and Review of the Literature', lecture given at *The 2nd International Congress of Yemenite Studies*, Princeton University (New Jersey/USA, 26–28 July 1992).

Varisco, Daniel Martin, 'Arzneikunde und Heilpflanzen im mittelalterlichen Jemen', in Werner Daum (ed.), *Jemen: 3000 Jahre Kunst und Kultur des Glücklichen Arabien* (Innsbruck: Pinguin; Frankfurt/Main: Umschau, 1987), 306–7.

Weir, Shelagh, *Qat in Yemen: Consumption and Social Change* (London: British Museum, 1985).

Zadoc, Moshe, *History and Customs of the Jews in the Yemen* [Hebrew] (Tel Aviv: Am Oved, 1967).

HONEY, COFFEE, AND TEA IN CULTURAL PRACTICES OF ḤAḌRAMAWT

Mikhail Rodionov

Based on both oral and written sources, as well as on data collected by the author during field research, this paper aims to discuss the symbolic roles of honey, coffee, and tea in local cultural use, including some healing practices.

1. Honey and Apiculture

As a specific local product, honey is the oldest of the three substances under examination. Indeed, the best honey in Yemen is reputed to come from Ḥaḍramawt, and the best in the region from Wādī Daw'an.[1] Wādī Laysar, the eastern branch of Wādī Daw'an, boasts a honey-producing area between the villages of al-Dūfa and al-Khayla al-Sharqiyya where, since the first half of the twentieth century, rich returnee emigrants have built ambitious houses. Bee-keeping is seen here as an indication of wealth, and honeycombs placed in round tins (Fig. 1) as the symbol of their native land, especially for Hadramis abroad.

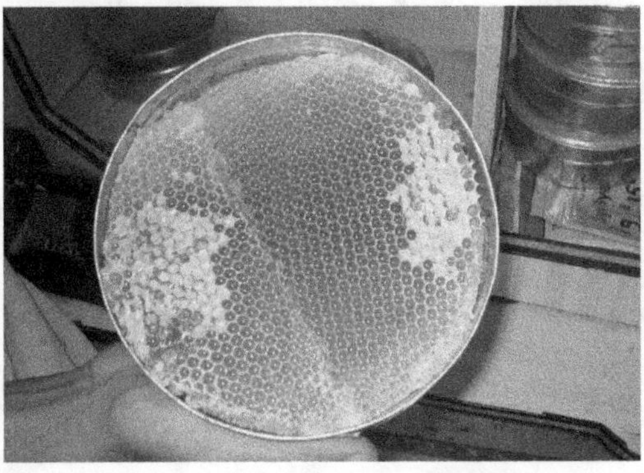

Figure 1. Honeycombs are considered a symbol of Ḥaḍramawt (al-Mukallā) (© Mikhail Rodionov, 2008)

[1] See Ingrams, 'Bee-Keeping'. Wādī Daw'an is the spelling confirmed by local scholars rather than 'Duw'an'.

Apiculture has a long history in Ḥaḍramawt, confirmed by the Greek author Strabo (d. *c.* 24 CE) in chapter 4 of his *Geography*,[2] and is to this day practised according to traditional methods, as elsewhere in Yemen.[3] Proof that such age-old techniques of bee-keeping are still employed is the use of simple, frameless, horizontal, bottle-shaped hives made of baked clay (Fig. 2)—a design used for many centuries. In the past, the hives were mounted in rows inside an outer wall of a house to assure their safety and to protect the bees from temperature extremes. Today the hives are placed on the flat roof of a house (sometimes on a low trestle), in the yard, in fields, or on mountain slopes near nectar-bearing plants. Occasionally, they are taken by truck to neighbouring valleys where greater opportunities for nectar collection are to be found.

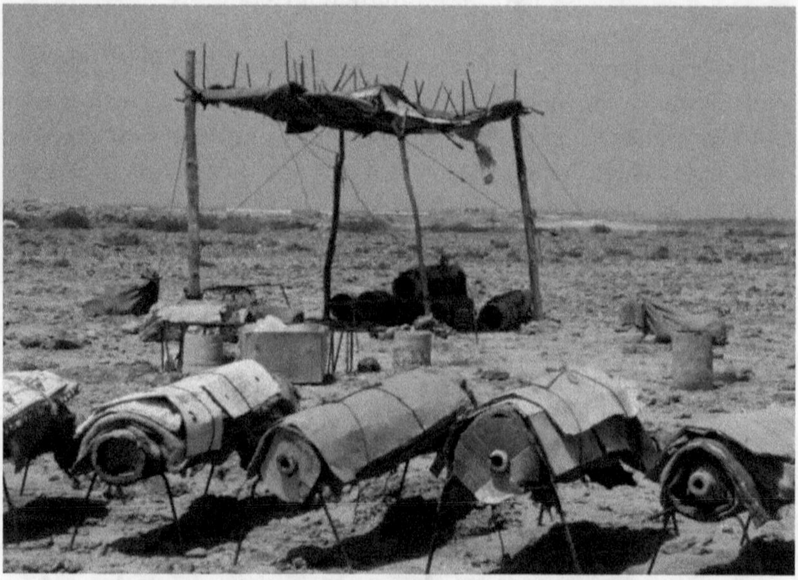

Figure 2. Horizontal bottle-shaped hives near al-Mukallā (© Hanne Schönig, 1992)

Local bee-keepers make a distinction between two high seasons, which accord with the periods when the main nectar-bearing plants are in bloom. The first is the time of the blooming of the *sumr* tree (*Acacia spirocarpa*). My informant ʿUmar al-Ḥabshī, a resident of al-Ghabra village in Wādī Dawʿan, points out that this season lasts fifty-two days, beginning with

[2] Strabo, *Geography*, Book 16.4.4; for more details, see Rodionov, *Ḥaḍramawt*, 107–10.
[3] See Canova, 'Api e apicoltori'.

the early-evening rising of the lunar mansion of al-Jabha (21 February) to the last days of the lunar mansion of (al-)ʿAwwā (14 April).[4] The other season is in October–December when the *ʿilb* tree (*Zizyphus spina-christi*) blossoms. A Western specialist in apiculture attests that this honey is the most expensive in the world.[5] Indeed, the honey produced during the second season—called *mariyya* or *ṣayfī*—is valued four times more than the honey of the earlier *sumr* period. In rainy years there is a third season, the *marbāʿī*, when flowering herbs provide the necessary nectar. Other local experts suggest slightly different time frames, which correlate with rainy seasons.[6]

The ownership of bees and hives is inherited, so one apiary can be owned by several members of a family. There are special 'bee judges' in Ḥaḍramawt who customarily adjudicate conflicts between bee-keepers. In the lower reaches of Wādī Dawʿan, the most authoritative of the judges in the 1990s was Mubārak Bin Shamlān, a resident of Wādī ʿAmd. Most experts in bee-keeping are members of tribes (*qabāʾil*), or occasionally they belong to the descendants of the Prophet, the *sāda*. The occupation is performed by males only, as in other Arab countries.[7]

As elsewhere in the Arab world, apiculture in Ḥaḍramawt is based on an authoritative written tradition. Local bee-keepers memorize verses from the quranic *sūra* "The Bee" (Q 16:68–9). In the Maktabat al-Aḥqāf public library in Tarīm one can examine various medieval treatises on honey, for example, Ms. 2735, ff. 241–67: *Tarqīq al-asal fī taṣfīq al-ʿasal* by Abū ʿAbdallāh Muḥammad b. Yaʿqūb b. Muḥammad al-Fayrūzābādī (d. 1414/15). In this work, whose title may be translated as 'The Refinement of a Reed in the Praise of Honey,' an Ibadite[8] scholar addresses in detail the excellent properties of honey created by God. Familiar to the *ḥaḍramī* scholars, this manuscript represents one of the few leftovers of the Ibadite influences in the traditional culture of Ḥaḍramawt (Fig. 3).

---

[4] Pellat, 'Anwāʾ', 523–4, provides a brief description of the significance of the lunar mansions in the agricultural almanac tradition of Arabia. See Kunitzsch, *Sternnomenklatur*, nos. 44 and 103a, for the astronomical identification of the two cited lunar mansions.

[5] Sergent, 'Le miel le plus cher du monde'.

[6] al-Ṣabbān, *al-Fallāḥūn*, 19–27, and id., *al-Shiʿr al-shaʿbī*, 11–19, 26–7.

[7] Canova, 'Api e miele', 69–85.

[8] A Muslim community outside the large branches of Sunni and Shiite Islam with distinct views on doctrine and caliphate. Ibadites are nowadays found mainly in Oman.

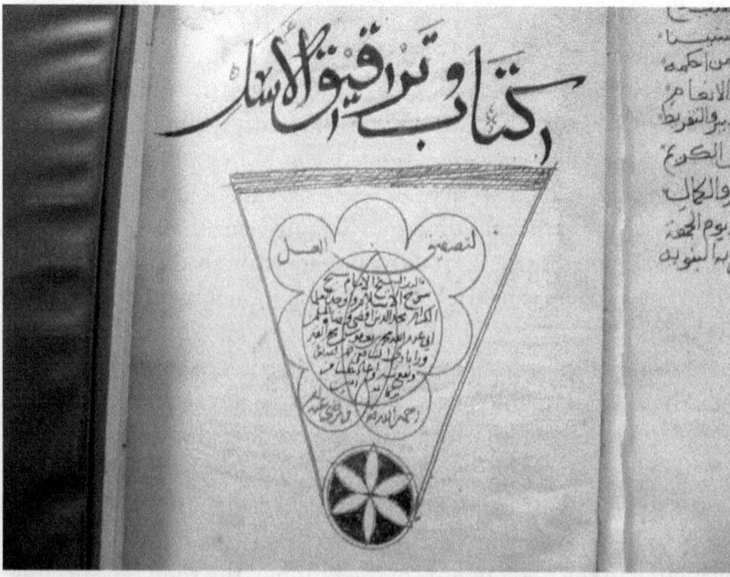

Figure 3. A medieval Ibadite treatise on honey: *Tarqīq al-asal fī taṣfīq al-ʿasal* [The Refinement of a Reed in the Praise of Honey] by Muḥammad b. Yaʿqūb al-Fayrūzābādī (d. 1414/15) (© Mikhail Rodionov)

This explains why honey has acquired widespread respect for its health-giving properties. Honey fortifies, heals wounds, treats gastritis, ulcers, liver and kidney diseases, and diabetes; when taken with meat it is an aphrodisiac.[9] It serves as distraction for a child during circumcision and as a good omen for newlyweds. Honey is a symbol of vital energy and fertility.

Currently, traditional Ḥaḍramawt bee-keeping is to a significant degree oriented toward the external market, but the main demand for local honey comes from *ḥaḍramī* emigrants working in the oil-rich countries of the Arabian Peninsula. Attempts were made as early as the 1930s to export Ḥaḍramawt honey, although at that time London experts considered the product uncompetitive in Great Britain as it "is a dextro-rotatory honey [...] a product of the 'honeydew' type,[10] which would account for its unusual flavour and odour."[11] Today there are several thousand beehives

---

[9] Rodionov, *Ḥaḍramawt*, 137–9.

[10] "Produced by the bee from secretions of leaves and sometimes from secretions deposited by insects" (Ingrams, *Aden Protectorate*, 54, n. 1).

[11] Ibid., 53–4.

in Ḥaḍramawt, and each vital bee colony produces from 8 to 16 kg per season, depending on weather conditions. Nowadays traditional honey shops flourish in Say'ūn, the Bā Yazīd being one of the most prosperous honey merchant families from the Wādī Ḥaḍramawt (Fig. 4). In al-Mukallā most of the honey shops are owned by members of the al-Huzaylī family who claim their descent from the Bedouin tribe of Banū Hudhayl, famous for their poems that describe a honey hunter who followed wild bees up to their rock nests and took the honeycombs—a practice that still survives in the southern regions of Oman.[12] The al-Huzaylī label their commodities as *al-ʿasal al-dawʿanī*, or the honey from Wādī Dawʿan, and distribute their product within Arab countries through the Lebanese company Effel. In 2008, the price for the round tin of honeycombs (about 4 pounds) varied from 1500 YR to 6000 YR, or $ 7.50 to $ 30 (Fig. 1). The international airport in al-Mukallā offers "Yemeni coffee" and "Doan [= Dawʿan] honey" in its shop. The renown of the Wādī Dawʿan honey is recognized in Ṣanʿā' too, although many of the honey shops in the capital do not specifically mention Dawʿan on their signboards.

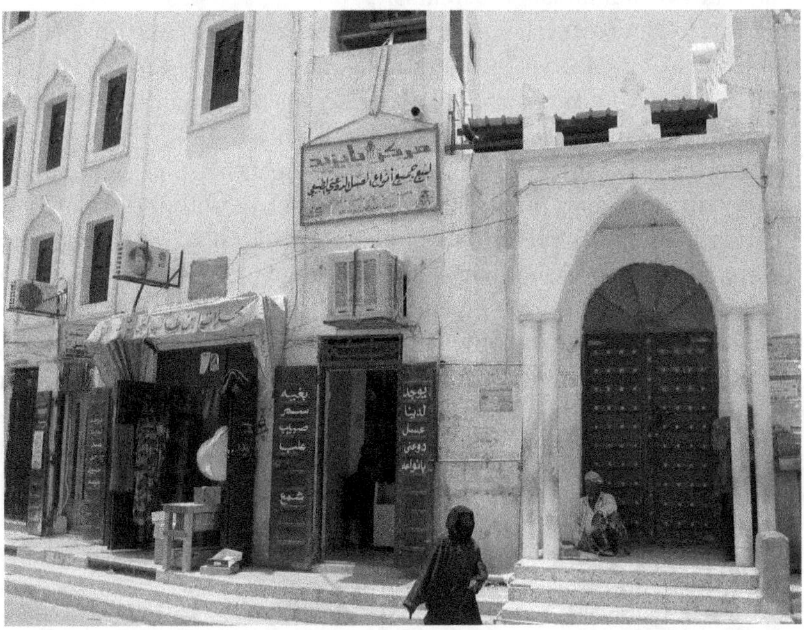

Figure 4. A honey shop of the Bā Yazīd family in Say'ūn (© Mikhail Rodionov, 2006)

[12] Canova, "Cacciatori di miele", 194–200.

2. Honey and Coffee in Local Medicine and Folklore

The perceived strengthening effect of honey is enhanced when it is taken with coffee, although in contrast to the local origin of honey, coffee came to the Ḥaḍramawt from outside and only arrived several centuries ago.[13] Local tradition connects coffee with the famous Sufi shaykh ʿAlī al-Shādhilī (d. 1418); they say the introduction of the beverage was one of his miracles. A kind of bitter coffee is even called here ʻal-Shādhilī,' as in the verse of the twentieth-century poet al-Shubayr Bā Yaʿshūt.[14]

My informant, Ḥusayn ʿAbdallāh Bin Shaykh Bū Bakr from Khuraykhar in Wādī Dawʿan, bee-keeper, bee judge, and one of the best experts in local medical traditions including cauterization (*kayy*), argues that the best healing properties are offered by *sharīkh*, a decoction of coffee husk flavoured with *zanjabīl* (ginger) and *hayl* (cardamom). *Sharīkh* fights heartburn and acts as a digestive after heavy and rich food. Cases of anaemia are treated with plain coffee and honey, flavoured with brown cane sugar (*sukkar aḥmar*). Ḥusayn also claims that fresh aloe sap with honey and oil treats pulmonary tuberculosis.

Local folklore extols honey in many ways. Rabīʿ ʿAwḍ Bin ʿUbaydallāh, a folk poet from Madūda in Wādī Ḥaḍramawt, in his *qaṣīda* "The Queen of the Trees" (*Malikat al-ashjār*) eulogizes the date palm, exclaiming that the beloved Ḥaḍramawt is deep in his heart and the date palm is the source of his inspiration and poetry.[15] In his personal communications with me in 2003 he compared this royal tree with the honey-bee, related even by its phonetic semblance: *al-nakhl* (date palms) with *al-naḥl* (bees); the sweetness of their products, he added, differs, but both dates and honey are given to us by God.

Local culture contrasts the sweetness of honey to bitterness (*qār*), like the contrast of life to violent death. This notion is reflected, for example, in the verse of a folk poet who lived in the first half of the twentieth century, Sālim Bin Jibrān from the al-Quza village in Wādī Dawʿan, who wrote: "*wa-l-qabwala mā ṭaʿamhā illā qār // mā shī muṣallaḥ min jubūhū*," or, "The nourishment of tribal arrogance is nothing but bitterness; // there is no honey in its hive."[16] The juxtaposition of honey/bitterness to life/death, one of the earliest in the mythic-poetic legacy of

---

[13] [Schönig], 'Mokka aus dem Jemen', 34–9.
[14] Rodionov, *Ḥaḍramawt*, 189.
[15] Bin ʿUbaydallāh, *Malikat al-ashjār*, 30.
[16] My field data, Hadramawt 1983.

Eurasia, is reflected, for example, in the great Indian epic poem Mahabharata.[17] Another word for bitterness, *baṣal* (onion), is used in local proverbs defining marriage as honey for a month, and onion for the rest of the time.

Honey and coffee feature in the wedding ceremony: the bride and the bridegroom have to drink coffee with honey in the evening of their first wedding night. This custom is observed by all members of traditional social strata in Ḥaḍramawt. The coffee set as a part of the dowry includes a clay frying pan (*miḥmās*, pl. *maḥāmīs*) to roast the coffee beans; a wooden mortar and pestle; a woven tray over which the coffee beans are spread so that every guest can smell and appreciate them; and a coffee pot (*dalla*, pl. *dalal*).[18] The coffee ceremony among both the Bedouin and settled populations has become a representation of traditional Arab hospitality.

At midday, the Hadramis prefer *sharīkh* as a refreshing hot beverage; this is made from coffee beans (*bunn*), coffee husks (*qishr*), and ground ginger. It is widely believed that *sharīkh* stimulates heart activity. Coffee with almonds and honey is served on Fridays and at weddings.

3. Coffee and Tea: Two Rivals[19]

Local scholars maintain that coffee has been known in Ḥaḍramawt since the mid-forteenth century, while tea was brought into the country by a Tarīm resident, Ḥāmid b. ʿAbdallāh al-Junayd, in the late nineteenth century.[20] However, it was only in the 1930s that cheap red and green tea from China and South East Asia appeared in Ḥaḍramawt. Since then tea has pushed coffee into the background. There are still people alive who remember this transition. Tea sets and samovars have become a part of the dowry and a common wedding gift. Actually, tea changed the everyday life and cultural practices of the Hadramis.

The central place in a tea set is occupied by the samovar, or tea urn, preserving its original Russian name (*samāwar* or *bukhārī*). Some Hadramis even know the name of Tula, the Russian town where samovars are manufactured, although some believe it to be a suburb of Bukhara.

---

17 Vassilkov, 'Parable of a Man'; cf. with the 'honey of poetry' of Scandinavian myths, Meletinskij, 'Miod poezii', 127–8.

18 al-Ṣabbān, *ʿĀdāt wa-taqālīd*, 152–6.

19 See Rodionov and Schönig, *The Hadramawt Documents*, 4.2 'Food and Beverages'.

20 al-Shāṭirī, *Adwār al-taʾrīkh*, 71; al-Ṣabbān, *ʿĀdāt wa-taqālīd*, 152, 156.

Today, it is not coffee, but tea with honey and ginger that is drunk before the wedding night. The cultural roles of these substances are flamboyantly expressed in local folklore, as shown in an unpublished essay of ʿAlī Bā Rajāʾ, a contemporary poet from Sayʾūn, and in other local writings.[21]

If local poetry equates honey to life and inspiration, in contrast to the bitterness of an empty bee-hive symbolizing death and tribal arrogance, coffee is praised for its invigorating effect by the great *ḥaḍramī* Sufi poet ʿUmar Bā Makhrama (d. 1546) who compared coffee (*qahwat al-bunn*) with the heavenly wine.[22] ʿAbd al-Ṣamad b. ʿAbdallāh Bā Kathīr (d. 1616) celebrates the culture of coffee drinking in his poetry[23] and ʿUmar b. Saqqāf al-Ṣāfī (d. 1802) dedicated his book *Tafrīḥ al-qulūb wa-tafrīj al-kurūb* [Delight of Hearts and Separation from Concerns] to coffee.[24] This pure beverage, they argued, when consumed by true connoisseurs, helps one comprehend with serenity both hidden and outward things. On the other hand, a number of Islamic scholars, particularly the *fuqahāʾ*, such as a resident of Wādī Dawʿan, ʿAlī b. Aḥmad b. Saʿīd Bā Ṣabrayn in the 1880s,[25] condemned private parties where men mixed with women and sang, danced, played chess, and sipped coffee.[26]

Robert Serjeant published a record of a dispute between coffee and tea in verse composed by Abū Ṣāliḥ ʿAbd al-Qādir b. ʿUmar b. Umbārak Bin Shaybān (d. 1923/4) from the Tamīm tribe, a *ḥaḍramī* emigrant to Surabaya, Indonesia.[27] This early twentieth-century poem entitled *Kitāb al-Basṭ wa-l-salwa lil-muḥāwara bayn al-shāy wa-l-qahwa* [The Book of Amusement and Fun in a Dispute Between Tea and Coffee] concludes that coffee is for elderly scholars, whereas tea is for younger merchants engaged in the pleasures of this life.

In the twentieth century, enthusiastic poets, such as ʿAlī b. Muḥammad b. Ḥusayn al-Ḥabshī (d. 1914/15), Saqqāf b. Muḥammad al-Saqqāf (d. 1972), Ḥusayn b. Muḥammad Bā Rajāʾ, and many others praised tea in Sufi terminology as the key to eternity, the honey of Salsabīl (a spring of

---

21 Serjeant, *Prose and Poetry*, 38–53 (of the Arabic text).

22 Bin ʿAqīl, *ʿUmar Bā Makhrama al-Saybānī*, 200–7.

23 al-Ṣabbān, *ʿAbd al-Ṣamad Bā Kathīr*, 174–83.

24 Bā Rajāʾ, *al-Shāy ʿinda shuʿarāʾ Sayʾūn*, 1–2, who quotes partially their bibliography.

25 Bā Ṣabrayn, *al-Jumal min al-muhimmāt al-dīniyya*, 11b–14a.

26 See Hattox, *Coffee*, chapter 4: 'Wine, Coffee and the Holy Law'.

27 Serjeant, *Prose and Poetry*, 38–53 (of the Arabic text); Rodionov, 'Spor dvukh napitkov', 380–4.

Paradise), and the universal medicine.[28] So in the contest for cultural predominance, coffee, related to the local Sufi tradition and criticized by the *fuqahā'*, surrendered its cultural role to tea that is regarded now as a symbol of modernity and enterprise. The partisans of tea, however, use the metaphors and arguments of their predecessors.

4. Conclusion

It is evident that clichés of the classical *khamriyyāt* genre of wine poems, over the course of time, have been successively transferred from wine to coffee and, finally, to tea with honey as a primordial concomitant attribute. Each beverage condemns the previous one and supersedes it in popularity, itself regarded as a unique, thrilling (if not magical) substance with renowned and extraordinary properties and special rules (*dasātīr*, sg. *dustūr*) of consumption.

The mystic concept of symbolic intoxication with heavenly wine is reflected in an honorific nickname *Sakrān* ('drunk' or 'high') that is still popular in Ḥaḍramawt. Among the local epithets associated with tea drinking one can find a humourous nickname given to the poet 'Umar Muḥammad Bā Kathīr (d. 1995)—*Barṭama*[29] that means he who talks like boiling water gurgling in a tea pot. This is an example of symbolic vocabulary as part of the cultural practices of South Arabia in which honey, coffee, and tea still play significant roles today.

Bibliography

Bā Rajā', 'Alī Aḥmad, *al-Shāy 'inda shu'arā' Say'ūn* (unpublished [Say'ūn, 2005?]).

Bā Ṣabrayn, 'Alī b. Aḥmad b. Sa'īd, *al-Jumal min al-muhimmāt al-dīniyya fī ba'ḍ al-murtakib min al-manāhī l-rabbāniyya* (Ms, Tarīm: Maktabat al-Aḥqāf, 1294 [1877–8]; *Fihrist Maktabat al-Aḥqāf*, 2, 221, *majmū'*, no. 2530/1, ff. 1–22).

Bin 'Aqīl, 'Abd al-Raḥmān Ja'far, *'Umar Bā Makhrama al-Saybānī, 884–952 h. Ḥayātuhu wa-taṣawwufuhu wa-shi'ruhu* (Damascus: Dār al-fikr, 2002).

Bin 'Ubaydallāh, Rabī' 'Awḍ, *Malikat al-ashjār* (Madūda, 2002).

Canova, Giovanni, 'Api e apicoltori nello Yemen orientale', *Quaderni di studi arabi*, 14 (1996), 179–93.

———, 'Api e miele tra sapere empirico, tradizione e conoscenza scientifica nel mondo arabo-islamico', *Quaderni di studi arabi, Studi e testi*, 3 (1999), 69–92.

———, '"Cacciatori di miele". Dalla poesia Huḏaylita alle pratiche tradizionali nel Dhofar (Oman)', *Quaderni di Studi Arabi*, 20–1 (2002–3), 185–206.

---

[28] Bā Rajā', *al-Shāy 'inda shu'arā' Say'ūn*, 5–9.

[29] Ibid., 3.

al-Fayrūzābādī, Abū ʿAbdallāh Muḥammad b. Yaʿqūb b. Muḥammad, *Tarqīq al-asal fī taṣfīq al-ʿasal* (Ms, Tarīm: Maktabat al-Aḥqāf, 3 Dhū l-Ḥijja 1065 [15 October 1655]; *Fihrist Maktabat al-Aḥqāf*, 2, 339, *majmūʿ*, no. 2735/12, ff. 241–67).

Fihrist Maktabat al-Aḥqāf lil-makhṭuṭāt bi-Tarīm (4 vols.; Sayʾūn: al-Markaz al-Yamanī lil-abḥāth al-thaqāfiyya wa-l-āthār wa-l-matāḥif, 1988).

Hattox, Ralph S., *Coffee and Coffeehouses: The Origins of a Social Beverage in the Medieval Near East* (Near Eastern Studies, 3; Washington: University of Washington Press, 2000).

Ingrams, W.H., *Aden Protectorate. A Report on the Social, Economic and Political Condition of the Hadhramaut* (London: H.M. Stationary Office, 1936).

———, 'Bee-Keeping in the Wadi Duʿan', *Man*, 37 (1937), 32.

Kunitzsch, Paul, *Untersuchungen zur Sternnomenklatur der Araber* (Wiesbaden: Harrassowitz, 1961).

Meletinskij, Eleazar M., 'Miod poezii' [The Honey of Poetry], in S.A. Tokorev (ed.), *Mify narodov mira* [Myths of the Peoples of the World] 2 (Moscow: Sovetskaya entsiklopediya, 1992), 127–8.

Pellat, Ch., 'Anwāʾ', *The Encyclopaedia of Islam* (New Edition), (I; Brill: Leiden, 1960), 523a–524a.

Rodionov, Mikhail, 'Spor dvukh napitkov (iz poezii Hadramauta)' [The Contest of Two Beverages (from the Ḥaḍramawt poetry)], in A.V. Sedov and I.M. Smilianskaya (eds.), *Arabia Vitalis. Arabskiy Vostok, Islam, drevniaya Araviya. Sbornik statey, posviashchennykh 60-letiyu V. Naumkina* [Arabia Vitalis. Arabian East, Islam, Ancient Arabia. Festschrift in Commemoration of the 60th Anniversary of V. Naumkin] (Moscow: The Orient Institute, Russian Academy of Sciences, 2005), 380–4.

———, *The Western Ḥaḍramawt: Ethnographic Field Research, 1983–91* (Orientwissenschaftliche Hefte, 24; Halle (Saale): OWZ, Martin-Luther-Universität Halle-Wittenberg, 2007).

Rodionov, Mikhail, and Schönig, Hanne, *The Hadramawt Documents, 1904–51: Family Life and Social Customs under the Last Sultans* (Beiruter Texte und Studien, 130; Würzburg: Ergon, 2011).

al-Ṣabbān, ʿAbd al-Qādir Muḥammad, *ʿAbd al-Ṣamad Bā Kathīr, shāʿir Ḥaḍramawt fī l-qarn al-ʿāshir al-hijrī* (al-Mukallā: al-Markaz al-Yamanī lil-abḥāth al-thaqāfiyya wa-l-āthār wa-l-matāḥif, 1979).

———, *ʿĀdāt wa-taqālīd bi-l-Aḥqāf* (Manshūrāt al-Markaz al-Yamanī lil-abḥāth al-thaqāfiyya wa-l-āthār wa-l-matāḥif farʿ m[uḥāfaẓat] Ḥaḍramawt, 12/1; al-Mukallā: [1400/1980]). (Photocopied stencil publication).

———, *al-Fallāḥūn wa-ʿādātuhum al-mihniyya* (Sayʾūn: al-Markaz al-Yamanī lil-abḥāth al-thaqāfiyya wa-l-āthār wa-l-matāḥif, 1983).

———, *al-Shiʿr al-shaʿbī maʿa l-muzāriʿīn* (Sayʾūn: Idārat al-thaqāfa wa-l-siyāḥa, 1984).

[Schönig, Hanne], 'Mokka aus dem Jemen: Das Schicksal einer Kaffeemetropole', in Heike Heklau and Hanne Schönig, *Von Mokka bis Muckefuck: Zur Botanik und Kulturgeschichte des Kaffees* (Halle/Saale: Martin-Luther-Universität Halle-Wittenberg, 2001), 31–49.

Serjeant, Robert Bertram, *Prose and Poetry from Ḥaḍramawt: South Arabian Poetry*: I (London: Taylor's Foreign Press, 1951).

al-Shāṭirī, Muḥammad b. Aḥmad b. ʿUmar, *Adwār al-taʾrīkh al-ḥaḍramī* (part 2; al-Mukallā: Maktab al-shaʿb, 1972).

Vassilkov, Yaroslav, 'Parable of a Man Hanging in a Tree and Its Archaic Background', *Jadavpur Journal of Comparative Literature*, 32 (1994–5), 38–51.

Internet Sources

Sergent, Thierry, 'Le miel le plus cher du monde est le Ziziphus spina-christi (jujubier sauvage)', <http://www.beekeeping.com/abeille-de-france/articles/yemen.htm>, accessed 14 February 2009.

FROM MEDICINAL PLANTS OF YEMEN TO THERAPEUTIC HERBAL DRUGS

Jacques Fleurentin

1. Project Definition

1.1. *Traditional Medicine in Yemen*

Traditional medicine in Yemen includes medical beliefs and practices determined by epidemiological, cultural, historical, and economic factors. A part of the work carried out in Yemen consisted of establishing an inventory of the medicinal plants used in traditional therapy. For that purpose, the author of this report spent two and a half years as a pharmacist working in the laboratory of the French Medical Mission in the Taʿizz Republican Hospital.

Working in close cooperation with anthropologist Cynthia Myntti and botanist John Wood, we undertook an ethnopharmacological survey of traditional medicine in Yemen. The approach adopted was fundamentally anthropological, with a discussion of the theoretical underpinnings of traditional medicine, an overview of the practitioners, and an assessment of the healing options as perceived by the local people. We then undertook a study of the historical sources to determine the cultural background of the practices, to identify the pre-Islamic (Greek, Indian, and Chinese) elements of the pharmacopoeia, as well as that of Arabic medicine.

1.2. *Conceptual Background*

Greek medicine began with Hippocrates around 400 BCE. Recognized as 'The Father of Medicine,' Hippocrates' humoural theory is based on four elements (earth, fire, water, air), four humours (blood, yellow bile, black bile, phlegm), and four qualities (hot, cold, dry, wet). These elements, humours, and qualities in various combinations compose an organism and characterize its personality or temperament. Good health is defined as an ideal condition in which equilibrium between the four humours is properly maintained in the body. Two famous authors, Dioscorides (1st century CE) with *De Materia Medica* describing 519 medicinal plants, and Galen

(d. after 203), 'The Father of Pharmacy,' are the most important sources of this tradition of medicine.

One starting point of medicine in the Islamic world is with the medical recommendations of the Prophet Muḥammad. 'The Prophet's' or 'Islamic' medicine combines medical content and religious belief. The Prophet's immediate successors, the first caliphs, expanded Islamic control over all of Arabia and beyond. This development was reinforced during the time of the Umayyad Dynasty (660–751) that was based in Damascus and established sovereignty over vast territories from the Pyrenees to Central Asia. The Abbasid Dynasty with its capital in Baghdad (751–1258) made significant contributions to the development of culture, the arts, and the sciences. Sponsorship of learning was also extended to north-western Africa (the Maghreb) and the Iberian Peninsula (al-Andalus). Many of the treatises of Greek and Ayurvedic medicine were translated into Arabic and thus became available to the Muslim scholars. Innovative new medical treatises were composed, including *The Comprehensive Book on Medicine* by Rhazes (d. *c.*925) and the *Canon of Medicine* by Avicenna (d. 1037). Ibn al-Bayṭār (d. 1248) wrote the *Treatise on Simples*, describing no less than 1500 drugs. The texts of classical Arabic medicine were eventually translated into Latin and provided the basis for European medicine.[1]

1.3. *Methodology*

The science of ethnopharmacology is the interdisciplinary investigation of the full set of medical approaches that use remedies of vegetable, animal, or mineral origin. It includes the relevant knowledge and practices that are implemented by vernacular cultures for therapeutic, curative, preventive, and diagnostic purposes.[2] Thus, ethnopharmacology is the study of traditional medicines and the corresponding pharmacopoeias with the help of numerous disciplines. It bridges the gap between practices from the past and modern scientific knowledge. At the same time, it serves as the meeting point between the humanities and the natural sciences—that is, ethnology, history, and linguistics on the one hand and botany, pharmacology, pharmacognosy, and medicine on the other. While it is respectful of traditional practices, ethnopharmacology is resolutely open to innovation.

---

1 See Fleurentin and Younos, 'Médecine islamique'.

2 Dos Santos and Fleurentin, 'L'ethnopharmacologie', 28.

Research in ethnopharmacology can be roughly subdivided in three stages:

a) *Fieldwork* is carried out with the purpose of making an inventory of the various forms of medical treatment, the different uses of medicinal plants and drugs of natural origin anywhere in the world, in both advanced and developing countries. Research activities include:

- Collecting information to gain full understanding of the traditional medical system, i.e. information on a culture's specific understanding of physiology, the causes of disease, therapy, classification of drugs and foodstuffs, and the position of traditional healers. This is basically the task of an anthropologist.[3]
- Compiling an inventory of traditional remedies (composed of ingredients of plant, animal, or mineral origin), which includes a herbarium and a drug collection, together with assembling data on preparation, posology (the study of the dosages of medicines), and therapeutic indications. This is the task of a pharmacist and an ethnobotanist.[4]
- Identifying the plants is the task of a botanist.[5]

b) The second stage involves *laboratory work*, using the sophisticated tools of modern pharmacology, chemistry, and biology, with the aim of attaining a better understanding of the agents involved in the therapeutic activity of these substances. Selection of the kind of scientific experimentation is necessarily guided by a remedy's traditional usage.

c) *Post-laboratory follow-up* aims at achieving sustainability. The goal is to assess the results of pharmaco-toxicological analysis, validate the efficiency of traditional therapies, and improve primary health care through the application of traditional medicines. In particular, sustainable production of herbal medicines using local resources can be promoted through establishing gardens where medicinal plants are cultivated and through preparing phytodrugs in local pharmacies.

---

[3] See Myntti, *Medicine*, for an example.

[4] Fleurentin, *Répertoire des pharmacopées traditionnelles*, provides the details of what is involved in the work.

[5] Wood's *Handbook* is the outcome of this particular research.

2. Scope of the Study

2.1. *Fieldwork in Yemen with Traditional Healers*

During fieldwork in Yemen (1977–9), interviews with traditional healers (and self-medicated people) were conducted in various regions in order to understand their practice and to identify the medicinal plants used in that part of the country.[6] The places of investigation included Taʿizz, Ṣanʿāʾ, Ṣaʿda, al-Turba, Ḥadda, Banī Ghāzī, Jabal Ṣabir, Jabal Ḥubaysh, Jabal Rayma, Sūq Wādī Zabab, Zabīd, Bayt al-Faqīh, al-Mukhā, al-Khūkha, al-Ḥudayda, Barʾāt, al-Buqaʿ, Wādī Umla, and Wādī Uṭla. Most traditional healers borrow freely from the medical theories developed in the past, including classical Greek humoural medicine, classical Arabic medicine, Islamic medicine, and local traditions. The following list indicates the type of expertise of healers:

2.1.1. *Traditional Healers Specializing in Classical Arabic Medicine*

These healers are generally literate males who have acquired their knowledge, skills, and wisdom from an older generation after long and rigorous apprenticeship. The medium used for transmission of this knowledge is handwritten texts handed down from generation to generation, as well as published books. Traditional healers are considered professionals who expect to receive remuneration for their services. The basic tenets they abide by are:

i. Any individual is unique, and this has a bearing on their health balance.
ii. The causes of imbalance and ill health are to be found in the environment (e.g. food, water, air). Treatment for the most part is based on the use of the recognized properties of specific medicinal plants. If the healer determines that some form of internal disequilibrium is the root-cause of the illness, he will treat the problem through the medium of allopathy, using plants that have properties to countervail the imbalance.

2.1.2. *Traditional Healers Who Combine a Simplified Humoural Tradition with Magico-religious Practice*

The healers listed below are persons who have specialized and have developed expertise in a specific aspect of medicine:

[6] See Fleurentin, Myntti, and Pelt, 'Traditional Healers'.

i. The bonesetter (*mujabbir*) is still found in rural communities.
ii. The traditional midwife (*muwallida*) is a central figure in child delivery. The services provided include activities from abdominal and back massage to repositioning the uterus after delivery.
iii. The bloodletter (*ḥajjām, muzayyin, ḥallāq*) and cautery (*makwā*) practitioner performs scarified cupping and cauterization. He may be a butcher or a barber. Cautery is a common treatment in Yemen for a wide range of conditions from stress and fear to localized internal pain.
iv. The amulet writer (*ṣāḥib al-kitāb*) claims that he receives special grace (*baraka*) and inspiration from God which enable him to write benedictory and protective charms.
v. The mystical healer (*ṣūfī*) has special healing powers that have been endowed through the establishment of a relationship with the genies (*jinn*) and provide the key to accurate diagnosis and cure.

2.1.3. *The Herbalists*

These persons have stalls in the perfume and spice sections of the markets and offer herbal, animal, and mineral drugs for sale. The herbal drugs are either derived from plants commonly cultivated in Yemen, or from species that have been imported from abroad.

2.2. *Textual Sources*

Yemen occupies the southern tip of the Arabian Peninsula; its cultural and religious identity has been formed for the last 1500 years almost exclusively by that of Islam. Its traditional medicine is therefore rooted strongly in classical Arabic medicine. One of the most significant works of Arabic pharmacopoeia is Ibn al-Bayṭār's *Treatise on Simples*.[7] Yet it is also interesting to trace the influences that ancient Greek and Indian texts have exerted on Arabic medicine. The most prominent example for Greek pharmacopoeia is Dioscorides' work *De Materia Medica*,[8] and for ancient Indian medicine it is the *Caraka-Saṃhitā*, originally written in Sanskrit.[9] These three pharmacopoeias serve as reference works that were checked with regard to whether or not the medicinal plants identified by the project were mentioned, and for which indications.

---

[7] See Ibn al-Bayṭār/Leclerc (trans.), *Traité*.
[8] See Matthiole, *Commentaire*.
[9] See Sharma (ed. and trans.), *Caraka-Saṃhitā*.

3. Results of the Fieldwork

3.1. *General Considerations*

Yemen is an invaluable cradle of biodiversity with five plants in particular: *qāt* is a species containing amphetamine-like substances; coffee, whose cultivation originated in Yemen, has become one of the top beverages in the world; aloe, now widely grown from China to America, is a plant native to Yemen; frankincense and myrrh provided one of the motivations for the Romans to try and gain full control over their production areas in Yemen. Yemen's biodiversity is extraordinary, not so much in terms of quantity (1750 plant species), but from the point of view of quality and the specific properties of some plants such as the examples given.

Traditional medicine in Yemen is highly original. Out of the 160 medicinal plants that were collected, identified, and analyzed by the project, 54% are mentioned by Ibn al-Bayṭār, 44% by Dioscorides, and 22% in the *Caraka-Saṃhitā*. But 36% are not recorded at all in these three reference works. Therefore a wide range of plants belongs specifically to the Yemeni pharmacopoeia. As well, a considerable number of therapeutic indications to which the plants are applied are unique to Yemen and unknown elsewhere.[10]

Starting in ancient times, there has been extensive cultural intermingling between the Arabic, Indian, and European medicines, as well as with Chinese medicine. However, it should be noted that while the influence of Arabic medicine is acknowledged as the basis of European medicine, its relationship with Chinese medicine has so far been poorly defined.

3.1.1. *Examples of Local Perception and Preoccupation with Health Care and Healing*

The two main objectives of traditional medicine are the maintenance of bodily purity and proper blood quantity. Illness is thus considered an accumulation of 'dirt,' i.e. humours that are considered harmful such as yellow bile, or a problem with blood quality. Blood is the main source of bodily strength, and the quantity of blood in a person's body should neither be too much nor too little. In the case of women, due to their reproductive functions, preoccupations concerning blood are closely related to adequate evacuation of what is considered 'bad' blood. Women can use the galls

[10] See Fleurentin, Mazars, and Pelt, 'Cultural Background'; eid., 'Additional Information on the Cultural Background'.

(*ʿafṣ*) collected from the infected leaves of *Quercus infectoria* as a vaginal antiseptic, or the seeds of *Lepidium sativum* (*ḥirf*) in the case of excessive menstruation.[11] Preventive measures consist of eating blood-producing foodstuffs such as fenugreek, sorghum, honey, and dates. Routine cleansing of the digestive system includes purgatives (e.g. senna, aloe) or diuretics (e.g. fennel).

3.1.2. *Relationship between the Medicinal Plants and Their Milieu*

The 160 medicinal plants that were identified by the project were classified according to their geographical origin and habitat: 22% of the medicinal plants are cultivated in Yemen, 62% grow wild, and 16% are imported from elsewhere. Except for the cultivated and the imported species, the healers and common people select medicinal plants growing wild in a variety of habitats—from the highlands of Yemen to the desert.[12]

3.1.3. *Medicinal Plants and Their Therapeutic Indications*

Medicinal plants were classified according to the main therapeutic indication for which they are used (Table 1). The predominance of dermatological infections in Yemen—and infectious diseases in general—is closely related to a lack of hygiene and preventive measures; this explains why anti-infective plants have priority amongst the plants prescribed. Analgesic plants form another significant group. The full list of indications gives a clear picture of the dominant pathological problems in Yemen: they are parasitic, pulmonary, urinary, and ocular.

3.2. *Medicinal Plants Whose Therapeutic Indications Were Confirmed through Laboratory Analysis*

In order to make an informed decision regarding effective and safe administration of the plants, close cooperation between ethnologists and pharmacologists is required. Following fieldwork, a number of plants were examined for their chemical, toxicological, and clinical characteristics.[13] In summary, we can say that the effectiveness of 75% of the traditional therapeutic indications has been confirmed through pharmacological evaluation in a ten-year period of research in our laboratory at the University of Metz, France.

---

[11] Fleurentin, 'Le sang', 188.

[12] Id. and Pelt, 'Repertory', 85–108; eid., 'Additional Information for a Repertory'.

[13] Fleurentin et al., 'Two Traditional Medicinal Plants'; Lanhers et al., 'Influence'.

Table 1. Main therapeutic indications for 160 medicinal plants of Yemen

Therapeutic indication	Number of plants	%
dermatology (antibacterial)	28	17.5
analgesia	12	7.5
urology	12	7.5
ophthalmology	12	7.5
gastroenterology and liver	12	7.5
pneumology	11	7
parasites	10	6
neurology	9	6
amulets	8	5
aphrodisiac	7	4
purgation, constipation	5	3
fever	5	3
haemostasis	4	2.5
others	25	16

3.2.1. *Examples of Plants for Internal Treatments*

Crepis rueppellii (*mūrār*)[14] is an herbaceous plant from Arabia and north-western tropical Africa and is considered the best medicine for liver disorders by traditional healers. It is used for hepatic syndromes, icterus, hepatitis, colitis in children, anaemia, and as an antispasmodic. Pharmacological investigation by the author[15] shows the following:

i. It stimulates bile flow (hypercholeresis), mainly the bile acid-dependent fraction.
ii. It has a hepato-protective effect against hepatitis as induced by ethanol in mice and by carbon tetrachloride in rats.
iii. It shows a curative effect against carbon tetrachloride induced hepatitis.
iv. It has synergetic effects when administered in association with *Anisotes trisulcus.*

Anisotes trisulcus (*madīḍ* or *ṣarab*)[16] is a small tree from Arabia; the leaves are used in infusions against hepatic disorder. In combination with the leaves of *Pulicaria orientalis*, it is recommended as a diuretic and against kidney stones and gallstones. Pharmacological investigation by the author[17] demonstrated an effect on the liver and the kidneys:

---

[14] Fleurentin, *Répertoire des pharmacopées traditionnelles*, 239.
[15] See above n. 14 and Fleurentin et al., 'Hepatoprotective Properties'.
[16] Fleurentin, *Répertoire des pharmacopées traditionnelles*, 230.
[17] See above n. 14 and Fleurentin et al., 'Hepatoprotective Properties'.

i. It stimulates bile flow (hypercholeresis), mainly the bile acid-dependent fraction.
ii. It has a hepato-protective effect against hepatitis induced by ethanol in mice and by carbon tetrachloride in rats.
iii. It shows a diuretic effect in rats, increasing sodium, potassium, and chloride excretion and calcium retention.

Trigonella foenum-graecum (*ḥulba*) is a Mediterranean medicinal herb. Pharmacological experiments confirm the traditional uses as an agent to stimulate appetite, lower blood sugar and cholesterol, and reduce kidney stone formation.[18]

3.2.2. *Examples of Plants for Treatment of Fractures or External Infections*

To treat open fractures, traditional healers use an antiseptic plaster combining aloe sap (*ṣabr*), myrrh (*murr*), and *mūmiyā*, a bituminous stone from Yemen. The properties of these plants have been widely demonstrated:

Aloe vera (= *A. barbadensis*) is endemic in Yemen. It produces a latex containing anthraquinones with laxative properties. The transparent gel from the leaves has several effects, from anti-inflammatory (methylchromone being active on cyclooxygenase) to healing and collagen stimulating. Since the gel contains polysaccharides, it also has immuno-modulating and anti-mutagenous properties, and it is both antibacterial and antifungal.[19]

Aloe fleurentinorum is a new endemic species discovered by the author (hence the species name). It was described by Lavranos and Newton in 1977.[20]

Myrrh is an oleo-gum resin from the bark of *Commiphora myrrha*. It is traditionally used as a disinfectant and to make plasters; it shows anti-inflammatory, opioid analgesic (furanoeudesma-1,3-diene, curzerene), bactericidal, and immuno-stimulating effects. Myrrh is also recommended in the European pharmacopoeia for external application to treat colds, diseases of the mouth, and wounds.[21]

---

18 Fleurentin, *Les plantes*, 174–5.
19 Eid., *Plantes médicinales*, 127.
20 Lavranos and Newton, 'Aloe fleurentinorum', 113.
21 Fleurentin, *Plantes médicinales*, 135.

3.2.3. *Medicinal Plants Specific to Yemen: Cultivated or Wild, Used in Yemen or Exported to Other Countries*

Catha edulis (*qāt*): already described by Peter Forskål in 1762.[22] The tree is cultivated in the mountains; its leaves contain natural amphetamine-like molecules (cathine and cathinone). The leaves are chewed in *qāt* sessions every afternoon throughout the country.

Boswellia sacra (*lubān* = frankincense): a gum resin obtained from the bark of the trunk. It is traditionally used in Yemen to treat asthma, aches, thoracic pains, and to repel *jinn*.[23] The healers in India prescribe the gum in cases of inflammatory diseases and, in Europe, in cases of respiratory diseases, toothache, and as a strengthener. Pharmacological experiments have demonstrated an anti-inflammatory effect in rat paw oedema (mediated by an inhibition of 5-lipoxygenase). The gum resin is also effective against haemorrhagic rectocolitis (Crohn's disease) with 350 mg administered three times per day vs. sulfasalazine; the active principles are the boswellic acids.[24]

Coffea arabica (*qahwa*, *bunn* = coffee):[25] cultivated in medium-altitude mountains; it is traditionally used in Yemen as a stimulant, against headaches and kidney stones. The properties of coffee are well known—it is a stimulant of the central nervous system, has a slightly diuretic effect and lipolytic action when used externally (as a cream).[26]

3.2.4. *Other Traditional Medicinal Plants*

Tribulus terrestris (*quṭba*): a tropical herb traditionally used in Yemen as an analgesic for urinary infection, an aphrodisiac, a diuretic, and for treatment of kidney stones. Pharmacological experiments demonstrate a diuretic effect, reduction of kidney stone growth in rats, and stimulation of erection in rats and in humans.[27]

Euphorbia hirta (*lubayn*): a tropical herb whose sap is used in Yemen against warts (and in Africa against dysentery). The pharmacological

---

22 Forskål, *Flora Aegyptiaco-Arabica*, 63. On *qāt*, see also Daniel Martin Varisco's chapter in this volume.

23 On the manifold uses of *Boswellia* spp., see Miranda Morris' chapter in this volume.

24 Fleurentin, *Plantes médicinales*, 81.

25 On coffee, see also Mikhail Rodionov's chapter in this volume.

26 Fleurentin, *Les plantes*, 51. For the history of the use of coffee as a medicine, see Hattox, *Coffee*, 61–71.

27 Weniger, Mortier, and Fleurentin, 'Tribulus terrestris'.

experiments show opioid analgesic, anti-inflammatory, antidiarrhoeal, and sedative effects.[28]

Plantago major (*bizr*): a ubiquitous herb whose crushed seeds are used in a massage against fever. Pharmacological investigation has displayed antihistaminic, anti-inflammatory, antibacterial, and antispasmodic effects.[29]

Thymus laevigatus (*zaʿtar*): an endemic plant traditionally used against parasitic worms and as an appetite stimulant. Antibacterial, antitussive, anti-inflammatory, and antispasmodic properties have also been established.[30]

Lavandula stoechas (*astāhīdus*): a Mediterranean herb traditionally used to treat cough, cold, bronchitis, and for diuresis. Antibacterial, diuretic, and choleretic properties have been demonstrated.[31]

Eucalyptus globulus (*kāfūr*): introduced from Australia, the plant is traditionally used for bronchopulmonary infections. Pharmacological evaluation confirms antibacterial, antitussive, and anti-inflammatory effects.[32]

3.2.5. *Medicinal Plants with Origins in Chinese Medicine*

Traditional Chinese medicine has a 2000-year-long history. The first formulary was *Shén nóng běn cǎo jīng* published during the Han Dynasty (221 BCE–220 CE) and the first pharmacopoeia was the revised *Materia Medica* by Su Jing during the Tang Dynasty (published 659). All of the plants listed below belong to the seventh edition of the Chinese pharmacopoeia.[33] The following plants originating in China are presently used in Yemen:[34]

Glycyrrhiza glabra (*sūs*): a plant from Central Asia that is used in China and Arabia for stomach ulcer and cough.[35]

Curcuma longa (*hurd*): an Indian plant administered in Ayurvedic medicine for its anti-inflammatory properties, in Chinese medicine for the circulation of *qī* (pre-menstrual syndrome symptoms and associated pain), and in Arabic medicine against stomach ulcers and to improve sight. Pharmacological investigation shows anti-inflammatory, hepato-protec-

28 Lanhers et al., 'Behavioral effects'; id. et al., 'Anti-inflammatory Properties'; id. et al., 'Neurophysiological Effects'.

29 Fleurentin, *Plantes médicinales*, 142–3.

30 Fleurentin, *Répertoire des pharmacopées traditionnelles*, 215.

31 Ibid., 200.

32 Fleurentin, *Plantes médicinales*, 44–5.

33 See Fleurentin, 'Pharmacopée chinoise'.

34 It should be noted that these plants were introduced to Europe through Arabic medicine.

35 Fleurentin, *Plantes médicinales*, 168–9.

tive, and anti-ulcer effects. Curcumin from the rhizome also inhibits *in vitro* cancer cell growth by inducing apoptosis (programmed cell death).[36]

Zingiber officinale (*zanjabīl*): an Indian plant applied in Chinese, Indian, and Arabic medicine against cough and nausea.[37]

Syzygium aromaticum (*zirr*, *qaranful*): from the Pacific Islands, used in Arabic medicine for diseases of the digestive tract and dysuria.[38]

4. Conclusion and Outlook

Yemen's biodiversity is extraordinary, not so much from a purely quantitative point of view—although 1,750 species makes an impressive list—but rather in terms of quality and the properties of a number of plants, such as frankincense (*Boswellia sacra*), aloe (*Aloe vera*, syn. *Aloe barbadensis*), and coffee (*Coffea arabica*). Some plant species are widely used all over the world, including senna (*Cassia senna*) and henna (*Lawsonia inermis*).

In 1978, the WHO conference in Alma Ata submitted a programme for the integration of traditional medicine into national health care schemes and a scientific evaluation of traditional herbal drugs.[39] Whereas considerable research has already been completed in Yemen,[40] a Yemeni national pharmacopoeia is still non-existent.

Fieldwork showed that thirty years ago the people themselves were still in possession of medical knowledge, particularly with regard to causality and treatment. Pharmacological experiments have demonstrated that many plants from classical Arabic medicine have valid, high potential for prevention and cure of diseases.

It would be beneficial for Yemen to consider preparing phytodrugs for the local pharmaceutical market from several plants such as *Plantago major* (antiallergic), *Tribulus terrestris* (aphrodisiac), *Trigonella foenum-graecum* (antidiabetic), *Eucalyptus globulus* and *Thymus laevigatus* (both antimicrobial), and *Lavandula stoechas* (sedative).

A future programme for medicinal plant development in Yemen should include:

---

36 Ibid., 164–5.

37 Fleurentin, *Les plantes*, 172–3.

38 Eid., *Plantes médicinales*, 130–1.

39 WHO, *Stratégie*, 65.

40 See, for example, Fleurentin, *Répertoire des pharmacopées traditionnelles*; id., *Guérisseurs*; Schopen, *Heilmittel*; Awadh Ali, Al-Rahwi, and Lindequist, 'Some Medicinal Plants'.

i. An inventory of plants supplying raw substances for the pharmaceutical industry.
ii. An inventory of plants providing essential oils.
iii. A study of endemic plants, including botanical, pharmaco-toxicological, and chemical assessment.
iv. Regulations on, and a definition of, the status of medicinal plants with the aim of structuring a pharmacopoeia in Yemen.
v. Enhanced development of phytodrugs, as for instance in France.[41]

The post-laboratory follow-up on ethnopharmacological fieldwork should lead to sustainable production of phytodrugs. In order to achieve this goal, it is first of all necessary to disseminate the research results (knowledge sharing). Those traditional plants that have proven therapeutic effects need to be cultivated in the country, preferably in gardens that are established for that purpose. Finally, the application of locally prepared herbal medicines in the primary health care system has to be promoted.

Bibliography

Awadh Ali, Nasser A., Al-Rahwi, Khaldoon, and Lindequist, Ulrike, 'Some Medicinal Plants Used in Yemeni Herbal Medicine to Treat Malaria', *African Journal of Traditional, Complementary and Alternative Medicines*, 1 (2004), 72–6.

Dos Santos, José, and Fleurentin, Jacques, 'L'ethnopharmacologie : Une approche pluridisciplinaire', in Jacques Fleurentin et al., *Ethnopharmacologie : Sources, Méthodes, Objectifs* (Paris : Société Française d'Ethnopharmacologie and Orstom, 1991), 26–39.

Fleurentin, Jacques, *Répertoire des pharmacopées traditionnelles du Yémen et étude pharmacologique de deux espèces à propriétés hépatorénales : Crepis rueppellii et Anisotes trisulcus* (PhD thesis, Université de Nancy, 1983).

———, 'Le sang et les plantes du sang dans la médecine traditionnelle du Yémen', *Savoir*, 1 (1988), 177–91.

———, *Guérisseurs et plantes médicinales du Yémen : Au pays de l'encens, de l'aloès et du café* (Paris : Karthala, 2004).

———, 'Les plantes de la pharmacopée chinoise', *Ethnopharmacologia*, 34 (2004), 23–33.

——— (photos Hayon, Jean-Claude), *Les plantes qui nous soignent : Traditions et thérapeutique* (Rennes : Ouest France, 2007).

——— (photos Hayon, Jean-Claude), *Plantes médicinales : Traditions et thérapeutique* (Rennes : Ouest France, 2008).

———, Mazars, Guy, and Pelt, Jean-Marie, 'Cultural Background of the Medicinal Plants of Yemen', *Journal of Ethnopharmacology*, 7 (1982), 183–203.

———, Mazars, Guy, and Pelt, Jean-Marie, 'Additional Information on the Cultural Background of Drugs and Medicinal Plants of Yemen', *Journal of Ethnopharmacology*, 8 (1983), 335–44.

---

41 Fleurentin, *Les plantes*, 11–12.

———, Myntti, Cynthia, and Pelt, Jean-Marie, 'Traditional Medicine and Traditional Healers in North Yemen', *Curare*, special volume 5 (1986), 133–44.

———, and Pelt, Jean-Marie, 'Repertory of Drugs and Medicinal Plants of Yemen', *Journal of Ethnopharmacology*, 6 (1982), 85–108.

———, and Pelt, Jean-Marie, 'Additional Information for a Repertory of Drugs and Medicinal Plants of Yemen', *Journal of Ethnopharmacology*, 8 (1983), 237–43.

———, and Younos, Chafique, 'La médecine islamique', *Encyclopédie des Médecines Naturelles (Phytothérapie—Aromathérapie)* 1 (1990), 1A7–40A7.

———, et al., 'Hepatoprotective Properties of *Crepis rueppellii* and *Anisotes trisulcus*: Two Traditional Medicinal Plants of Yemen', *Journal of Ethnopharmacology*, 16 (1986), 105–11.

Forskål, Petrus/Niebuhr, Carsten (ed.), *Flora Aegyptiaco-Arabica. Sive descriptiones plantarum, quas per Aegyptum inferiorem et Arabiam felicem detexit* (Hauniae [Copenhagen]: Möller, 1775).

Hattox, Ralph S., *Coffee and Coffeehouses: The Origins of a Social Beverage in the Medieval Near East* (Seattle: University of Washington Press, reprint 1988 [1985]).

Ibn al-Bayṭār, ʿAbdallāh Ibn Aḥmad/Leclerc, Lucien (trans.), *Traité des simples par Ibn el-Beïthar* (3 vols.; Paris : Imprimerie nationale, 1877–83).

Lanhers, Marie-Claire, Bertrand, Isabelle, Fleurentin, Jacques, Lehr, Paul R., and Pelt, Jean-Marie, 'Influence of *Anisotes trisulcus* and *Crepis rueppellii* Extracts on Sites of Bile Formation in the Rat', *Arzneimittel-Forschung—Drug Research*, 36 (1986), 826–9.

———, Fleurentin, Jacques, Cabalion, Pierre, Rolland, Alain, Dorfman, Pierre, Misslin, René, and Pelt, Jean-Marie, 'Behavioral Effects of *Euphorbia hirta* L.: Sedative and Anxiolytic Properties', *Journal of Ethnopharmacology*, 29 (1990), 189–98.

———, Fleurentin, Jacques, Dorfman, Pierre, Mortier, François, and Pelt, Jean-Marie, 'Analgesic, Antipyretic and Anti-Inflammatory Properties of *Euphorbia hirta*', *Planta Medica*, 57 (1991), 225–32.

———, Fleurentin, Jacques, Dorfman, Pierre, Misslin, René, and Mortier, François, 'Neurophysiological effects of *Euphorbia hirta* L.', *Phytotherapy Research*, 10/8 (1996), 670–6.

Lavranos, John, and Newton, Len, 'Aloe fleurentinorum', *Cactus and Succulent Journal*, 49 (1977), 113.

Matthiole, Pierre A., *Commentaire sur les six livres de Ped. Dioscoride* (Lyon : Rouillé, 1572).

Myntti, Cynthia, *Medicine in Its Social Context: Observation from Rural North Yemen* (PhD thesis, The London School of Economics, 1982).

Schopen, Armin, *Traditionnelle Heilmittel in Jemen* (Wiesbaden: Steiner, 1983).

Sharma, Priyavrat (ed. and trans.), *Caraka-Saṃhitā* (2 vols.; Jaikrishnadas Ayurveda Series, 36; Varanasi: Chaukhambha Orientalia, 1983).

Weniger, Bernard, Mortier, François, and Fleurentin, Jacques, 'Tribulus terrestris', *Ethnopharmacologia*, 30 (2003), 14–29.

Wood, John R.I., *A Handbook of the Yemen Flora* (Kew: Royal Botanic Gardens, 1997).

Internet Sources

WHO (Organisation Mondiale de la Santé), *Stratégie de l'OMS pour la Médecine Traditionnelle pour 2002–2005* (2002) <http://apps.who.int/medicinedocs/fr/d/Js2298f/>, accessed 6 November 2010.

THE MIRACULOUS PLANT *ḤALQA* (*CYPHOSTEMMA DIGITATUM*): FROM GRANDMOTHER'S KITCHEN IN YEMEN'S SOUTH-WESTERN HIGHLANDS TO MODERN MEDICINAL AND CULINARY APPLICATIONS[1]

Mohammed Al-Duais and Gottfried Jetschke

Yemen's rich ethnobotanical heritage is due in part to the country's remarkable biodiversity, but also to the creativity of the Yemenis with their plant resources and to exchange with both neighbouring and more distant parts of the world. Specific ethnobotanical applications for many plants that are not indigenous to Yemen originate in that country and were transmitted from there to other areas. Among these plants are agarwood, coffee, and *qāt*.[2] As an example, the strong Yemeni ethnobotanical influence on Chinese medicine has been traced and illustrated by Jacques Fleurentin.[3]

The present chapter focuses on a particular aspect of creativity that has amazed one of the authors (M. Al-D.) since childhood—namely the regular use of a plant called *ḥalqa* (*Cyphostemma digitatum* Forsk. (Vitaceae)) by his grandmother in her kitchen for a variety of culinary and medicinal purposes. This is even more surprising because the plant seems to be rather toxic if consumed in non-processed form. The traditional processing of *ḥalqa* involves boiling clean leaves for about half an hour under pressure or overnight in a traditional oven to obtain a thick paste. This is subsequently formed into discs, 8 cm to 12 cm in diameter (Fig. 1) that are then dried in the sun. The discs can later be used as a food additive (e.g. for soups) or for medicinal application.

[1] We would like to thank all the farmers and traditional healers in the south-western highlands of Yemen who shared with us their comprehensive understanding of *ḥalqa* and its culinary and medicinal applications. They are the ones who gave us guidance for tracing the plant in nature. Many thanks go to the German Academic Exchange Service (Deutscher Akademischer Austauschdienst, DAAD) for financing the research that forms the basis of this chapter as part of the doctoral study of M. Al-D. at Jena University, Germany, and to Ibb University, Yemen, for allowing him to take a leave of absence to complete the study. We also thank the many colleagues who helped us with the various aspects of the biochemical analysis. Finally, a warm thank-you to the organizers of the very productive workshop in Halle.

[2] See Mikhail Rodionov's and Daniel Martin Varisco's chapters in this volume.

[3] Fleurentin, *Guérisseurs*, 23; Fleurentin and Pelt, 'Repertory'.

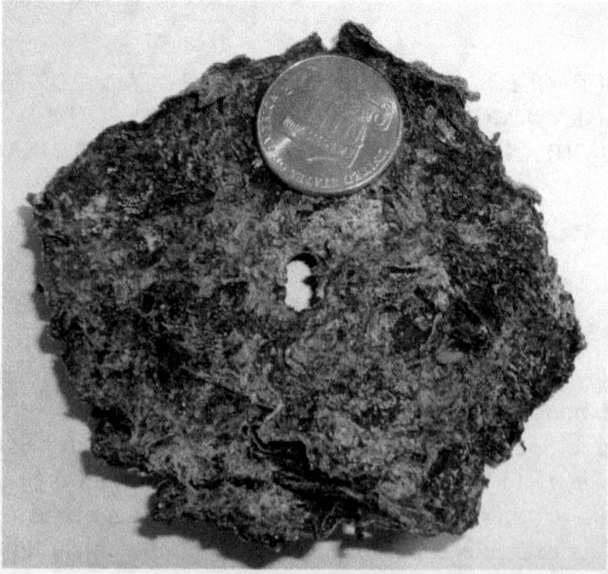

Figure 1. Discs of *ḥalqa* are typically 8 cm to 12 cm in diameter (© Mohammed Al-Duais)

Cyphostemma digitatum is a perennial, climbing, succulent undershrub with compound fleshy leaves and tendrils. The leaves are petiolate and digitately 3- to 5-foliolate; the leaflets are ovate and dentate. The plant flowers in pedunculate, axillary, flat-topped inflorescences, in which the central flowers open first, followed by the peripheral ones. Fruits are one-seeded, red, fleshy berries (Fig. 2). *C. digitatum* grows at altitudes of 1400 m to 2500 m, often on cliffs, and with a preference for shaded, stony places such as gullies and terrace walls. It is usually associated with plants of the genera *Acacia*, *Agave*, *Clematis*, and *Euphorbia*, and with *Senecio hadiensis*.[4]

The thirteenth-century Rasulid ruler al-Malik al-Muẓaffar (d. 1295) gives a detailed description of the plant, its ecology, and use in his treatise on *materia medica*, *al-Muʿtamad fī l-adwiya al-mufrada* [The Reliable Source on Simple Medicines].[5] The author characterizes the plant as a climber, similar to the grapevine, and mentions that it grows in marginal rocky lands.[6] He also states some interesting details about the preparation and

---

[4] Wood, *Handbook*, 18.

[5] See Ingrid Hehmeyer's chapter in this volume for the suggestion that the author of the work was, in fact, al-Malik al-Muẓaffar's son, al-Ashraf ʿUmar.

[6] al-Malik al-Muẓaffar/al-Saqqā (ed.), *al-Muʿtamad*, 90.

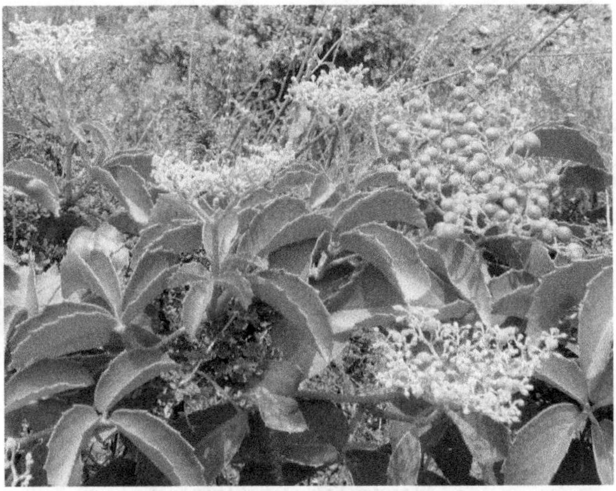

Figure 2. Mature *ḥalqa* plant with inflorescences, fruits, and fleshy leaves, ready to be harvested (north of Ibb) (© Gottfried Jetschke)

use of the plant, such as the fact that the leaves are acidic and should be cooked with meat. He further notes that the cleaned leaves may be simmered in water, and that—after pressing the leaves—the acidic extract can be mixed with *ʿuṣfur* (safflower, *Carthamus tinctorius*). This liquid's properties are described as being more beneficial than those of pomegranate juice. A mixture of the acidic extract and *ʿuṣfur* can also be dried (the text does not describe how, but one may assume a similar process as the one outlined above for the *ḥalqa* discs). The dried compound is said to be useful against vomiting and as an analgesic to treat irritation after vomiting. The author even gives another method of preparation—heating the leaves in the embers of a traditional baking oven, called *tannūr*, until they are black and dry. These are then homogenized with water at a ratio of 1:6 and the liquid is recommended as a remedy to treat vomiting, heartburn after vomiting, and asthma.[7]

Although knowledge about *ḥalqa* seems to be largely limited to the south-western highlands of Yemen, one can observe a recent increase in demand for the processed form beyond that area. Individuals and whole family enterprises are involved in intensive harvesting (and processing) of the plant, even in remote areas. In addition, the export of *ḥalqa* to places outside Yemen has increased dramatically. Overexploitation of the

[7] Ibid., 90.

plant resources is the result, and many source areas have already become devoid of *C. digitatum*. This observation has led the authors to the hypothesis that *ḥalqa* may constitute an important natural resource in Yemen, whose biochemical and ecological properties merit investigation. The four-year project (2005–9) was thus motivated by personal interest in the scientific validation of the culinary and medicinal potency of the *ḥalqa* plant and concern about the threat of its extinction. The aims of the project were to study *C. digitatum* as a culinary and medicinal species through biochemical analysis; to evaluate the plant's ecological requirements through extended field observations; and to recommend measures for a sustainable use of *C. digitatum*. Additional information as well as colour photographs can be found in a separate publication.[8]

1. Materials and Methods

1.1. *Collection of Information*

The existing information had to be gathered by asking local informants a number of basic questions, such as: Where can we find this overexploited species? How long has it been known and used in the region? How is the plant used and for which purposes? Is there any known toxicity associated with the plant? Is there any large-scale commercial harvesting by local inhabitants of the region or by people from other areas and if so, why? What is the market for the end product and where is it traded? Is the end product pure, or is it mixed with other plants? What is the current state of growth of the plant in the region compared with the past? Where can one find typical source areas where the plant is still growing abundantly? This and related information was collected with the help of a questionnaire (see Appendix 1) during meetings with local informants that included people who harvest, consume, and trade *ḥalqa*, as well as traditional healers (Fig. 3). Thus we were able to gain comprehensive ethnocultural and socioeconomic information from people throughout the south-western highlands of Yemen.

[8] Jetschke, 'Tradition trifft moderne Wissenschaft'.

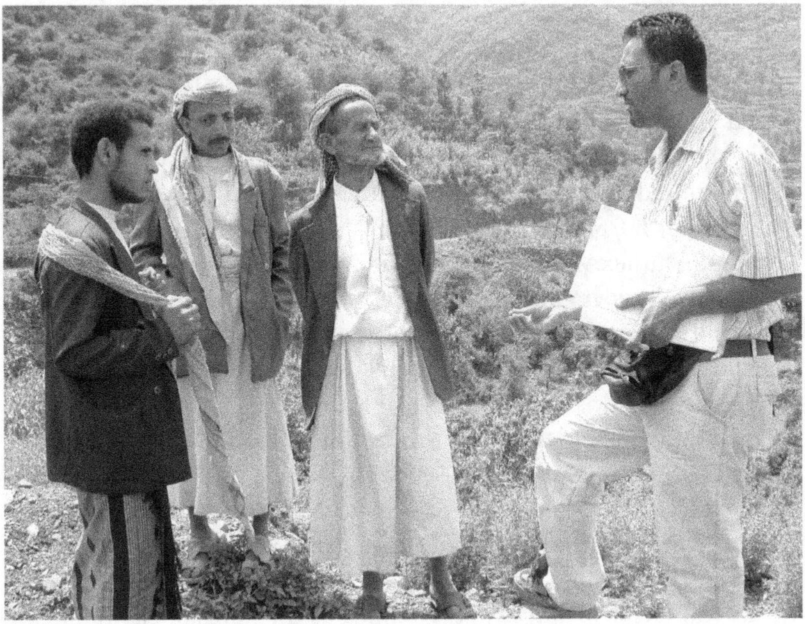

Figure 3. Interview with local informants (east of Ibb) (© Gottfried Jetschke, 2007)

1.2. *Ecological Field Data*

Three field surveys (2005–7) were each conducted in August and September, the months following the late-summer rains in the south-western Yemeni highlands and therefore the time when vegetation growth peaks in the area. The surveys covered a large region in the governorates of Ibb and Taʿizz and some neighbouring areas. In 2005, we focused on the acquisition of phytosociological data to understand the ecological requirements of *C. digitatum*, and to classify its main harbouring vegetation units according to species composition. At fourteen typical sites, vegetation data were recorded in detail to compile a comprehensive list of all plant species growing together with *C. digitatum*, and to estimate their local abundance. Plot locations were subjectively chosen in areas with relatively homogeneous and intact natural vegetation and as far away from human impact as possible. Sampling areas were predetermined as 10 m x 10 m plots according to the 'minimal sampling area method' that involves finding the minimal size of a representative plot that contains nearly all species of a particular vegetation unit. Estimates of vegetation cover were obtained using the 'centralized replicate sampling procedure'[9] with the standard Braun-Blanquet cover-abundance scale. This is an easy-to-use field method in which the local amount of a species is estimated—and classified—either based on numbers of specimens, if populations are small ('abundance'; scale 1, 2–5, 6–50 specimens), or, if populations are large, based on percentage of ground cover of the species ('dominance'; scale 5–25%, 25–50%, 50–75%, >75%). Site conditions such as slope, aspect, geology, soil type, soil depth, surface water availability, and human influence were recorded, together with geographical coordinates and altitude (GPS, ±8 m precision). This kind of standardized recording of vegetation is called 'relevé' in phytosociology and comprises the basic unit for subsequent classification according to floristic similarities.

In addition, while travelling through the area, at locations that were chosen rather randomly, the presence or absence (within a range of vision of about 100 m to 200 m) of *Cyphostemma digitatum* specimens was recorded, together with the above-mentioned site conditions, coordinates, and altitude. These data were needed to characterize the so-called 'realized ecological niche' of *ḥalqa* that is defined as the range of environmental factors under which the target plant can grow and establish itself in spite of natural competition with other plants for resources such as light, water, or nutrients.

Since almost nothing was known about the ecology of *ḥalqa* in published scientific literature, in 2005 we were mainly led by previous personal experience and by information collected over the course of our first field survey. In the years 2006 and 2007, however, we had already gained considerable experience. We had also obtained the first results from computer-based modelling of the species' potential occurrence. Thus, besides some randomly chosen locations, specific areas were visited that required expanding the original study region around Taʿizz and Ibb. Altogether we compiled eighty-nine complete phytosociological relevé data *sensu* Braun-Blanquet and simple presence/absence data of *C. digitatum* from about 1100 locations.

1.3. *Sample Preparation*

Fresh leaves of *ḥalqa* were collected in August 2006 in the Baʿdān district of the south-western highlands, a remote area away from any substantial

[9] Mueller-Dombois and Ellenberg, *Aims and Methods*, 43.

human impact. A voucher sample was given to the Agricultural Research Centre in Taʿizz. Preparation of the plant material for chemical analysis followed the household recipes in order to obtain the product in its typical form. One part of the clean leaves was boiled under pressure for 30 minutes, then the water was removed and the leaf mass stirred with a wooden spoon. As soon as the mass thickened, the paste was scooped out onto flat plates and formed into discs (8 cm to 12 cm in diameter) that were dried in the sun (covered with mesh) at an average temperature of 30°C during the day. The discs were turned every day until completely dry. We refer to the discs as the 'processed' sample. Another part of the collected fresh leaves was dried in an oven at 40°C for 90 minutes and is referred to as 'raw' sample. Samples were packed in dark, airtight containers and stored at ambient temperature for three to five months before use.

1.4. *Biochemical Analysis*

The main aim of the biochemical analysis was to investigate how household processing influences the biochemical properties of the plant material, and in particular how it eliminates its toxicity. In preparation of laboratory analysis, both the 'raw' and the 'processed' samples were milled with a mechanical mill (Cyclotec mill, 1 mm mesh). Extracts from both kinds of samples were obtained using ethanol and water, respectively. The total phenolic content of the extracts was quantified using the Folin-Ciocalteu method (also called Gallic Acid Equivalent Method) that measures the amount of a particular chemical substance needed to inhibit oxidation of the reagent. The specific antioxidant capacity was analyzed by laboratory methods that are sensitive to different compounds.[10] As for the vitamins and carotenoids, analysis was based on reversed-phase high-performance liquid chromatography (HPLC) that is routinely used to identify, quantify, and purify the individual components of a mixture. Volatile compounds (that are important for aroma and flavour) were extracted by solid phase microextraction and analyzed by gas chromatography.

1.5. *Statistical Analysis and Modelling*

Vegetation data from the eighty-nine relevés were analyzed by multivariate statistical methods, including cluster analysis, indicator species analysis,

---

10 A detailed description is beyond the scope of this chapter, but can be found in Al-Duais et al., 'Antioxidant Capacity', 815–16.

and non-metric multidimensional scaling. Cluster analysis is a method of a computer-assisted, nested classification of samples through the similarity of observed traits; in our case through the similarity in species composition and abundance. Indicator species analysis involves the search for particular species that are closely related to corresponding clusters, hence being characteristic of a particular plant community. Non-metric, multidimensional scaling is an indirect ordination technique to illustrate the relationships between samples in species composition space. The accuracy of the obtained classification was evaluated by multi-response permutation procedure (using PC-ORD software).[11] The presence/absence data for *ḥalqa* itself and for its harbouring plant communities were analyzed by nonparametric multiplicative regression (NPMR) with HyperNiche software.[12] Geographical Information System (GIS) software was used to construct predictive maps of the potential distribution of *C. digitatum* in Yemen.

2. Results

2.1. *Ethnobotany and Ethnomedicine*

During the fieldwork, an interesting picture about the existing knowledge of *ḥalqa* emerged. While in some areas the plant was grown in private gardens for regular use, in other more remote regions in the northern parts of the study area the plant was sometimes completely unknown. In some areas, only older people were able to lead us to places where *ḥalqa* grew, while in other cases, even children knew what we were looking for. In the southernmost part of our research area, mainly in the Taʿizz region, the plant species was often documented as absent due to intensive and commercial exploitation. Based on our visits to many regions and interviews with numerous people, we obtained an impressive list of culinary and medicinal applications, together with their recipes for preparation. A selection of examples is given in Table 1. It seems that *ḥalqa* is first of all a food

[11] For details, see McCune and Mefford, *PC-ORD: Multivariate Analysis*.

[12] McCune, *Nonparametric Multiplicative Regression*, 1–52; id., 'Non-parametric Habitat Models'. NPMR is a numerical smoothing procedure to derive the realized niche of a plant species, i.e. the quantitative response (here: probability of occurrence) of the species to the most influential environmental factors. Roughly speaking, a window of fixed width is moved through the range of environmental variables such that the proportion of presence observations ('response') can be estimated and smoothed as a function of these explaining variables ('predictors').

flavouring, and as such it is a main ingredient of the traditional Yemeni meat broth (*maraq*). Besides that, *ḥalqa* was described to us as being used medicinally to treat gastroenteritis, fatigue, vomiting, headache, and malaria, and generally for the promotion of good health. Preparation of an acidic drink to treat heartburn and asthma as described in al-Malik al-Muẓaffar's thirteenth-century work on *materia medica*[13] was not documented during the field surveys. Today one of *ḥalqa*'s main medicinal applications is to prevent vomiting. Its use as an analgesic was predominantly documented in the Ibb governorate, especially in the districts of Mudhaykhira, Baʿdān, al-Shiʿir, and al-Jaʿāshin.

2.2. *Bioactivity*

Biochemical analysis revealed that *C. digitatum* has a considerable antioxidant capacity and content of phenolic compounds (total phenolic content of 1.41 g/100 g in the 'raw' and 0.80 g/100 g in the 'processed' water extracts). The antioxidant capacity was found to be higher than that of asparagus (0.49 g/100 g and 0.45 g/100 g, respectively), broccoli, red pepper, white onion, snap bean, tomato, white cabbage, carrot, and peas—if measured by the same methods.[14] The compounds resulting in the remarkably high antioxidant capacity were investigated and quantified: *C. digitatum* contains reasonable quantities of vitamin C (49.5 mg/100 g in the 'raw' and 20.3 mg/100 g in the 'processed' form), vitamin E (82.7 mg/100 g and 101.2 mg/100 g, respectively, including β- and γ-tocotrienol forms that are very rare in nature), provitamin A (2.49 RE/100 g and 2.40 RE/100 g, respectively), and carotenoids (42.2 mg/100 g and 15.0 mg/100 g, respectively). Compared to other green, leafy vegetables, all of these bioactive compounds were found in high quantities.[15] It is also not surprising that an aroma test identified twenty-three favourable aroma-active compounds.[16]

---

13 al-Malik al-Muẓaffar/al-Saqqā (ed.), *al-Muʿtamad*, 90.

14 Al-Duais et al., 'Antioxidant Capacity'.

15 Al-Duais et al., 'Contents of Vitamin C'.

16 Al-Duais and Bartzsch, 'Key Aroma Components'.

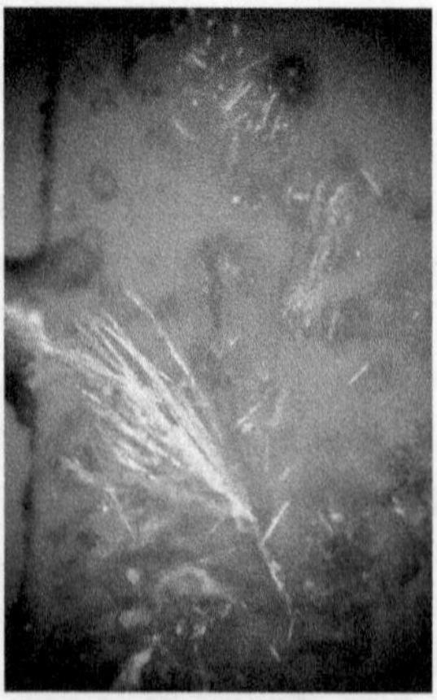

Figure 4. Spiny crystals (presumably composed of calcium oxalate) on the dry leaves of *C. digitatum*, photographed under the polarized light microscope (magnification: 100×) (© Mohammed Al-Duais)

However, it became clear that household processing results in a significant reduction of the quantities of most bioactive compounds; only vitamin E was enhanced. This situation can only be improved if a less destructive method of preparation of the fresh plant material is found. Hence, one of our tasks was to analyze the source of the toxicity of the fresh leaves, and how it is eliminated by household processing. Investigations showed that the toxicity is not of a chemical nature, but caused mechanically by microscopic spiny crystals (presumably composed of calcium oxalate) on the leaves (Fig. 4).

2.3. *Phytosociology*

Because of the lack of existing ecological studies about *C. digitatum*, the dialogue with local people provided important background information and guidance for discovering and characterizing the habitats that normally harbour the species. The field survey method (following the Braun-Blanquet approach) and the subsequent data analysis (by multivariate statistics) enabled us to classify the accompanying vegetation into seven different plant communities. This extends the description given by Ahmed Al-Hubaishi and Klaus Müller-Hohenstein[17] and Wood considerably.[18] Each

[17] Al-Hubaishi and Müller-Hohenstein, *Vegetation of Yemen*, 69–92.
[18] Wood, *Handbook*, 18.

community can be characterized by a few typical indicator species. Two of these communities were mainly found at altitudes between 1000 m and 1800 m. They belong to the higher zone of frost-free vegetation, and can be fairly well recognized by presence of the tree species *Acacia etbaica* and *Acacia mellifera*, and a rather low grass cover. The third community marks a transitional zone, while four of the seven communities were mainly found above 1800 m, extending to 2600 m and higher, where vegetation is rather frequently exposed to frost. The latter four host the tree species *Acacia gerrardii*, *Euphorbia parciramulosa* and *Acacia origena* and exhibit a higher grass cover. These seven communities can be recognized easily in the field and follow a typical sequence with increasing altitude. Contrary to previous estimates by Al-Hubaishi and Müller-Hohenstein[19] and Wood,[20] we were able to show that the borderline between the higher, frost-free vegetation and the vegetation exposed to frost is located around 1800 m.

2.4. *Ecology and Predictive Modelling*

Based on presence/absence data from about 1100 locations of *ḥalqa* and their main abiotic conditions, a response function of the species *C. digitatum* (and its harbouring communities) to environmental conditions was derived statistically. It shows that *C. digitatum* has a rather broad ecological amplitude and can be found from an elevation of 1000 m to even 3000 m. The optimum of occurrence is around 2000 m. Annual rainfall (mainly determined through elevation) and the temperature during the driest quarter of the year (winter) were the most influential climatic variables. Predictive probability maps of potential occurrence of *C. digitatum* were constructed. Based on these, some areas of potential occurrence were visited to validate the map. As a result, several new places have been identified where *C. digitatum* grows naturally, some of them in the northern parts of the study area where *ḥalqa* is much less known.

3. Discussion

Our fieldwork demonstrates that there is substantial and diverse local knowledge about *ḥalqa*.[21] Most locals were eager to answer the question-

19 Al-Hubaishi and Müller-Hohenstein, *Vegetation of Yemen*, 77.

20 Wood, *Handbook*, 18.

21 It should be pointed out that this local knowledge also includes other plants with culinary and medicinal applications.

naire and wanted to know our purpose for collecting the information. Interestingly, the ways of using *ḥalqa* were quite diverse across the region we visited. This was particularly the case with regard to the methods of preparation. Knowledge was less common the further we moved north. We also found many additional applications that are not mentioned in al-Malik al-Muẓaffar's treatise on *materia medica*.[22] This suggests some shift or modification of use since the thirteenth century, or even the discovery of new applications.

Ours is the first scientific work to show the importance of leaves from a plant belonging to the family of Vitaceae (the grape family of flowering plants) as a rich source of antioxidants and phenolic compounds, compared to the intensive research that has been conducted on members of other families, such as Labiatae (the mint family), Compositae (the aster, daisy or composite family), Leguminosae (the pea family), Geraniaceae (the cranesbill family), and Rosaceae (the rose family).[23] Due to the high antioxidant capacity and content of phenolic compounds of *C. digitatum*, the species is clearly an important new source of functional food ingredients. Any concerns about harmful consequences may be disregarded, since the plant (in its processed form) has been regularly consumed for generations without any noticeable side effects or acute or chronic toxicity. Because *ḥalqa* is easily accessible and cheap, it might soon become a competitive source of phytonutrients, if its effectiveness and use can be promoted to the general public.

It is estimated that there are about 76,000 blind people in Yemen, i.e. 35 blind per 10,000 inhabitants, most of them living in rural areas.[24] A study from the early 1990s on children between 1 and 5 years of age in western Yemen found that about 2.2% of the children were suffering from xerophthalmia (abnormal dryness of the eye due to a deficiency of tears).[25] If untreated, xerophthalmia can ultimately lead to blindness. Xerophthalmia (and night blindness as well) is caused by severe vitamin A deficiency. The results from the study are alarming, demonstrating that xerophthalmia and vitamin A deficiency are among the major health problems in western Yemen.[26] It is our strong recommendation that *ḥalqa* be used as a food supplement to combat this problem.[27]

---

22 al-Malik al-Muẓaffar/al-Saqqā (ed.), *al-Muʿtamad*, 90.
23 Al-Duais et al., 'Antioxidant Capacity'.
24 Al-Akily and Bamashmus, 'Causes of Blindness'; Ghaleb, 'Blindness on the Increase'.
25 Rosen et al., 'Vitamin A Deficiency'.
26 Ibid.
27 Al-Duais et al., 'Contents of Vitamin C'.

The main sources of vitamin E are animal fat, plant oils, and green, leafy vegetables, with the latter being particularly rich in vitamin E. Intake of fats and oils can be replaced by a diet rich in green, leafy vegetables. *C. digitatum* could also become a significant food supplement for people suffering from fat and oil malabsorption that can lead to vitamin E deficiency.

The carotenoids lutein and zeaxanthin and some other antioxidants are very susceptible to oxidative degradation by heat. Thus, in order to maximize their dietary intake and bioavailability, we are currently exploring a modification of the cooking and processing practices of *C. digitatum* to reduce such losses of carotenoids as much as possible, and to increase their bioavailability. Specifically, this involves crushing the dried plant material with a high pressure mill. The expected effect is the destruction of the spiny crystals that cause the toxicity of the fresh leaves. Short heating times in a microwave oven instead of lengthy cooking may also reduce the losses.

C. digitatum has the potential of being a resource for the extraction of pure vitamin E for the pharmaceutical, cosmetic, and food industries. This would require large-scale cultivation of the species. Research on the potential for antifungal activity of *C. digitatum* is at an early stage.

These various findings confirm that historical and ethnobotanical knowledge can be a valuable source of information about culinary and medicinal applications of Yemeni plants. Not all of the alleged beneficial properties of *ḥalqa* in ethnomedicine have yet been proven. For instance, although we received reports that *ḥalqa* is used against malaria, no such effect could be determined by specialists from the Swiss Tropical Institute in Basel.[28] However, there are promising indications that its effectiveness against sleeping sickness, which has similar symptoms, may be proven by us in the future.

Due to the help of many local people we were able to establish the ecological conditions under which the plant *ḥalqa* potentially occurs in nature. Our observations showed that *C. digitatum* is a very tolerant species, with a rather broad ecological range. It is closely associated with some other widespread species, and can be found within a set of well-distinguished plant communities that can be easily recognized by a few indicator species. These vegetation units cover the higher, frost-free zones, and the lower frost zone of the south-western highlands of Yemen. Early steps,

---

[28] Personal communication with Matthias Hamburger, Institute of Pharmaceutical Biology, University of Basel (June 2009).

though, of modelling the potential occurrence of *C. digitatum* in Yemen did not seem to be successful. The explanation for these initial problems was quite simple. Our data were flawed because many locations in the Ta'izz region, where the plant was recorded as absent, were, in fact, only pseudo-absence points due to overexploitation of *ḥalqa*: the typical indicator species known from other areas were still observable. A combination of these characteristic plant communities with predictive modelling gave much better projections of potential occurrence and finally enabled us to find intact *C. digitatum* populations in remote places with similar ecological conditions.

The broad ecological niche of *C. digitatum* suggests the potential for successful re-introduction of the species through seeds and cuttings in regions that have been overexploited in the past. Adding *ḥalqa* to the list of endangered species might reduce intensive commercial harvesting as it would be illegal. This would also give time for a well-planned, systematic and large-scale re-introduction to be established. However, the enforcement of such a label on a local level might be a challenge for the rather weak central government of Yemen. Another way of expanding the availability of the plant and its usage would be to promote its cultivation in people's private gardens, together with an educational programme instructing people on *ḥalqa*'s many culinary and medicinal benefits.

Overall, our project has increased knowledge about *C. digitatum*—one of the most intensively harvested wild species of Arabia. Furthermore, during our studies it has become clear that ethnobotanical research, which usually has a historical component, can reveal valuable resources, even though knowledge of them may have been lost in modern times. Comprehensive study of a particular plant, including its botany, ecology, history, and its culinary, medicinal, and commercial use can open up valuable information for today's world. In addition, this broad approach is the only one that permits appreciation of a plant in its entirety. Needless to say, regarding *ḥalqa*, there is still a lot to be learned.

Bibliography

Al-Akily, Saleh A., and Bamashmus, Mahfouth A., 'Causes of Blindness among Adult Yemenis: A Hospital-based Study', *Middle East and African Journal of Ophthalmology*, 15 (2008), 3–6.

Al-Duais, Mohammed, *Vegetation Ecology and Ethnobotany of* Cyphostemma digitatum *in the Western Highlands in Yemen* (PhD thesis, Institute of Ecology, University of Jena, Germany, 2009).

Al-Duais, Mohammed, and Bartzsch, Christine, 'Search for the Key Aroma Compounds in *Cyphostemma digitatum* before and after Processing', Submitted to *Journal of Food Chemistry and Toxicology* (2009).

———, Hohbein, Juliane, Werner, Susanne, Böhm, Volker, and Jetschke, Gottfried, 'Contents of Vitamin C, Carotenoids, Tocopherols and Tocotrienols in the Subtropical Plant Species *Cyphostemma digitatum* as Affected by Processing', *Journal of Agricultural and Food Chemistry*, 57 (2011), 5420–7.

———, Müller, Lars, Böhm, Volker, and Jetschke, Gottfried, 'Antioxidant Capacity and Total Phenolics of *Cyphostemma digitatum* before and after Processing: Use of Different Assays', *European Food Research and Technology*, 228 (2009), 813–21.

Fleurentin, Jacques, *Guérisseurs et plantes médicinales du Yémen : Au pays de l'encens, de l'aloès et du café* (Paris : Karthala, 2004).

———, and Pelt, Jean-Marie, 'Repertory of Drugs and Medicinal Plants of Yemen', *Journal of Ethnopharmacology*, 6 (1982), 85–108.

Al-Hubaishi, Ahmed, and Müller-Hohenstein, Klaus, *An Introduction to the Vegetation of Yemen* (Eschborn: Deutsche Gesellschaft für Technische Zusammenarbeit, 1984).

Jetschke, Gottfried, 'Tradition trifft moderne Wissenschaft: Zur Biochemie und Ökologie der Pflanzenart "Halka" (*Cyphostemma digitatum*)', *Jemen-Report*, 41/1–2 (2010), 20–4.

al-Malik al-Muẓaffar Yūsuf b. ʿUmar al-Ghassānī al-Turkmānī/al-Saqqā, Muṣṭafā (ed.), *al-Muʿtamad fī l-adwiya al-mufrada* (Beirut: Dār al-qalam, 2004).

McCune, Bruce, 'Non-parametric Habitat Models with Automatic Interactions', *Journal of Vegetation Science*, 17/6 (2006), 819–30.

———, and Mefford, Michael J., *PC-ORD: Multivariate Analysis of Ecological Data. Version 4. User's Guide* (Gleneden Beach, OR: MjM Software Design, 1999).

Mueller-Dombois, Dieter, and Ellenberg, Heinz, *Aims and Methods of Vegetation Ecology* (New York: Wiley, 1974).

Rosen, David S., Al-Sharif, Z., Bashir, M., Al-Shabooti, A., and Pizzarello, Louis D., 'Vitamin A Deficiency and Xerophthalmia in Western Yemen' (Helen Keller International Publication), *European Journal of Clinical Nutrition*, 50/1 (1996), 54–7.

Wood, John R.I., *A Handbook of the Yemen Flora* (Kew: Royal Botanic Gardens, 1997).

Internet Sources

Ghaleb, Thuria, 'Blindness on the Increase in Yemen', *Yemen Observer* 2007 (18 September 2007) <http://www.yobserver.com/sports-health-and-lifestyle/10012961.html>, accessed 20 January 2011.

McCune, Bruce, *Nonparametric Multiplicative Regression for Habitat Modeling* (2009) <http://www.pcord.com/NPMRintro.pdf>, accessed 21 March 2010.

Table 1. Examples of typical methods of preparation and use of *C. digitatum*

Governorate / Region	Preparation and use
Taʿizz / Jabal Ṣabir and Bilād al-Ḥayqī	Throughout the area, *ḥalqa* is prepared on a commercial scale mixed with *ḥalaṣ* (*Cissus rotundifolia*) and *ʿuthrub* (*Rumex nervosus*). The dried discs are sold afterwards—dishonestly—as a pure *ḥalqa* product.
Taʿizz / Jabal Ṣabir and Bilād al-Ḥayqī, al-Ḍāliʿ / Jabal Juḥāf	Discs prepared of pure *ḥalqa* are powdered and used for salads and other dishes.
Taʿizz / al-Misrākh	Fresh, cleaned leaves of *ḥalqa* are milled and cooked with garlic and black pepper and used to treat malaria symptoms.
Taʿizz / Sharʿab, Ibb / al-ʿUdayn	Fresh, cleaned leaves of *ḥalqa* are cooked with spices, garlic, onion, and ghee (*samn*) and eaten with bread or *ʿaṣīd* (sorghum porridge).
al-Ḍāliʿ / al-ʿAwd	Branches of fresh *ḥalqa* are thrown into the fire of a traditional oven (*tannūr*) to add a special flavour to the sorghum bread.
Ibb / Mudhaykhira – al-Jawāliḥ (a subregion of Mudhaykhira)	Fresh, cleaned leaves of *ḥalqa* are cooked overnight in the *tannūr* with hot peppers, garlic, and thyme. The mixture is then formed into discs, dried, and stored for use.
Ibb / Mudhaykhira, Baʿdān, al-Shiʿir, and al-Jaʿāshin	In addition to its culinary use as a spice and food flavouring, *ḥalqa* discs are used medicinally to prevent vomiting, as an analgesic, and for the general promotion of good health.
Ibb / Ṣuhbān	Fresh, cleaned leaves of *ḥalqa* are cooked with potatoes, spices, garlic, onion, and ghee (*samn*). The mixture is eaten with bread.
Dhamār / al-Manār	Fresh, cleaned leaves of *ḥalqa* are cooked overnight in the *tannūr* to a thick paste. This is applied externally to skin abscesses to promote healing.
Rayma / al-Salafiyya	Fresh leaves of *ḥalqa* are used for cleaning silver and antiques.
Ḥajja / Ḥuṣn ʿAzzān	Fresh, cleaned leaves of *ḥalqa* are eaten after boiling them with milk.

Appendix 1: Questionnaire for Collection of Ethnocultural and Socio-economic Information

Date | / / |

Governorate | |

District | | Village | |

Name of informant | | Sex | | Age | |

Profession | |

(1) Where can we find *ḥalqa* in this region?

(2) Where can we find a typical source area where the plant is still abundant?

(3) How long has *ḥalqa* been known and used in the region?

(4) How do you use the plant, for which purposes, and how frequently?

(5) Is it used as a pure product, or mixed with other plants (if yes, which ones)?

(6) Is there any large-scale commercial harvesting by local inhabitants of the region, or by people from other areas?

(7) What is the current state of growth of the plant in the region compared with the past?

(8) What is the market for the end product and where is it traded?

(9) Is there any known toxicity associated with the plant?

(10) Any other information about *ḥalqa*?

A PHARMACIST'S VIEW OF THE POTENTIAL VALUE TO MODERN MEDICINE OF PLANTS AND FUNGI USED BY TRADITIONAL MEDICINE IN YEMEN[1]

Ulrike Lindequist

An interest in drugs derived from natural sources and the utilization of plants for pharmaceutical purposes is increasing all over the world. Over 60% of anticancer drugs currently in use have been isolated from natural sources, including plants, marine organisms, or microorganisms, or are related to them.[2] Nearly all antibiotics have their origin in natural sources. Famous examples for natural compounds that have been licensed as drugs are the cytostatic paclitaxel, from *Taxus* species, or the antimalaria drug artemisinin, from *Artemisia annua*. As well as isolated substances, plant extracts are also used in the treatment of various diseases, e.g. extracts from *Valeriana officinalis* for sleeping disorders, or *Thymus* extracts for cough. Nevertheless, there are still many diseases that cannot be treated successfully. The occurrence of drug resistances and of new illnesses intensifies the problem and therefore there is a great need for new drugs worldwide. Plants from the ethnomedicine of many developing countries, such as Yemen, can be an important source for the potential development of new drugs.

Herbal medicine represents one of the most important fields of traditional medicine in Yemen, especially in the rural areas. Thus, phytotherapy is practised by a large proportion of Yemen's population for the

---

[1] We are very thankful to Professors Ramzi Mothana and Nasser A. Awadh Ali, University of Ṣanʿāʾ, and Mohamed Al-Fatimi and Samira Abdullah Mahmood, University of Aden, for the very fruitful and pleasant collaboration in all parts of this work. Without their initiative and their practical as well as theoretical input this work could not have been done. Besides this, we wish to acknowledge the named Yemeni Universities, as well as the German Academic Exchange Service (Deutscher Akademischer Austauschdienst, DAAD) and the Humboldt Foundation, for financial support for the visit of the Yemeni scientists to the University of Greifswald. We are also indebted to the Yemeni inhabitants for sharing their herbal medicine expertise with us, and to all our colleagues and students in Yemen and Germany who have supported this work. Especially we wish to thank Professor Hanns Kreisel and PD Dr. Peter König, University of Greifswald, for their valuable support in tackling all the taxonomical problems, and Professor Patrick Bednarski, University of Greifswald, for revision of the English.

[2] Newman, Cragg, and Snader, 'Natural Products'.

treatment of several physical, physiological, mental, and social ailments. To promote the proper application of herbal medicine and to determine the potential of the traditionally used plants as sources for new drugs, it is essential to study them in a more intensified and scientific manner with the help of modern biological and chemical methods. Since 1997, in collaboration with our Yemeni colleagues we have studied a broad spectrum of plants from the inventory of traditional Yemeni ethnomedicine in order to identify interesting biological activities and bioactive components. Because of the increasing need for new antibiotics and antitumour drugs worldwide, plants with antimicrobial and cytostatic/cytotoxic activities have been the centre of our attention. The initiation of the projects, as well as the collection of plants and the recording of traditional experiences, was carried out by our Yemeni colleagues and their students: Prof. Ramzi A.A. Mothana, University of Ṣan'ā', Prof. Nasser A. Awadh Ali, University of Ṣan'ā', Prof. Mohamed Al-Fatimi, University of Aden, and Prof. Samira Abdullah Mahmood, University of Aden. These Yemeni scientists are responsible for much of the practical and theoretical work of the project (see cited papers).

In addition to plants, larger fungi were also included in our investigations. Knowledge about the occurrence, taxonomy, chemistry, pharmacology, and application of Yemeni fungi is very limited. Following the collection of a few larger fungi in Yemen during the nineteenth century, there was a long break of about eighty years in the scientific investigation of the larger fungi of Yemen. Because of the increasing importance of fungi as 'medicinal mushrooms' and as a source of biologically active compounds, our Yemeni colleagues—mainly Prof. Mohamed Al-Fatimi—directed their attention not only towards plants, but also to fungi. They collected larger fungi in several regions of North and South Yemen, and on the island of Soqotra. The taxonomic identification has been carried out by Prof. Hanns Kreisel at the University of Greifswald.[3] Judging from the data currently available, it has been concluded that the macromycete flora of Yemen is mainly a tropical one, composed of pantropic and paleotropic taxa and a few elements that Yemen has in common either with central and southern Africa or with south-western and central Asia.[4] Some results of our screening investigations of Yemeni plants and fungi are summarized below. In addition, selected examples are reported in more detail.

---

3 Kreisel and Al-Fatimi, 'Basidiomycetes'.

4 Eid., 'Further Basidiomycetes'.

1. Screening Investigations

1.1. *Plants*

The selection of plants for evaluation was based firstly on traditional use for the treatment of infectious and other diseases, secondly on their availability, and thirdly on the level of knowledge about these plants. A typical questionnaire for the description of the collected plants and their application, as used by the Yemeni scientists during their collecting excursions, is attached at the end of this contribution. Plants known for their traditional use in Yemeni ethnomedicine were collected from different localities in Yemen and were identified by the collaborating Yemeni scientists. Among them are a number of plants from the island of Soqotra; some of these are endemic to this island known for its unique and rich flora. Sample specimens of the investigated plants are stored in the herbariums of the universities in Ṣanʿāʾ and Aden. To date 184 different plant species have been investigated. After drying the parts of the plants that are used by indigenous people (leaves, flowers, fruits, or roots), these parts were then extracted with organic solvents of different polarity. In total, extracts of 108 plant species (about 60% of the whole number tested) showed one or more remarkable biological activities. In many cases the results of the biological screening validates the use of the plants in traditional Yemeni medicine.

1.1.1. *Antimicrobial Activities*

All extracts were tested for antimicrobial activities against the gram-positive bacteria *Staphylococcus aureus*, *Micrococcus flavus*, and *Bacillus atrophaeus*, as well as against the gram-negative bacteria *Pseudomonas aeruginosa* and *Escherichia coli*. *Staphylococcus aureus* can cause severe inflammations or poisoning by food. *Micrococcus flavus* and *Bacillus atrophaeus* are non-pathogenic representatives of gram-positive bacteria. They are therefore very easy to handle in the laboratory. *Pseudomonas aeruginosa* and *Escherichia coli* are responsible for infections of the urinary tract, gastrointestinal tract, or wounds.

The main test organism among the fungi was the yeast *Candida maltosa*. It represents pathogenic yeast species like *Candida albicans*. Additionally, some extracts were tested against other human pathogenic fungal strains, e.g. *Trichophyton* and *Aspergillus*. Fungal infections occur very often in immune-compromised patients, e.g. in tumour patients or after transplantations. They cause chronic exanthemas and inflammations of skin and mucous membranes.

The activities against gram-positive strains were mostly stronger than those against the gram-negative bacteria. Most remarkable were the activities of some extracts against methicillin-resistant strains of *Staphylococcus aureus* (MRSA). Such strains cannot be inhibited by common antibiotics and are responsible for severe nosocomial infections (infections acquired in hospitals). Strong *in vitro* activity against MRSA (inhibition zones in the agar diffusion assay > 20 mm) was exhibited, for example, by the methanolic extracts of *Meriandra bengalensis*, *Pulicaria inuloides*, *Tarchonanthus camphoratus*,[5] *Lippia citriodora*, and *Plectranthus hadiensis*.[6]

The growth of *Pseudomonas aeruginosa*, a gram-negative bacterium, was reduced, for example, by *Cupressus sempervirens*[7] and *Thymus laevigatus*. *Th. laevigatus* is also interesting because of its activity against a broad spectrum of human pathogenic fungi, e.g. *Aspergillus fumigatus*, *Candida albicans*, and *Trichophyton mentagrophytes*.[8] Antifungal activity against several pathogenic fungi was also exhibited by *Azima tetracantha*, *Sansevieria ehrenbergii*, and *Solanum incanum*.[9] The plants with pronounced antimicrobial activities are summarized in Table 1.

1.1.2. *Antiviral Activities*

In contrast to bacterial and fungal diseases, infections caused by viruses cannot be treated with antibiotics. Therefore new antiviral drugs are urgently needed. We tested the plant extracts against influenza A virus (the cause of influenza A), and herpes simplex type I virus (responsible for herpes labialis, which is characterized by formation of painful blisters on the lips). Viruses need host cells for their replication. Influenza A virus was propagated in canine kidney cells—so-called MDCK cells (Madin-Darbin canine kidney)—and herpes simplex type I virus in African green monkey kidney cells—so-called Vero cells. Nine percent of the tested extracts obtained from 25 different plant species exhibited remarkable antiviral activities against both or one of the test viruses in non-cytotoxic concentrations. For influenza A virus, the highest activities were observed for aqueous extracts of *Boswellia ameero*, *Boswellia elongata*, *Fagonia luntii*, and *Jatropha unicostata*, as well as for methanolic extracts of *Boswellia elongata*, *Dracaena*

[5] Mothana et al., 'Evaluation'.
[6] Id. et al., 'Phytochemical Screening'.
[7] Id. et al., 'Evaluation'.
[8] Al-Fatimi et al., 'Radical Scavenging Activities'.
[9] Id. et al., 'Selected Medicinal Plants'.

cinnabari, *Exacum affine*, *Jatropha unicostata*, and *Kalanchoe farinacea* (50% inhibition concentrations, IC_{50}, ranging from 0.7 to 3.1 µg/mL). The most marked effects against herpes simplex type I virus were estimated for the methanol extracts of *Boswellia elongata*, *Buxus hildebrandtii*, and *Euryops arabicus* with IC_{50} values of 0.35 µg/mL.[10]

1.1.3. *Cytotoxic Activities*

To exclude undesirable side effects, all extracts were investigated for possible cytotoxic activities against FL cells—fibroblast-like cells (a 'normal' cell line). On the other hand, there is a great need for drugs with cytotoxic effects against cancer cells. Therefore we also tested many extracts against human tumour cells. In an investigation of methanol extracts from twenty four plants for *in vitro* cytotoxic potency against two lung cancers, two bladder carcinomas, and one breast cancer cell line, the extracts of *Buxus hildebrandtii*, *Dendrosicyos socotrana*, *Dracaena cinnabari*, *Withania adunensis*, and *Withania riebeckii* exhibited high activity against the growth of all tumour cell lines, with IC_{50} values ranging between 0.29 and 5.54 µg/mL.[11] Also extracts from *Centaurothamnus maximus*, *Costus arabicus*, *Cupressus sempervirens*, *Dichrocephala integrifolia*, *Euphorbia schimperi*, *Gomphocarpus fruticosus*, *Kanahia laniflora*, *Meriandra bengalensis*, *Pulicaria inuloides*, *Solanum glabratum*, *Tarchonanthus camphoratus*, and *Vernonia leopoldii* showed cytotoxic activities against several tumour cell lines with IC_{50} values lower than 50 µg/mL.[12] All plants with notable cytotoxic activities are listed in Table 1.

1.1.4. *Antioxidative Activities*

It is well known that reactive oxygen species (ROS) are able to damage cellular constituents such as DNA, proteins, and lipids, and they act as secondary messengers in inflammation. Some ROS are radicals, such as hydroxyl radical and superoxide radical. Antioxidants can scavenge ROS and can also reduce inflammation pathways. The use of antioxidants may be useful in the treatment or prophylaxis of certain diseases, e.g. arteriosclerosis, stroke, and cancers. Thus there is much interest in identifying natural antioxidants, i.e., substances that can destroy ROS. Plants with strong radical scavenging properties determined in the DPPH assay are summarized in Table 1. DPPH (2,2-diphenyl-1-picrylhydrazyl radical) is a

---

10 Mothana et al., 'Antiviral Activity'.
11 Id. et al., 'Anticancer Potential'.
12 Eid., 'Evaluation'.

stable radical and is violet coloured. Radical scavengers reduce the radical to the yellow coloured 2,2-diphenyl-1-picrylhydrazin. The colour change can be measured by spectrophotometric methods. Plants with strong effects, comparable to the activity of ascorbic acid, are for example *Acalypha fruticosa*, *Actiniopteris semiflabellata*, *Verbascum bottae*,[13] *Acacia asak*, and *Solanum nigrum*.[14]

1.1.5. *Antimalaria Activities*

Malaria is one of the most serious health problems in Yemen. Approximately 60% of the population live in areas with malaria risk, and *Plasmodium falciparum* accounts for more than 90% of the malaria cases.[15] The disease is caused by *Plasmodium* species of microorganisms. It is associated with considerable morbidity and mortality and significant social and economic impact. Development of drug resistance and the lack of a vaccine strengthen the need for new antimalaria drugs.

In a pilot study, Dr. Awadh Ali and his students interviewed 492 inhabitants of thirteen villages located on the coastal plain of four Yemeni provinces. They reported the use of nineteen plants belonging to fourteen families for the treatment of malaria, each with the local name, methods of preparation and parts used. The traditional use of *Anisotes trisulcus*, *Cissus rotundifolia*, *Citrullus colocynthis*, *Dodonaea viscosa*, *Plantago major*, and *Tamarindus indica* for the treatment of malaria has been reported for the first time.[16] In experimental testing, the antiplasmodial activities with IC_{50} values lower than 4 µg/mL were found for water extracts of *Acalypha fruticosa*, *Azadirachta indica* and *Dendrosicyos socotrana*.[17]

1.1.6. *Enzyme Inhibiting Activities*

The methanolic extracts of twenty medicinal plants from the island of Soqotra, selected according to traditional use and availability, were screened with respect to their inhibitory potency against the peptidases angiotensin converting enzyme (ACE), neutral endopeptidase (NEP), and aminopeptidase N (APN). The enzymes are involved in the metabolism of peptide hormones regulating blood pressure and other physiological parameters. Inhibitors of these enzymes are of interest for the treatment of

---

13 Mothana et al., 'Phytochemical Screening'.
14 Al-Fatimi et al., 'Selected Medicinal Plants'.
15 *National Malaria Control Program, Annual Report.*
16 Awadh Ali, Al-Rahwi, and Lindequist, 'Medicine to Treat Malaria'.
17 Alshawsh et al., 'Assessment of Antimalarial Activity'.

patients with hypertension and congestive heart failure. *Boswellia elongata, Cissus hamaderohensis,* and *Kalanchoe farinacea* inhibited all three enzymes. The most active extract was prepared from *K. farinacea.*[18] The essential oil of *Boswellia socotrana* showed stronger anticholinesterase activity than the essential oils of *Boswellia elongata* and *Boswellia ameero.* Acetylcholinesterase is responsible for the hydrolysis of the neurotransmitter acetylcholine. Inhibitors of this enzyme are of interest for the treatment of Alzheimer's disease and other illnesses.[19]

1.2. *Fungi*

So far, twenty-three species of Yemeni basidiomycetes have been extracted with different organic solvents, and screened for their *in vitro* antimicrobial, cytotoxic, and antioxidant activities. The highest antibacterial activity was demonstrated for extracts of *Agaricus* spp., *Coriolopsis caperata, Ganoderma colossus, Ganoderma resinaceum, Phellorinia herculeana,* and *Tulostoma obesum.* Strong antioxidative effects employing the DPPH assay were exhibited by methanol extracts of *Ganoderma resinaceum, Inonotus ochroporus, Phellinus rimosus,* and *Phellorinia herculeana.* No extract showed notable cytotoxicity against FL cells.[20]

2. Selected Examples

2.1. *Podaxis pistillaris*

The fungus *Podaxis pistillaris* (L. Pers.) Morse agg. (Basidiomycetes) is indigenous to the semi-deserts of Africa, Asia, Australia, and America. In Yemen it can be found in arid zones. No species of this genus have yet been identified in Europe. The fruiting bodies of *P. pistillaris* are used in some parts of Yemen for the treatment of skin diseases. We produced mycelial cultures of this mushroom and extracted the mycelium and the culture medium. In particular, the ethyl acetate extract from the culture medium exhibited strong antibacterial activity against *Staphylococcus aureus, Escherichia coli,* and other bacterial strains. With the help of bioactivity-guided isolation, it was possible to isolate three epidithiodiketopiperazines—epicorazine A, B, and C—from the culture medium. These

---

18 Oleski et al., 'Inhibitory Activity'.
19 Awadh Ali et al., 'Soqotraen *Boswellia* Species'.
20 Al-Fatimi et al., 'Selected Basidiomycetes'.

compounds had not previously been reported as constituents of *P. pistillaris*. It is assumed that the identified compounds contribute to the antibacterial activity of the extract. These results confirm the ethnomedicinal use of this mushroom. However, due to the possible side effects of the epicorazines, the drug should be applied with caution.[21]

2.2. *Meriandra bengalensis*

Meriandra bengalensis (Roxb.) Benth. (Labiatae) is an aromatic shrub that grows up to 2 m high on rocky hills at altitudes between 2000 m and 2800 m in the high plateaus of Yemen. An infusion of the plant is used mainly as an antiseptic agent for wounds and for the treatment of urinary tract infections. During our screening work, strong cytotoxic, antimicrobial, and antioxidative *in vitro* activities were found in extracts from this plant.[22] With the help of bioactivity-guided isolation, four abietane diterpenoids were isolated from the methanolic extract of the roots of this plant. Two diterpenoids were reported for the first time in this plant species. The compounds possess potent cytotoxic effect against three human cancer cell lines (lung, bladder, and breast cancer) as well as antibacterial effect against *Staphylococcus aureus*, *Bacillus atrophaeus*, and *Micrococcus flavus*.[23]

2.3. *Catha edulis*[24]

Catha edulis Forsk. (Celastraceae), or *qāt*, is an evergreen shrub, that grows at high altitudes. It is one of the most famous plants in Yemen; the chewing of *qāt* leaves is a deep-rooted social and cultural tradition. People chew the fresh leaves for their stimulant and pleasurable effects that are mainly attributed to the compound cathinone. An enormous amount of data has been published on the pharmacology, toxicology, and chemistry of *qāt*.[25]

We investigated the effect of *C. edulis* on some important parameters of the metabolic syndrome by using rats that show symptoms of metabolic disorders. Feeding them *qāt* leaves reduced important parameters of the metabolic syndrome, such as body weight, triglyceride levels, blood glucose concentrations, and the leptin contents of the animals. The results

---

[21] Id. et al., '*Podaxis pistillaris*'.
[22] Mothana et al., 'Evaluation'.
[23] Id. et al., '*Meriandera benghalensis*'.
[24] See also Daniel Martin Varisco's chapter in this volume.
[25] Al-Hebshi and Skaug, 'Khat'; Al-Motarreb, Baker, and Broadley, 'Khat'.

need confirmation from human studies but already they could be helpful in evaluating the risks and/or potential of *qāt* for human health.[26]

3. Conclusion and Outlook

The results of our studies substantiate the fact that plants and fungi used in traditional Yemeni medicine offer an enormous potential for health care in Yemeni communities. In addition, they provide exceptional possibilities for the discovery of new chemical structures with interesting pharmacological activities; those already discovered in these plants are in most cases in agreement with their traditional uses.

It may be concluded from this study that biological screening forms a good basis for the bioactivity-guided isolation and structure elucidation of bioactive compounds from the extracts. This is demonstrated by the examples of *Podaxis pistillaris* and *Meriandra bengalensis.* To explore the full potential of Yemeni plants and fungi, further pharmacological and toxicological tests—including *in vivo* investigations and mode of action studies—are required. Sustainable production and pharmaceutical quality of the herbal drugs have to be ensured.

Finally, it should be emphasized that the exploration of potential Yemeni medicinal plants and fungi can contribute not only to the improvement of health in the indigenous people, but also to the economic development and conservation of natural and cultural resources of the country.

Bibliography

Alshawsh, Mohammed A., Mothana, Ramzi A., Al-shamahy, Hassan A., Alsllami, Salah F., and Lindequist, Ulrike, 'Assessment of Antimalarial Activity against Plasmodium Falciparum and Phytochemical Screening of Some Yemeni Medicinal Plants', *Evidence-based Complementary and Alternative Medicine*, 6 (2009), 453–6.

Awadh Ali, Nasser A., Al-Rahwi, Khaldoon, and Lindequist, Ulrike, 'Some Medicinal Plants Used in Yemeni Herbal Medicine to Treat Malaria', *African Journal of Traditional, Complementary and Alternative Medicines*, 1 (2004), 72–6.

Awadh Ali et al., 'Screening of Yemeni Medicinal Plants' = Awadh Ali, Nasser A., Jülich, Wolf-Dieter, Kusnick, Carolina, and Lindequist, Ulrike, 'Screening of Yemeni Medicinal Plants for Antibacterial and Cytotoxic Activities', *Journal of Ethnopharmacology*, 74 (2001), 173–79.

———, 'Soqotraen Plants' = Awadh Ali, Nasser A., Mothana, Ramzi A.A., Ghaleb, Nasr Abdo, and Lindequist, Ulrike, 'Screening of Traditionally Used Endemic Soqotraen

26 Mahmood and Lindequist, 'Catha edulis Forsk'.

Plants for Cytotoxic Activity', *African Journal of Traditional, Complementary and Alternative Medicines*, 4 (2007), 529–31.

———, 'Soqotraen *Boswellia* Species' = Awadh Ali, Nasser A., Wurster, Martina, Arnold, Norbert, Teichert, Axel, Schmidt, Jürgen, Lindequist, Ulrike, and Wessjohann, Ludger, 'Chemical Composition and Biological Activities of Essential Oils from the Oleogum Resins of Three Endemic Soqotraen *Boswellia* Species', *Records of Natural Products*, 2 (2008), 6–12.

———, 'Essential Oil' = Awadh Ali, Nasser A., Wurster, Martina, Arnold, Norbert, Lindequist, Ulrike, and Wessjohan, Ludger, 'Essential Oil Composition from Oleogum Resin of Soqotraen *Commiphora kua*', *Records of Natural Products*, 2 (2008), 70–5.

———, 'Chemical Composition' = Awadh Ali, Nasser A., Wurster, Martina, Arnold, Norbert, Lindequist, Ulrike, and Wessjohan, Ludger, 'Chemical Composition of the Essential Oil of *Teucrium yemense* Deflers', *Records of Natural Products*, 2 (2008), 25–32.

al-Dubaʿī, ʿAbd al-Raḥmān S., and al-Khulaydī, ʿAbd al-Walī A., *al-Nabātāt al-ṭibbiyya wa-l-ʿiṭriyya fī l-Yaman* [Medicinal and Aromatic Plants in Yemen] (Ṣanʿāʾ: Markaz ʿUbādī lil-dirāsāt wa-l-nashr, 1996).

Al-Fatimi et al., 'Selected Basidiomycetes' = Al-Fatimi, Mohamed, Wurster, Martina, Kreisel, Hanns, and Lindequist, Ulrike, 'Antimicrobial, Cytotoxic and Antioxidant Activity of Selected Basidiomycetes from Yemen', *Pharmazie*, 60 (2005), 776–80.

———, '*Podaxis pistillaris*' = Al-Fatimi, Mohamed, Jülich, Wolf-Dieter, Jansen, Rolf, and Lindequist, Ulrike, 'Bioactive Components of the Traditionally Used Mushroom *Podaxis pistillaris*', *Evidence-based Complementary and Alternative Medicine*, 3 (2006), 87–92.

———, 'Selected Medicinal Plants' = Al-Fatimi, Mohamed, Wurster, Martina, Schröder, Gudrun, and Lindequist, Ulrike, 'Antioxidant, Antimicrobial and Cytotoxic Activities of Selected Medicinal Plants from Yemen', *Journal of Ethnopharmacology*, 111 (2007), 657–66.

———, 'Radical Scavenging Activities' = Al-Fatimi, Mohamed, Wurster, Martina, Schröder, Gudrun, and Lindequist, Ulrike, '*In vitro* Antimicrobial, Cytotoxic and Radical Scavenging Activities and Chemical Constituents of the Endemic *Thymus laevigatus* (Vahl)', *Records of Natural Products*, 4 (2010), 49–63.

Fleurentin, Jacques, and Pelt, Jean-Marie, 'Repertory of Drugs and Medicinal Plants of Yemen', *Journal of Ethnopharmacology*, 6 (1982), 85–108.

Al-Hebshi, Nezar N., and Skaug, Nils, 'Khat (*Catha edulis*): An Updated Review', *Addiction Biology*, 10 (2005), 299–307.

Kreisel, Hanns, and Al-Fatimi, Mohamed, 'Basidiomycetes and Larger Ascomycetes from Yemen', *Feddes Repertorium*, 115 (2004), 547–61.

———, 'Further Basidiomycetes from Yemen', *Feddes Repertorium*, 119 (2008), 463–83.

Mahmood, Samira Abdulla, and Lindequist, Ulrike, 'A Pilot Study on the Effect of *Catha edulis* Frosk. [*sic*], (Celastraceae) on Metabolic Syndrome in WOKW Rats', *African Journal of Traditional, Complementary and Alternative Medicines*, 5 (2008), 271–7.

Al-Motarreb, Ahmed, Baker, Kathryn, and Broadley, Kenneth J., 'Khat: Pharmacological and Medical Aspects and Its Social Use in Yemen', *Phytotherapy Research*, 16 (2002), 403–13.

Mothana, Ramzi A.A., and Lindequist, Ulrike, 'Antimicrobial Activity of Some Medicinal Plants of the Island Soqotra', *Journal of Ethnopharmacology*, 96 (2005), 177–81.

Mothana et al., 'Antiviral Activity' = Mothana, Ramzi A.A., Mentel, Renate, Reiss, Christiane, and Lindequist, Ulrike, 'Phytochemical Screening and Antiviral Activity of some Medicinal Plants from the Island Soqotra', *Phytotherapy Research*, 20 (2006), 298–302.

———, 'Anticancer Potential' = Mothana, Ramzi A.A., Grünert, Renate, Lindequist, Ulrike, and Bednarski, Patrick J., 'Study of the Anticancer Potential of Yemeni Plants Used in Folk Medicine', *Pharmazie*, 62 (2007), 305–7.

———, 'Phytochemical Screening' = Mothana, Ramzi A.A., Abdo, Salah A.A., Hasson, Sidgi, Faisal, Althawab M.N., Alaghbari, Sama A.Z., and Lindequist, Ulrike, 'Antimicrobial, Antioxidant and Cytotoxic Activities and Phytochemical Screening of Some Yemeni Medicinal Plants', *Evidence-based Complementary and Alternative Medicine*, 7(2010), 323–30.

———, 'Evaluation' = Mothana, Ramzi A.A., Grünert, Renate, Bednarski, Patrick J., and Lindequist, Ulrike, 'Evaluation of the *in vitro* Anticancer, Antimicrobial, and Antioxidant Activities of Some Yemeni Plants Used in Folk Medicine', *Pharmazie*, 64 (2009), 260–8.

———, 'Selected Yemeni Medicinal Plants' = Mothana, Ramzi A.A., Lindequist, Ulrike, Grünert, Renate, and Bednarski, Patrick J., 'Studies of the in vitro Anticancer, Antimicrobial and Antioxidant Potentials of Selected Yemeni Medicinal Plants from the Island Soqotra', *BMB Complementary and Alternative Medicine*, 9 (2009), 7–18.

———, '*Meriandera* [*sic*] *benghalensis*' = Mothana, Ramzi A.A., Jansen, Rolf, Grünert, Renate, Bednarski, Patrick J., and Lindequist, Ulrike, 'Antimicrobial and Cytotoxic Abietane Diterpenoids from the Roots of *Meriandera benghalensis* (Roxb.) Benth', *Pharmazie*, 64 (2009), 613–15.

National Malaria Control Program, Annual Report, ([Ṣanʿāʾ]: Ministry of Public Health and Poplulation, 2002).

Newman, David J., Cragg, Gordon M., and Snader, Kenneth M., 'Natural Products as Sources of New Drugs over the Period 1981–2002', *Journal of Natural Products*, 66 (2003), 1022–37.

Oleski, Anike, Lindequist, Ulrike, Mothana, Ramzi A.A., and Melzig, Matthias F., 'Screening of Selected Arabian Medicinal Plant Extracts for Inhibitory Activity Against Peptidases', *Pharmazie*, 61 (2006), 359–61.

Schopen, Armin, *Traditionelle Heilmittel in Jemen* (Wiesbaden: Steiner, 1983).

Questionnaire[1]

date: collectionYMP[2] no.:

1. **Locality:**
   district: village:
   distance and direction from major town:
   habitat:
2. **Type of plant:**

tree	☐	herb	☐	parasite	☐
shrub	☐	liana	☐	aquatic	☐

3. **For trees:**
   height & bulk:
   bark description:
   cutting for sap:
4. **Flower colour:**
5. **Fruit description:**
6. **Smell:**
7. **Latex present:**
8. **Attacked by insects etc.:**
9. **Provisional identification:**
10. **Vernacular name:**
11. **Name of traditional healer:**
12. **Preparation of remedy:**

    plant part: fresh: dried:

    amount taken:

    crushed: powdered:

    mixed with water (amount): mixed with cold water:

boiled: doused with boiling water:

mixed with other vehicle (amount):

other preparation:

13. **Dose and regimen:**

14. **Disease treated:**

15. **Plant used together with the following plants:**

vernacular name or YMP-number:

part of plant:

amount of plant part taken in preparation, or other details, if preparation differs from description in no. 12 above:

16. **Additional notes (e.g. side effects):**

[1] Example of a questionnaire for gathering ethnobotanical data provided by Prof. Nasser A. Awadh Ali (translated into English from the Arabic version that was used in the field survey).

[2] YMP: Yemeni Medicinal Plants collection, Department of Pharmacognosy, Ṣan'āʾ University

Table 1. Plants investigated bearing remarkable antimicrobial, cytotoxic, and/or radical scavenging activ (published results only; for details, see referred literature)

Plant species	Plant family	Traditional use[1]	Anti-mi activity[2]
Acacia asak	Leguminosae	gastric ulcer, skin diseases	x
Acacia nilotica	Leguminosae	cough, wounds, pharyngitis, bronchitis, diabetes	x
Acacia pennivenia	Leguminosae	mastitis (as paste for local application)	x
Acacia tortilis	Leguminosae	stomach ache, dyspepsia	x
Acalypha fruticosa	Euphorbiaceae	skin diseases, malaria, wounds	x
Acanthospermum hispidum	Compositae	unknown	
Actiniopteris semiflabellata	Pteridophyta	wounds, burns	
Aloe perryi	Aloaceae	eye infection, wounds	x
Azima tetracantha	Salvadoraceae	rheumatism, cough	x
Ballochia atro-virgata	Acanthaceae	unknown	
Boswellia ameero	Burseraceae	common cold, bronchitis, asthma, rheumatism	x
Boswellia dioscorides	Burseraceae	common cold, bronchitis, asthma, rheumatism	x
Boswellia elongata	Burseraceae	common cold, bronchitis, asthma, rheumatism	x
Boswellia socotrana	Burseraceae	common cold, bronchitis, asthma, rheumatism	x
Buxus hildebrandtii	Buxaceae	malaria	x
Cadaba farinosa	Capparaceae	urinary infection, haemorrhoids	x
Calotropis procera	Asclepiadaceae	skin infection	
Centaurea pseudosinaica	Compositae	wounds, kidney diseases	x
Centaurothamnus maximus	Compositae	wounds	x
Chenopodium ambrosioides	Chenopodia-ceae	worm infestation, skin and kidney diseases	
Chenopodium murale	Chenopodia-ceae	skin infection	
Commiphora foliacea	Burseraceae	skin infection, wounds	x
Commiphora kua	Burseraceae	face and skin infection, cough, bronchitis	x
Commiphora ornifolia	Burseraceae	skin infection, diarrhoea, dysentery, emmenagogue	x
Commiphora parvifolia	Burseraceae	skin infection, diarrhoea, dysentery, menstrual pains	x
Costus arabicus	Zingiberaceae	cancer	
Cupressus sempervirens	Cupressaceae	cough, wounds, diarrhoea, haemorrhoids	x
Dendrosicyos socotrana	Cucurbitaceae	constipation	
Dichrocephala integrifolia	Compositae	wounds	
Dodonaea viscosa	Sapindaceae	malaria, wounds, burns	x
Dracaena cinnabari	Dracaenaceae	gingivitis, wounds, colic	
Enicostema verticillare	Gentianaceae	diabetes	x
Euclea divinorum	Ebenaceae	oral care, toothache, fungal diseases, wounds	x
Euphorbia schimperi	Euphorbiaceae	skin infection, warts	
Euphorbia socotrana	Euphorbiaceae	skin diseases, wounds	x
Eureiandra balfourii	Curcubitaceae	unknown	
Fagonia luntii	Zygophyllaceae	skin infection, burns	x
Ficus vasta	Moraceae	cough	x
Gomphocarpus fruticosus	Apocynaceae	heart diseases	
Gossypium areysiamum	Malvaceae	wounds, dermatitis	x

Cytotoxic activity[3]	Radical scavenging activity[4]	References
	x	Al-Fatimi et al., 'Selected Medicinal Plants'.
		Al-Fatimi et al., 'Selected Medicinal Plants'.
	x	Mothana et al., 'Selected Yemeni Medicinal Plants'.
		Al-Fatimi et al., 'Selected Medicinal Plants'.
x	x	Mothana et al., 'Phytochemical Screening'.
x		Mothana et al., 'Selected Yemeni Medicinal Plants'.
	x	Mothana et al., 'Phytochemical Screening'.
		Awadh Ali et al., 'Screening of Yemeni Medicinal Plants'.
		Al-Fatimi et al., 'Selected Medicinal Plants'.
x		Mothana et al., 'Selected Yemeni Medicinal Plants'.
		Mothana and Lindequist, 'Antimicrobial Activity'.
x	x	Mothana et al., 'Selected Yemeni Medicinal Plants'.
		Mothana and Lindequist, 'Antimicrobial Activity'.
x	x	Awadh Ali et al., 'Soqotraen Plants'; id. et al., 'Soqotraen *Boswellia* Species';
		Mothana et al., 'Selected Yemeni Medicinal Plants'.
x		Mothana and Lindequist, 'Antimicrobial Activity'; Mothana et al., 'Anticancer Potential'.
		Al-Fatimi et al., 'Selected Medicinal Plants'.
x		Awadh Ali et al., 'Screening of Yemeni Medicinal Plants'.
		Mothana et al., 'Phytochemical Screening'.
x		Mothana et al., 'Evaluation'.
		Mothana et al., 'Evaluation'.
	x	Awadh Ali et al., 'Screening of Yemeni Medicinal Plants'.
		Al-Fatimi et al., 'Selected Medicinal Plants'.
x		Al-Fatimi et al., 'Selected Medicinal Plants'; Awadh Ali et al. 'Essential Oil'.
x	x	Awadh Ali et al., 'Soqotraen Plants'; Mothana et al., 'Selected Yemeni Medicinal Plants'.
		Mothana and Lindequist, 'Antimicrobial Activity'.
x		Mothana et al., 'Evaluation'.
x		Mothana et al., 'Evaluation'.
x		Mothana et al., 'Anticancer Potential'.
x		Mothana et al., 'Evaluation'.
	x	Mothana et al., 'Phytochemical Screening'.
x		Mothana et al., 'Anticancer Potential'.
		Mothana et al., 'Evaluation'.
		Mothana et al., 'Selected Yemeni Medicinal Plants'.
x		Mothana et al., 'Evaluation'.
x		Mothana et al., 'Selected Yemeni Medicinal Plants'.
x		Awadh Ali et al., 'Soqotraen Plants'; Mothana et al., 'Selected Yemeni Medicinal Plants'.
		Al-Fatimi et al., 'Selected Medicinal Plants'.
		Al-Fatimi et al., 'Selected Medicinal Plants'.
x		Mothana et al., 'Evaluation'.
		Al-Fatimi et al., 'Selected Medicinal Plants'.

Table 1. Continued.

Plant species	Plant family	Traditional use[1]	Anti-micro activity[2]
Indigofera oblongifolia	Leguminosae	urinary tract infection, cough	x
Iris albicans	Iridaceae	rheumatism, gout	
Jatropha unicostata	Euphorbiaceae	wounds, eczema, scabies	x
Jatropha variegata	Euphorbiaceae	wound infection, haemorrhage	x
Kalanchoe farinacea	Crassulaceae	tissue injuries, enlarged ganglia, peptic ulcer	x
Kanahia laniflora	Asclepiadaceae	tumours, skin diseases, scabies, itching	
Lawsonia inermis	Lythraceae	skin infection, wounds	x
Leucas samhaensis	Labiatae	cough, common cold	x
Leucas virgata	Labiatae	heartburn, dyspepsia	x
Lippia citriodora	Verbenaceae	colic, dyspepsia, common cold, sleep disorder	x
Meriandra bengalensis	Labiatae	wound, skin and urinary tract infection	x
Nepeta deflersiana	Labiatae	wound infection, rheumatism, fever, colic	x
Ocimum forskolei	Labiatae	fever, skin infection, skin care	x
Plectranthus hadiensis	Labiatae	skin infection, haemorrhage	x
Plicosepalus curviflorus	Loranthaceae	cancer	x
Pulicaria inuloides	Compositae	wounds	x
Pulicaria orientalis	Compositae	gastrointestinal tract pains, fever	
Pulicaria stephanocarpa	Compositae	unknown	x
Punica protopunica	Punicaceae	worm infestation, peptic ulcer, diarrhoea, dysentery	x
Rhus thyrsiflora	Anacardiaceae	anorexia, articular pain, general weakness	x
Sansevieria ehrenbergii	Dracaenaceae	warts, skin infection	x
Solanum glabratum	Solanaceae	nephrocystitis, urolithiasis, syphilis, scabies, cough, haemorrhoids	
Solanum incanum	Solanaceae	toothache, skin diseases	
Solanum nigrum	Solanaceae	skin infection, diarrhoea, cough, haemorrhage	x
Tamarindus indica	Leguminosae	skin infection, insects	x
Tarchonanthus camphoratus	Compositae	wounds, urinary tract infections	x
Teucrium socotranum	Labiatae	dyspepsia, halitosis	x
Teucrium yemense	Labiatae	kidney diseases, rheumatism	x
Thymus laevigatus	Labiatae	cough, tonsillitis, pharyngitis, dyspepsia	x
Tragia pungens	Euphorbiaceae	allergy, skin diseases	x
Tribulus terrestris	Zygophyllaceae	urolithiasis, dysuria	
Verbascum bottae	Scrophulariaceae	cough, skin diseases, rheumatism	x
Vernonia leopoldii	Compositae	cough, colic, skin diseases	x
Withania adunensis	Solanaceae	inflammation, wounds, rheumatism	x
Withania riebeckii	Solanaceae	inflammation, wounds, rheumatism	x
Withania somnifera	Solanaceae	burns, wounds	
Zizyphus spina-christi	Rhamnaceae	skin diseases, wounds	x

[1] Information about traditional use has been taken from Fleurentin and Pelt, 'Repertory', Schopen, *Heilmittel*, al-Dubaʿī and al-Khulaydī, *al-Nabātāt al-ṭibbiyya*, and local people in Yemen.

[2] Antimicrobial activities against different bacterial strains and against *Candida maltosa* were determined in agar diffusion assay, and mostly in microdilution assay (for description of methods, see cited literature).

Cytotoxic activity[3]	Radical scavenging activity[4]	References
		Awadh Ali et al., 'Screening of Yemeni Medicinal Plants'.
x		Mothana et al., 'Phytochemical Screening'.
x		Mothana and Lindequist, 'Antimicrobial Activity';
		Mothana et al., 'Anticancer Potential'.
		Mothana et al., 'Phytochemical Screening'.
		Mothana and Lindequist, 'Antimicrobial Activity'.
x		Mothana et al., 'Evaluation'.
		Awadh Ali et al., 'Screening of Yemeni Medicinal Plants'.
		Mothana et al., 'Selected Yemeni Medicinal Plants'.
		Mothana et al., 'Selected Yemeni Medicinal Plants'.
x		Mothana et al., 'Phytochemical Screening'.
x		Awadh Ali et al., 'Screening of Yemeni Medicinal Plants';
		Mothana et al., 'Evaluation';
		id. et al., '*Meriandera benghalensis*'.
		Mothana et al., 'Evaluation'.
		Al-Fatimi et al., 'Selected Medicinal Plants'.
	x	Mothana et al., 'Phytochemical Screening'.
x	x	Al-Fatimi et al., 'Selected Medicinal Plants'.
x		Mothana et al., 'Evaluation'.
x		Awadh Ali et al., 'Screening of Yemeni Medicinal Plants'.
		Mothana and Lindequist, 'Antimicrobial Activity'.
x		Mothana and Lindequist, 'Antimicrobial Activity';
		Mothana et al., 'Anticancer Potential'.
		Mothana et al., 'Selected Yemeni Medicinal Plants'.
x		Al-Fatimi et al., 'Selected Medicinal Plants'.
x		Mothana et al., 'Evaluation'.
x		Al-Fatimi et al., 'Selected Medicinal Plants'.
	x	Al-Fatimi et al., 'Selected Medicinal Plants'.
x		Al-Fatimi et al., 'Selected Medicinal Plants'.
x		Mothana et al., 'Evaluation'.
		Mothana et al., 'Selected Yemeni Medicinal Plants'.
		Awadh Ali et al., 'Chemical Composition';
		Mothana et al., 'Evaluation'.
x	x	Al-Fatimi et al., 'Radical Scavenging activities'.
x	x	Mothana et al., 'Phytochemical Screening'.
x		Awadh Ali et al., 'Screening of Yemeni Medicinal Plants'.
	x	Mothana et al., 'Phytochemical Screening'.
x		Mothana et al., 'Evaluation'.
x		Mothana and Lindequist, 'Antimicrobial Activity';
		Mothana et al., 'Anticancer Potential'.
x		Mothana and Lindequist, 'Antimicrobial Activity';
		Mothana et al., 'Anticancer Potential'.
x		Awadh Ali et al., 'Screening of Yemeni Medicinal Plants'.
		Awadh Ali et al., 'Screening of Yemeni Medicinal Plants'.

3 Cytotoxic activities were determined in neutral red assay and/or MTT assay (for description of methods, see cited literature).

4 Radical scavenging activities were determined by DPPH assay (for description of methods, see cited literature).

HEALTH ISSUES IN THE MOUNTAINS OF YEMEN: HEALING PRACTICES AS PART OF FARMERS' TRADITIONAL KNOWLEDGE[1]

Amin Al-Hakimi, Anhar Ya'ni, and Frédéric Pelat

The medicinal properties of plants have no value without the knowledge to identify and make use of the plants, and this knowledge is ineffective without people to keep it alive and make it available for all. This chapter discusses the specific linkages that many mountain Yemeni farming communities have developed with their particular agro-ecosystems to make use of wild and cultivated plants for their daily healing needs. The authors are involved in sustainable agricultural development founded on indigenous knowledge and local genetic resources, and their objective here is to highlight the intimate relationship between the traditional Yemeni farmer and his environment in which the 'man-plant' linkage in a quite natural and almost unconscious character remains an essential, but very fragile, keystone.

1. Agro-ecosystems in the Highlands of Yemen

The western part of Yemen is dominated by the high mountain range running from the Saudi border in the north to the Gulf of Aden in the south. From a height of 700 m in the foothills and rising to more than 3,600 m (with Jabal al-Nabī Shuʿayb reaching 3,670 m west of Ṣanʿāʾ), the Yemeni highlands constitute unique ecological and social agro-ecosystems that are quite distinct from those in other regions of the country. Unlike the coastal and high-altitude valleys or the plains and plateaus where in recent decades well irrigation has spread rapidly and in an uncontrolled way, these regions have managed to conserve agricultural practices that mostly rely on rainfall (from 200 mm annually to more than 800–1,000 mm, depending on the region.) Traditionally the upper escarpments were managed as community rangeland or forest, where many wild plants have been conserved and were used for multiple purposes, whereas the slopes have

[1] Scientific names of plants were revised by Abdul Wali Ahmed Al Khulaidi and Daniel Martin Varisco.

been shaped into terraced areas.[2] These operate as huge water catchments and optimize the use of the rather limited amount of land. They also capture precious water run-off, and thus prevent erosion and destructive floods in the lower-lying areas. The resulting dry to semi-dry, and even semi-wet, agro-ecosystems have generated and sheltered a significant diversity of wild plants and crops, which have been adapted empirically over time by farmers and have resulted in a system that is sustainable. The farmers have preserved edible wild plants and herbs along the terraces, and these are made use of regularly because of their dietary or medicinal properties, or are taken as a complementary or alternative diet during periods of drought. Each high-altitude escarpment is thus an 'agro-ecosystem,' as defined by Jean Lebel: "[it is] simply a coherent geographical and functional entity where agricultural production takes place. Agro-ecosystems consist of living and non-living components and their interactions."[3] They correspond to the 'steep to very steep lands' category used by the Food and Agriculture Organization of the United Nations (FAO) classification of agro-ecological zoning.[4]

Ecosystems are based on complex socio-cultural, economic, health, and ecological dynamics in terms of both time and space. Natural processes and human activities influence these dynamics, and they can create stresses that may have an impact on human health and ecosystem sustainability. The integrated 'EcoHealth approach' promoted by the Canadian International Development and Research Centre (IDRC)[5] seeks to address and improve human health through better management of ecosystems (or 'agro-ecosystems' when talking about the rain-fed terraces)—'healthy communities in healthy ecosystems.' For this purpose, EcoHealth does not focus only on the social and environmental variables that influence individual risk factors, but also identifies a web of ecologically-based factors that influence human health. This requires a holistic understanding of health, placed at the centre of the system, while equally recognizing economic, social, and environmental components.

---

2 According to Tony Wilkinson, terraced farming on steep to very steep slopes has been practised for more than 4,000 years ('Settlement', 185).

3 Lebel, *Health*, 41.

4 FAO, 'Terrastat Database'.

5 See the website <http://www.idrc.ca/ecohealth> for more information on IDRC Ecosystems and Human Health Program.

Terraced rain-fed farming, of variable local importance, occurs in some fourteen governorates[6] from the north to the south of the country. Today it covers only 1.25% of Yemen—around 660,000 ha—as noted by the Socio-Economic Development Plan for Poverty Reduction (2006–10), based on a 2002 governmental study assessing land degradation.[7] However, a few decades ago, the area was greater. This type of subsistence farming, including the breeding of small livestock, is still practised in more than half of the available arable land. It occupies nearly two thirds of the active workers[8] and has led to a concentration of some 20–30% of the entire population in these regions.[9] Population density reaches extreme levels, ranging from 500 to 900 inhabitants per km². Human demands are high and exert enormous pressure on natural resources. These regions also have the highest poverty rates in Yemen.

2. Examples of Plant-based Healing Practices[10]

It was through the authors' field research in the rain-fed mountain areas that the real wealth of the farming communities became apparent—the female and male farmers' knowledge of medicinal plants and their experience in using them. They are proud to share their expertise with anyone who shows an interest in it and who appreciates it.

The expertise of female and male farmers in using plants for self-medication varies from one area to another, a result of different environmental and climatic conditions determining the natural vegetation and the potential for cropping systems. However, a similar medicinal practice using the same plant, or a variety of it, can be found in regions at some distance from each other, as is the case for fennel (*Foeniculum vulgare*), for example. Fennel seeds are used to treat stomach ache by communities from the region of Taʿizz in the southern highlands to the Ṣanʿāʾ highlands, some 300 km to the north.

---

6 These governorates are: Ṣaʿda, Ḥajja, ʿAmrān, Ṣanʿāʾ, al-Maḥwīt, al-Ḥudayda, Rayma, Dhamār, Ibb, Taʿizz, al-Bayḍāʾ, al-Ḍāliʿ, Laḥj, and Abyān.

7 Ministry of Planning & International Cooperation, *Socio-Economic Development Plan*, 47.

8 Ward, *Yemen*, 1.

9 Personal estimations based on national statistics on population and agriculture.

10 See the tables below for more details on all recorded examples quoted in this paragraph and in the whole chapter.

The range of treatments for any kind of pain or disease may rely on locally available wild plants or on crops specifically cultivated by farmers. Rural people believe that no plants (including weeds and wild plants) are useless, as each one might have a potential medicinal application. This includes the smallest and seemingly insignificant herb as well as big trees, such as *Acacia etbaica*, that are cultivated for the wood they supply as a fuel and for the leaves that are used to treat stomach ache. In the same way, nearly all crops—cereals, legumes, tubers, fruits, vegetables, herbs, spices—are considered to have positive impacts on health, and in traditional recipes both nutritional and medicinal benefits play a role.

A preliminary inventory of some of the practices recorded by the authors reveals that diverse plant parts are used. Although in some instances the entire plant is included in a preparation, in others a single plant part might be isolated for use. Seeds of the African juniper (*Juniperus procera*) are used to treat toothache, while leaves of the coffee bush (from the numerous *Coffea arabica* varieties) are included in preparations to remedy anaemia. The fibre in the pods of *Flemingia congesta* is applied to women's faces as a sunscreen, while the fruits of okra (*Abelmoschus esculentus*) are used to treat stomach ache, and the sap of *Ficus cordata* serves as a collyrium to treat wounds in eyes. In the opinion of the farmers, seeds, leaves, stems, roots, fruits, saps, oils, and even the tiniest parts of the plants such as the stigma, are all of potential value. Some plants have more benefits than others, with more than one of their parts being used medicinally. This is the case with dock (*Rumex nervosus*): the leaves and stems can be boiled to make a beverage to treat diarrhoea, acid indigestion (dyspepsia), or malaria, and the leaves alone can be eaten to remedy periodontal infections.

2.1. *Field Data on Wild and Cultivated Plants*

The following two tables compile some of the data collected during fieldwork and projects, including participatory workshops with farmers, where such issues were raised spontaneously (although the workshops did not specifically focus on the medicinal usage of wild or cultivated plants).

Table 1 lists some wild plants and herbs, their scientific, vernacular, and English names (where known or identified correctly), examples of the healing practices, and the part(s) of the plant used. The information in this table came from workshops organized specifically for women as part of the *Women and Coping Strategies for Adaptation to Climate Change Using*

Agro-biodiversity Resources in the Rain-fed Highlands of Yemen study, commissioned by the World Bank in 2008.[11]

Table 2 displays the same information, but with more details about the regions where it was recorded, and focusing on cultivated plants. Unlike Table 1, Table 2 documents information provided by both male and female farmers at numerous participatory meetings which were conducted from 2004 onwards in various regions of Yemen as part of various field projects.[12]

Table 1. Traditional healing knowledge using wild plants from different rural areas of Yemen (source: female informants)

#	Scientific name	Vernacular name	English name	Healing practices and part(s) of the plant used
1	*Acacia etbaica*	*qaraḍ*	acacia	Leaves are crushed and mixed with water and taken orally to reduce stomach pain.
2	*Aloe* spp.	*ṣabr*	aloe	Plants are charred on the fire to produce a wet poultice that is used externally on fractures or as a wound disinfectant.
3	*Buddleja polystachya*	*ʿafār*	butterfly bush	With plants nos. 5, 14, and 21 it is boiled to make a beverage to treat kidney stones and infections.
4	*Capparis cartilaginea*	*raṣf*		Plants are boiled for external application on painful knees.
5	*Cynodon dactylon*	*wabal*	Bermuda grass	With plants nos. 3, 14, and 21 it is boiled to make a beverage to treat kidney stones and infections.
6	*Cyphostemma digitatum*	*ḥalqa*		Leaves are boiled and crushed and taken orally to treat the symptoms of malaria.
7	*Ficus cordata*	*athab*	African fig	Seeds are used to treat toothache. They also serve to sweeten coffee or to make an incense-like perfume.
8	*Ficus vasta*	*ṭālūq*	fig	Plant is used with olive oil as a treatment for inflamed tonsils.

[11] Consultancy conducted by Amin Al-Hakimi and Anhar Ya'ni in several rural regions of Yemen (Al-Hakimi and Ya'ni, *Women and Coping Strategies*).

[12] The authors' specific programme of projects on these issues started in late 2004 with the "Capacity Building in Sustainable Agriculture, by Building on Indigenous Knowledge and Genetic Resources to Improve Sustainable Rain-fed Agriculture in Yemen" workshops that led to the creation of YASAD, the Yemeni Association for Sustainable Agriculture Development in 2007. The first projects were implemented under the authors' leadership in the Yemeni Genetic Resources Centre (YGRC) at Ṣanʿāʾ University, and all others, including the current studies, form part of a partnership between YASAD and the French NGO Iddeales (Initiatives de Développement Durable et Equitable sur la base d'Actions Locales et d'Echanges de Savoirs). See the bibliography for some project reports used in this chapter.

Table 1. Continued.

#	Scientific name	Vernacular name	English name	Healing practices and part(s) of the plant used
9	*Hypoestes forskalei*	*ṣūrab*	Polka dot plant	Plant is used as an insect repellent.
10	*Jatropha dhofarica*	*ābkī*	jatropha	Plant is used to treat nosebleed.
11	*Jatropha spinosa*	*dumāʿ, dimaʿ*	jatropha	Drops of sap from the stems are applied on wounds.
12	*Juniperus procera*	*furūsh, ʿarʿar*	(East) African juniper	Seeds are used to treat toothache. They also serve to sweeten coffee or to make an incense-like perfume.
13	*Lawsonia inermis*	*ḥinnāʾ*	henna	Plant is used to anoint someone with heatstroke.
14	*Linum usitatissimum*	*mūma*	flax	With plants nos. 3, 5, and 21 it is boiled to make a beverage to treat kidney stones and infections.
15	*Meriandra bengalensis*	*ḍarū*		Leaves are boiled to make a beverage to treat kidney gravel and kidney stones.
16	*Pulicaria undulata*	*jathjāth*		Plant is used as an insect repellent in livestock shelters.
17	*Rumex nervosus*	*ʿuthrub*	dock, sorrel	Leaves and stems are boiled to make a beverage to treat diarrhoea, acid indigestion (dyspepsia) or malaria. Leaves can be eaten to treat periodontal infections.
18	*Ruta chalepensis*	*shadhāb*	fringed rue	Leaves are mixed with sesame oil, and drops of the mixture are applied to treat earache.
19	*Selaginella yemensis*	*ḥaka*		Plant is used to absorb humidity.
20	*Tapinanthus globiferus*	*hidāl*		Plant is cut, crushed, and mixed with milk to make a beverage to treat nosebleed.
21	*Tribulus terrestris*	*quṭba*	caltrop	With plants no. 3, 5, and 14 it is boiled to make a beverage to treat kidney stones and infections.
22	*Withania somnifera*	*ʿubab*	Indian ginseng, winter cherry	Leaves are used on wounds.

Table 2. Traditional healing knowledge using cultivated plants from different rural areas of Yemen (source: male and female informants)

#	Scientific name	Vernacular name	English name	Healing practices and part(s) of the plant used	Regions
1	*Abelmoschus* (or *Hibiscus*) *esculentus*	*bāmiyā*	okra	Soaked fruits are used to treat stomach ache.	Ṣan'ā'
2	*Allium cepa*	*baṣal*	onion	Plant is used to treat colds.	Ta'izz
3	*Allium porrum*	*karrāth*	leek	The dew is collected and used as eyeliner to treat eye problems.	Ṣan'ā' (Old City)
4	*Allium sativum*	*thūm*	garlic	Plant is used to reduce blood pressure.	Ṣan'ā' and Ta'izz
5	*Ammi copticum*	*khalla, nakhwa*	bishop's weed	Seeds are used to treat stomach ache.	Ta'izz
6	*Brassica nigra*	*khardal aswad*	black mustard	Oil from the seeds is used to treat colds.	Ṣan'ā'
7	*Carica papaya*	*babāya, 'anb*	papaya	Fresh seeds are used against parasitic worms.	Ta'izz
8	*Carthamus tinctorius*	*'uṣfur, qarṭam*	safflower	Flowers are used as a sunscreen.	Ta'izz
9	*Ceratonia siliqua*	*kharnūb*	carob	Dried pods are used to treat diarrhoea.	Ta'izz
10	*Citrullus colocynthis*	*ḥanẓal*	colocynth	The fruit is used to treat haemorrhoids.	Ṣan'ā'
11	*Citrus limon*	*laymūn*	lemon	The fruit is used to treat fever.	Ta'izz
12	*Cuminum cyminum*	*kammūn*	cumin	Seeds are used to treat flatulence.	Ta'izz
13	*Curcuma longa*	*hurud*	curcuma, turmeric	Rhizomes are used as a paste to protect the face from the sun.	Ta'izz and Tihāma
14	*Coffea arabica*	*bunn*	coffee	Leaves are used to treat anaemia.	al-Maḥwīt
15	*Eleusine coracana*	*ṭahf*	finger millet	Grains are fed to malnourished infants.	Shabwa
16	*Flemingia congesta*	*wars*		The fibrous material in the pods is used as a sunscreen.	Ta'izz and Yāfi'
17	*Foeniculum vulgare* (or *Anethum foeniculum*)	*shammar*	fennel	Seeds are used to treat stomach ache.	Ta'izz and Ṣan'ā'
18	*Hordeum distichon*	*sha'īr thanā'ī al-ṣaff*	two-rowed barley	Grains are used to treat kidney gravel and kidney stones.	Ta'izz
19	*Hyphaene thebaica*	*bahsh, ṭārī*	doum palm	Sap is used against parasitic worms.	Aden
20	*Lawsonia inermis*	*ḥinnā'*	henna	Leaves are used to treat fevers.	Ta'izz and Ṣan'ā'
21	*Lepidium sativum*	*ḥilf, rashād*	garden cress	Seeds are used to treat fractures.	Ta'izz and Ṣan'ā'
22	*Linum usitatissimum*	*mūma*	flax	Seeds are used to treat kidney gravel and kidney stones.	Ṣan'ā' and Ta'izz
23	*Mentha piperita*	*na'na'*	mint	Leaves are used to treat stomach ache.	Ṣan'ā'

Table 2. Continued.

#	Scientific name	Vernacular name	English name	Healing practices and part(s) of the plant used	Regions
24	*Nigella sativa*	*ḥabba sawdāʾ*	black cumin	Seeds are used to treat a sore throat.	Ṣanʿāʾ
25	*Papaver somniferum*	*khashkhāsh*	poppy	Seeds are used to treat toothache.	Taʿizz
26	*Pimpinella anisum*	*yānisūn*	anise	Seeds are used to treat stomach ache.	Ṣanʿāʾ
27	*Prunus persica*	*firsak*	peach	Leaves are used against parasitic worms.	Ṣanʿāʾ
28	*Punica granatum*	*rummān*	pomegranate	Epicarp (peel) is used against stomach ulcers.	Ṣanʿāʾ
29	*Raphanus sativus*	*fijl*	radish	Seeds are used to promote male fertility.	Taʿizz
30	*Ricinus communis*	*kharūʿ*	castor oil plant	Seeds are used as a laxative.	Taʿizz
31	*Saccharum officinarum*	*qaṣab sukkar, maḍḍār*	sugar cane	Cane sugar is used against anaemia.	Taʿizz
32	*Sesamum indicum*	*jiljilān, simsim*	sesame	Leaves are used to treat stomach ache.	Tihāma
33	*Thymus laevigatus*	*zaʿtar*	thyme	Leaves are used to treat stomach ache.	Ṣanʿāʾ
34	*Triticum dicoccum*	*burr ʿalas, qamḥ nashawī*	wheat (emmer)	Grains of this local variety of wheat are used to treat injuries and fractures.	Ṣanʿāʾ
35	*Zea mays*	*dhura shāmiyya*	maize (corn)	Stigmas are used to treat kidney gravel and kidney stones.	Taʿizz
36	*Zingiber officinale*	*zanjabīl*	ginger	Roots are used to strengthen the stomach.	Ṣanʿāʾ
37	*Ziziphus lotus*	*sidr barrī*	nabk	Small seedlings are used to strengthen the body.	Taʿizz and Yāfiʿ

2.2. *Using Plants in Response to Everyday and Chronic Human Health Issues*

In the farming communities a very pragmatic way of responding to human health needs can be observed. Preparations, decoctions, and recipes are recommended to prevent, alleviate or even cure a wide range of medical problems. These can be everyday health issues, such as minor pain, toothache, fever, or nosebleed, as well as potentially more severe ailments, such as wounds, fractures, or kidney stones. Some of the health problems addressed are chronic ones, recognized as being common in remote regions, and intimately linked to the very poor socio-economic conditions of their rural communities.

For instance, a visitor suffering from an ailment such as stomach ache, if far from any health care facility, might be advised by a local Yemeni farmer to drink a beverage made from the crushed leaves of the *Acacia etbaica* tree. Another remedy involves ingesting sesame leaves (*Sesamum indicum*), or, in regions where this species is cultivated, a handful of okra fruit (*Abelmoschus esculentus*) soaked in water.

maṭīṭ is another example of a traditional recipe in which a local variety of barley is mixed with onions to mitigate dizziness, although a simple barley porridge is said to have the same effect in some cases.[13] It is not unusual to combine several plants and/or plant products. For instance, parts of *Buddleja polystachya*, *Tribulus terrestris*, *Cynodon dactylon*, and *Linum usitatissimum* can be boiled together to prepare a beverage taken to remedy kidney stones and infections. It is said that the medicinal benefits of all four plants are enhanced when used together.

Intestinal parasites, a major health problem, can affect more than 80% of the population in some places, in various degrees of severity and independent of age. *Ascaris* spp. and *Giardia* spp. are among those parasites that infest people.[14] As an initial response, worms such as *Ascaris* are evacuated by taking fresh papaya seeds or leaves from an endemic peach tree. According to the World Health Organization, malaria is one of the most serious health problems in Yemen today,[15] with approximately 60% of the population living in areas with malaria transmission. Political instability, in addition to climatic changes and heavy rainfall, contributed to malaria epidemics in 1996 and 1998. Among the farming communities the symptoms of malaria are traditionally lessened by ingesting boiled leaves of *Cyphostemma digitatum*.[16]

Plant-based healing practices are also used to treat another major preoccupation of the population—fertility and fecundity. Infant mortality remains very high in Yemen, as illustrated by the latest Arab Human Development Report: the under-five mortality rate reached 102 (per 1,000 live births) in 2005,[17] 46% of the children under the age of five were underweight in 2003,[18] and the maternal mortality rate was one of the high-

---

13 See the cookbook by Yaʿnī et al., *al-Wajabāt al-taqlīdiyya*, for details on these recipes: *maʿṣūba* (38), *maṭīṭ* (56), and more.

14 These are results from the EcoHealth Project conducted by the authors on traditional food systems in Ibb rural communities (Al-Hakimi et al., *Health and Dietary Diversity*).

15 WHO, <http://www.who.int/malaria/publications/country-profiles/profile_yem_en.pdf>.

16 See Mohammed al-Duais' and Gottfried Jetschke's chapter in this volume.

17 UNDP, *Arab Human Development Report*, 150.

18 Ibid., 136.

Table 3. Traditional healing knowledge using wild and cultivated plants from different rural areas of Yemen for treating animal ailments (source: female informants)

#	Scientific name	Vernacular name	English name	Healing practices and part of the plant used
1	*Aristolochia bracteolata*	*lawwīʿiyya*	birthwort, pipevine	Plant is given with *Sorghum bicolor* grains to animals suffering from bloat (a distended stomach).
2	*Calotropis procera*	*ʿushar*	apple of Sodom	Drops of plant sap are used to treat swellings.
3	*Cissus rotundifolia*	*ʿalfaq*	Arabian wax cissus	Plant is boiled and given to livestock to reduce stomach pain.
4	*Cyphostemma digitatum*	*ḥalqa*		Plant is boiled with salt to make a beverage given to stimulate an animal's appetite.
5	*Gomphocarpus fruticosus*	*sabīʿa*	milkweed	Plants are applied to the body of cow afflicted by heatstroke.
6	*Hordeum vulgare*	*shaʿīr*	barley	Plant is given together with *Trigonella foenum-graecum* to livestock suffering from constipation.
7	*Psiadia punctulata*	*fataḥ*		Plant is used to treat fractures in animals.
8	*Sorghum bicolor*	*gharab*	dark variety of sorghum	See no. 1.
9	*Trigonella foenum-graecum*	*ḥulba*	fenugreek	See no. 6.

est in the world, at 430 (per 100,000 live births) in 2005.[19] Finger millet (*Eleusine coracana*) is fed to infants to improve their health. In some regions, a woman about to give birth is given a special dish called *maʿṣūba* consisting of a local variety of wheat mixed with some fenugreek and animal fat. This, with soup and the meat of a young chicken, is given for one month prior to the anticipated birth. Milk production in a young mother is increased by eating the grain from the darker cultivars of sorghum, 'red sorghum.' The overall health of pregnant women is strengthened by taking barley-based porridge. Male infertility is treated with radish seeds.

Other healing practices in these mountain areas are related to diseases caused by the natural environment and climate. Numerous preparations address fevers and colds as well as problems related to environmental factors, such as sun, heat, dust, humidity, altitude, or insects. For instance, women from the Taʿizz and Yāfiʿ regions use the fibrous material in the pods of *Flemingia congesta* as a sunscreen, while flowers of safflower (*Carthamus tinctorius*) are used instead by women from other Taʿizz com-

[19] Ibid., 150.

munities. Both plants give a distinctive yellowish colour to the face. Traditional gardeners from the Old City of Ṣan'ā' recorded using the sap of *Ficus* spp. to treat irritations of the eye caused by dust and air pollution, while for more severe problems of the eye, such as wounds, they applied the dew collected from leek plants (*Allium porrum*). Dizziness caused by high altitude, another affliction of people living in the Yemeni mountains, is said to be lessened by a barley-based diet, and humidity indoors is reduced by *Selaginella yemensis*. Plants such as the *Hypoestes forskalei* provide useful insect repellents.

2.3. *Using Plants in Response to Animal Health Problems*

Animals are considered a part of the 'extended family' and caring for livestock is a matter of perpetual concern for the rural population. It is women who are mostly responsible for livestock rearing, and they mostly possess knowledge specific to treating sick animals. Table 3 summarizes some of the plants and associated practices which were mentioned by rural women during participatory workshops held within the same framework as described above (see Table 1). Pain, loss of appetite, fractures, and constipation are some of the problems mentioned. Some plants are used for both humans and animals, whereas the application of others is restricted to animals.

3. Indigenous Knowledge

Knowledge of medicinal plants forms part of the wider pool of empirical, holistic, and very practical systems of knowledge developed by the traditional mountain communities of farmers that allows them to use, manage, and conserve their environment. It is thus part of a local plant expertise that is used for more purposes than medication alone. Indigenous knowledge can be defined as the knowledge that people in a given community have developed, and continue to develop, over time.[20] It is based on experience, often tested over centuries, and is adapted to the local culture and environment. It is not static, but dynamic and changing. It is not confined to tribal groups or the original inhabitants of an area, nor is it confined to rural people. Other names for indigenous knowledge (or closely related concepts) are 'local knowledge,' 'indigenous technical knowledge', and

20 See the World Bank action framework on indigenous knowledge: *Connaissances autochtones pour le développement*.

'traditional knowledge.' In our current case, a more specific term might be 'farmers' knowledge,' because most of the communities concerned consist of farmers who possess a holistic approach to the various aspects of their daily life, including plants, their medicinal properties, and health issues.

This specific knowledge is thus quite complex and relies on various fields of indigenous knowledge, from botany and plant classification (e.g. vernacular names given to wild plants or to various distinctive characteristics that distinguish between local varieties of the same species), to ecology (e.g. the ability to determine the best location for a plant to grow, or the best soil in which to plant a specific variety), and to the associated healing practices. It may include dexterity in preparing decoctions, as well as sufficient experience with human or veterinary medicine to make it possible to diagnose a problem, to target the symptoms or the causes, and to identify the best healing approach. Despite the number of disciplines involved, this knowledge has been accessible to most farmers for centuries. Both female and male farmers possess it, with some gender specificity and complementarity (e.g. women focusing on veterinary knowledge). In addition, women might take a more 'practical' approach than men because they are the ones who prepare the medicines. Such knowledge is transmitted orally across the generations.

Jacques Fleurentin has pointed out the enormous breadth of Yemenis' knowledge of medicinal plants. He observed that "in rural areas, everyone was able to list in his/her surrounding environment or at the herbalist's office some twenty medicinal plants that he/she would use properly to treat common problems such as diarrhoea or skin infections."[21] The authors' recent experience confirms Fleurentin's observation and even widens the scope to include broader health and nutritional values of cultivated plants and their local varieties. Traditional rural recipes based on local landraces of cereals and legumes are indeed associated with good flavour and high energy and nutritional values. As an illustration, local wheat and barley varieties grown under rain-fed conditions, tested in the field, and analyzed in labs, revealed noteworthy nutritional values.[22] Local wheat landraces appeared to be better sources of minerals, fibre, and proteins than any so-called 'improved' wheat introduced into local farming systems, or than the imported refined flours that have become available

---

21 Fleurentin, *Guérisseurs*, 99 (translation by the authors). See also Jacques Fleurentin's chapter in this volume.

22 Those are results from the EcoHealth Project conducted by the authors on traditional food systems in Ibb rural communities (Al-Hakimi et al., *Health and Dietary Diversity*).

in markets in recent years. Local barley grains generally contain even higher rates of minerals than local wheats. Farmers' conception of health is intimately linked to the notion of a good diet protecting against ill health, and to the local origin of the crops. The Yemeni term *baladī*,[23] is used for such local crops, and is seen as an incontestable label of good quality, ecological production, and excellent flavour.

Collecting medicinal plants is often part of the daily routine—one task among many integrated into the schedule of a family member. This became evident in the field workshops when people talked about their daily work. While it was not possible to conduct a documentation session focusing on plants and their traditional medicinal applications, nevertheless the participants raised the topic regularly throughout workshops held with the aim of recording a typical rural daily schedule. For instance, a woman describing the time she spent collecting wood from the village pastures added that she took advantage of being at that place by collecting specimens of the common birthwort or pipevine (*Aristolochia bracteolata*) that she would later mix with grains of *Sorghum bicolor* and administer to her only cow suffering from pain resulting from bloat. In another case, an old man said that when he got hurt while ploughing far from his house, he was always happy to find a specimen of one of the numerous varieties of the Yemeni aloe (*Aloe* spp.), the sap of which serves as an emergency disinfectant.

4. Conclusion

This chapter has highlighted farmers' knowledge of wild and cultivated plants and their medicinal applications. The farmers have practised sustainable subsistence rain-fed farming for centuries. Yet today, many of the 150 plant species recorded by some studies as existing throughout Yemeni agricultural history—most of which were still used in the early 1970s—have become extinct. This is due to rapid and dramatic transformations in farming practice, as well as to social change.[24] For instance, even though landraces and old cultivars have recognized nutritional and medicinal benefits, in addition to being perfectly adapted to the mountainous environment in which they grow (characterized by high altitude and recurring droughts), their very existence is now endangered. It is high time to raise awareness

23 Literal meaning: originating from the country or the region.

24 Al-Hakimi, 'Traditional Farming Systems', 121.

of farmers' crucial role in food production and conservation of their agro-ecosystems, and to appreciate their unique knowledge and experience of the health-related properties of plants. What is even more urgently needed is to document the farmers' orally transmitted knowledge—as a significant part of Yemen's intangible cultural heritage[25]—and to safeguard the plants before they vanish forever, together with developing a strategy to protect the intellectual property rights of local communities. Otherwise there is a great danger that powerful international industrial groups might reap the profits of exploiting this expertise.

Bibliography

Fleurentin, Jacques, *Guérisseurs et plantes médicinales du Yémen : Au pays de l'encens, de l'aloès et du café* (Paris : Karthala, 2004).

Al-Hakimi, Amin A.S., 'Traditional Farming Systems and Their Role in Developing and Sustaining Agriculture in the Republic of Yemen', in Amin Al-Hakimi and Frédéric Pelat (eds.), *Indigenous Knowledge and Sustainable Agriculture in Yemen* (Les Cahiers du Cefas, 3; Ṣan'ā': Centre Français d'Archéologie et de Sciences Sociales de Sanaa, 2003), 121–6.

———, and Ya'ni, Anhar, *Women and Coping Strategies for Adaptation to Climate Change Using Agro-biodiversity Resources in the Rain-fed Highlands of Yemen* (Ṣan'ā': Report Prepared for the World Bank, 2008).

———, Al-Qubati, Adnan, Al Hagami, Adel, Saed, Sadeq S., Othman, Mokhtar D., Al Samawi, Ahmed, Yaani, Anhar A., and Pelat, Frédéric, *Health and Dietary Diversity in Yemen: Traditional Yemeni Rural Diets and Local Food Systems: Enhancing Contributions to Health and the Environment* (unpublished final report: EcoHealth Project, Ṣan'ā' 2008).

Wilkinson, Tony, 'Settlement, Soil Erosion and Terraced Agriculture in Highland Yemen: A Preliminary Statement', *Proceedings of the Seminar for Arabian Studies*, 29 (1999), 183–91.

Ya'nī, Anhar 'Abd al-Karīm, al-Ḥakīmī, Amīn, Pelat, Frédéric, al-Qubāṭī, Adnān, 'Uthman, Mukhtār D., Sharaf, Ṣādiq, and al-Samāwī, Aḥmad, *al-Wajabāt al-taqlīdiyya al-rīfiyya al-yamaniyya* (Traditional Recipes from Rural Yemen) (Ṣan'ā': Dār Jāmi'at Ṣan'ā' lil-ṭibā'a wa-l-nashr, 2008).

[25] The edition of the first cookbook on traditional recipes from rural regions of Yemen in 2008 by the current authors (Ya'nī et al., *al-Wajabāt al-taqlīdiyya*) formed an important first step. The book documents and disseminates orally transmitted indigenous knowledge on cooking, while at the same time promoting health-related benefits of local landraces and wild plants as part of traditional food preparations.

Internet Sources[26]

FAO (= Food and Agriculture Organization of the United Nations), 'Terrastat Database', 2010, <http://www.fao.org/ag/agl/agll/terrastat/wsrout1.asp?countrysel=YEM&search2=Show+all+statistics+!>

Lebel, Jean, *Health, an Ecosystem Approach* (Ottawa: International Development Research Centre, 2003), <http://www.idrc.ca/openebooks/012-8>

Ministry of Planning & International Cooperation, Republic of Yemen, *Socio-Economic Development Plan for Poverty Reduction (2006–2010)*, October 2006, <http://www.undp.org.ye/reports/ *DPPR.pdf*>

UNDP, *Arab Human Development Report* (UNDP Document, New York, 2009), <http://hdr.undp.org/ en/reports/regionalreports/arabstates/ahdr2009e.pdf>

[World Bank] Centre pour la Gestion de l'Information et de la Connaissance, Région Afrique, Banque Mondiale, *Connaissances autochtones pour le développement : Un cadre pour l'action* (Novembre 1998), <http://www.worldbank.org/afr/ik/ikrepfr.pdf>

Ward, C., *Yemen, Agricultural Strategy Note. Report no. 17973-YEM* (Washington DC: World Bank, 1998), <http://www-wds.worldbank.org/servlet/WDSContentServer/WDSP/IB/1999/09/14/000094946_9906260530330/Rendered/PDF/multi_page.pdf />

WHO (World Health Organization):
<http://www.who.int/malaria/publications/country-profiles/ profile_yem_en.pdf>
<http://www.idrc.ca/ecohealth

[26] All websites were accessed during July and August 2010.

INDICES[*]

INDEX OF PLANTS AND FUNGI[1]

MSA = Modern South Arabian[2]

---

* Prepared by H. Schönig.

[1] The taxonomy is given according to the current use after David J. Mabberley, *Mabberley's Plant-book: A Portable Dictionary of Plants, Their Classification and Uses* (3rd edn.; Cambridge: Cambridge University Press, 2008).

[2] For details and the respective dialect, see Miranda Morris' chapter in this volume.

INDEX OF NAMES[1]

All names are given in alphabetical order, disregarding the Arabic article al-, Al-.

[1] Includes proper names, geographical names and toponyms, nationalities, languages, dynasties, etc.

INDEX OF TOPICS AND KEYWORDS

www.ingramcontent.com/pod-product-compliance
Lightning Source LLC
LaVergne TN
LVHW010657300926
849161LV00005B/1147
* 9 7 8 9 0 0 4 2 2 1 5 0 5 *